ROTATOR CUFF DISORDERS: BASIC SCIENCE & CLINICAL MEDICINE

ROTATOR CUFF DISORDERS: BASIC SCIENCE & CLINICAL MEDICINE

NICOLA MAFFULLI MD MS PhD FRCS(Orth)
Centre for Sports and Exercise Medicine, Barts and the London School of Medicine and Dentistry, Mile End Hospital, London, UK

JOHN P FURIA MD
SUN Orthopedics and Sports Medicine, Chief Executive Officer, Evangelical Community Hospital Ambulatory Surgical Center, Lewisburg, Pennsylvania, USA

JP medical publishers

London • St Louis • Panama City • New Delhi

Published by JP Medical Ltd, 83 Victoria Street, London, SW1H 0HW, UK
Tel: +44 (0)20 3170 8910 Fax: +44 (0)20 3008 6180
Email: info@jpmedpub.com Web: www.jpmedpub.com

ISBN: 978-1-907816-08-6

British Library Cataloguing in Publication Data
A catalogue record for this book is available from the British Library

Library of Congress Cataloging in Publication Data
A catalog record for this book is available from the Library of Congress

JP Medical Ltd is a subsidiary of Jaypee Brothers Medical Publishers (P) Ltd, New Delhi, India.

Publisher: Richard Furn
Development Editors: Gavin Smith, Alison Whitehouse
Design: Designers Collective Ltd

Typeset, printed and bound in India.

Preface

Millions suffer from shoulder pain. Few understand why, and that's not good. Finally, we have a solution.

Rotator Cuff Disorders: Basic Science and Clinical Medicine was written to help physicians, health care professionals, and most importantly shoulder pain sufferers understand and correct their problem. The book is comprehensive, supported by the highest level of scientific evidence, and with chapter contributions from experienced leaders, filled with practical advice.

Unlike other texts, *Rotator Cuff Disorders: Basic Science and Clinical Medicine* was written in a 'quick-read' format. Our goal was to create a concise, practical and user-friendly guide. Each chapter is loaded with the pearls, 'tips and tricks' and sound clinical advice derived from years of experience.

The basic science, pathophysiology and genetic aspects of rotator cuff disease are presented clearly. The ideas are crisp and blunt. The principles are interwoven with case reports to make the material applicable to the clinical setting.

It is our hope that this text will foster enhanced clinical and scientific interest in the disorders of the shoulder. The foundation for an adequate appreciation of shoulder injury, pathophysiology, and treatment is established by making the material clinically relevant. We believe this integrated approach will facilitate decision making and ultimately patient care.

With concise descriptions, abundant clinical reports, easy-to-understand illustrations, and a touch of humor, *Rotator Cuff Disorders: Basic Science and Clinical Medicine* is 'an easy read', a book that can be digested in several hours, and one that will serve as a 'go-to' guide for years to come.

Nicola Maffulli
John P Furia
January 2012

Contents

Preface v

Contributors ix

Acknowledgements xi

Chapter 1
Rotator cuff: anatomy and embryology 1

Chapter 2
Surgical anatomy and rotator cuff tear pattern 9

Chapter 3
Why does the rotator cuff fail? The pathophysiology of rotator cuff disease 15

Chapter 4
Epidemiology and genetic basis of rotator cuff pathology 25

Chapter 5
Rotator cuff biomechanics 29

Chapter 6
Examination of the shoulder for rotator cuff disease 41

Chapter 7
Imaging of the rotator cuff 55

Chapter 8
Partial rotator cuff tears 63

Chapter 9
The overhead athlete 75

Chapter 10
SLAP lesions and tendinopathy of the long head of biceps 87

Chapter 11
Full-thickness rotator cuff tears 99

Chapter 12
Subscapularis tears 107

Chapter 13
Rotator cuff arthropathy and glenohumeral arthritis: prevention and treatment 117

Chapter 14
Single-row versus double-row rotator cuff repair 131

Chapter 15
Growth factors and tendon healing 137

Chapter 16
Rotator cuff orthobiologics 145

Chapter 17
Augmentation of massive rotator cuff tears 151

Chapter 18
Platelet-rich plasma: does it help tendon healing? 157

Chapter 19
Outcome measures 167

Chapter 20
Tissue engineering: the future of rotator cuff repair surgery 175

Index 181

Contributors

Jeffrey S Abrams MD
Clinical Professor of Orthopaedic Surgery
Seton Hall University
Attending Physician, University Medical Center at Princeton
Princeton, NJ
USA

Jesse Affonso MD
Orthopaedic Surgeon
Cape Cod Orthopaedics and Sports Medicine
Hyannis, MAUSA

Asheesh Bedi MD
Assistant Professor
Medsport
Department of Orthopedic Surgery
University of Michigan
Ann Arbor, MI
USA

Javier Beltran MD
Chairman, Department of Radiology
Maimonides Medical Center
Brooklyn, NY
USA

Alessandra Berton MD
Resident in Trauma and Orthopaedic Surgery
Campus Bio-Medico University of Rome
Rome
Italy

Fabrizio Campi MD
Shoulder and Elbow Orthopedic Surgeon
Unit of Shoulder and Elbow Surgery
"D. Cervesi" Hospital
Cattolica, Rimini
Italy

Michael R Carmont FRCS(Tr&Orth), FFSEM(UK), Dip SEM GB&I
Consultant Trauma and Orthopaedic Surgeon
Department of Orthopaedic Surgery
Princess Royal Hospital
Telford, Shropshire
UK

Alessandro Castagna MD
Shoulder Unit
IRCCS Humanitas Institute
Milan
Italy

Eugenio Cesari MD
Shoulder and Elbow Orthopedic Surgeon
Unit of Shoulder and Elbow Surgery
"D. Cervesi" Hospital
Cattolica, Rimini
Italy

Marco Conti MD, PhD
Shoulder Unit
IRCCS Humanitas Institute
Milan
Italy

Angelo Del Buono MD
Orthopaedic Surgeon
Department of Orthopaedic and
Trauma Surgery
Campus Bio-Medico University of Rome
Rome
Italy

Vincenzo Denaro MD
Professor of Orthopaedic Surgery
Department of Orthopaedic and
Trauma Surgery
Campus Bio-Medico University of Rome
Rome
Italy

Joshua S Dines MD
Assistant Professor of Orthopedic Surgery
Weill Cornell Medical College
Sports Medicine and Shoulder Service
The Hospital for Special Surgery
New York, NY
USA

Gianluca Falcone MD
Consultant Orthopaedic Surgeon
Department of Orthopaedics
Hand and Upper Extremity Service
Casa di Cura Villa Valeria
Rome
Italy

Francisco Forriol MD, PhD
Professor of Orthopaedic Surgery
Department of Medicine and Surgery
CEU University
School of Medicine
Madrid
Spain

Francesco Franceschi MD
Orthopaedic Surgeon
Department of Orthopaedic and Trauma Surgery
Campus Bio-Medico University of Rome
Rome
Italy

Michael Thomas Freehill MD
Fellow in Orthopaedic Surgery
Department of Orthopaedic Surgery
Shoulder Service
Harvard University
Boston, MA
USA

John P Furia MD
SUN Orthopedics and Sports Medicine
Chief Executive Officer
Evangelical Community Hospital Ambulatory Surgical Center
Lewisburg, Pennsylvania
USA

Raffaele Garofalo MD
Shoulder Service
Department of Orthopaedic Surgery
"F. Miulli" Hospital
Acquaviva delle Fonti, Bari
Italy

Juan Garzon-Muvdi MD
Clinical Research Fellow
Division of Shoulder Surgery
Department of Orthopaedic Surgery
The Johns Hopkins University
Baltimore, MD
USA

Varand Ghazikhanian MD, MS
Clinical Fellow in Musculoskeletal Imaging and Intervention
Department of Radiology
Brigham and Women's Hospital
Boston, MA
USA

Robert J Gillespie MD
Assistant Professor of Orthopaedic Surgery
Shoulder and Elbow Division
Department of Orthopaedic Surgery
University Hospitals Case Medical Center
Cleveland, OH
USA

Andrea Grasso MD
Senior attending and Surgeon in Chief Orthopaedics
Department of Orthopaedic Surgery
Casa di Cura Villa Valeria
Rome
Italy

Zakary A Knutson MD
Attending Surgeon, Oklahoma Sports and Orthopedics Institute
Clinical Professor, University of Oklahoma Department of Orthopedic Surgery and Rehabilitation
Norman, OK
USA

Robert B Kohen MD
Orthopaedic Sports Medicine Surgeon
Detroit Medical Center, Sports Medicine
Associate Team Physician, Detroit Red Wings
Farmington Hills, MI
USA

Ifedayo O Kuye BA
Medical Student
Harvard Medical School
Boston, MA
USA

Alfredo Lamberti MD
Resident in Trauma and Orthopaedic Surgery
Department of Orthopaedic and Trauma Surgery
Campus Bio-Medico University of Rome
Rome
Italy

Umile Giuseppe Longo MD, MS
Specialist in Trauma and Orthopaedic Surgery
Department of Orthopaedic and Trauma Surgery
Campus Bio-Medico University of Rome
Rome
Italy

Edward G McFarland MD
Wayne H Lewis Professor of Shoulder Surgery
Co-Director, Division of Shoulder Surgery
Vice-Chairman, Department of Orthopaedic Surgery
The Johns Hopkins University
Baltimore, MD
USA

Nicola Maffulli MD, MS, PhD, FRCS (Orth)
Centre for Sports and Exercise Medicine
Barts and The London School of Medicine and Dentistry
Mile End Hospital
London
UK

Omer Mei-Dan MD
Assistant Professor
University of Colorado School of Medicine
Department of Orthopaedics
Division of Sports Medicine
Aurora, CO
USA

James T Monica MD
Orthopaedic Surgeon
University Orthopaedic Associates, LLC
New Jersey
USA

Francesco Oliva MD, PhD
Full Specialist in Orthopaedics and Traumatology
Department of Orthopaedics and Traumatology
University of Rome "Tor Vergata" School of Medicine
Rome
Italy

Leonardo Osti MD
Clinical Instructor, Residency Program
University of Ferrara
Chief, Arthroscopy and Sports Medicine Unit
Hesperia Hospital
Modena
Italy

Paolo Paladini MD
Shoulder and Elbow Orthopedic Surgeon
Unit of Shoulder and Elbow Surgery
"D. Cervesi" Hospital
Cattolica, Rimini
Italy

Rocco Papalia MD, PhD
Orthopaedic Surgeon
Department of Orthopaedic and Trauma Surgery
Campus Bio-Medico University of Rome
Rome
Italy

Steve A Petersen MD
Associate Professor
Department of Orthopaedic Surgery
The Johns Hopkins University
Baltimore, MD
USA

Giuseppe Porcellini MD
Professor of Shoulder and Elbow Surgery
Unit of Shoulder and Elbow Surgery
"D. Cervesi" Hospital
Cattolica, Rimini
Italy

Neema Pourtaheri MD
Chief Resident in Orthopaedic Surgery
Department of Orthopaedics
Seton Hall University
School of Health and Medical Sciences
St Joseph's Regional Medical Center
New Jersey
USA

Scott A Rodeo MD
Co-Chief, Sports Medicine and Shoulder Service
Professor, Orthopaedic Surgery
Weill Medical College of Cornell University
Attending Orthopaedic Surgeon
The Hospital for Special Surgery
Associate Team Physician,
New York Giants Football
New York, NY
USA

Marc R Safran MD
Professor, Orthopaedic Surgery
Associate Director, Sports Medicine
Team Physician
Department of Orthopaedic Surgery
Stanford University
California
USA

Matteo Salvatore MD
Consultant Orthopaedic Surgeon
Department of Orthopaedics
Shoulder and Knee Service
Casa di Cura Villa Valeria
Rome
Italy

Anthony J Scillia MD
Chief Resident in Orthopaedic Surgery
Department of Orthopaedics
Seton Hall University
School of Health and Medical Sciences
St Joseph's Regional Medical Center
New Jersey
USA

Stephen J Snyder MD
Southern California Orthopedic Institute
Simi Valley, CA
USA

Filippo Spiezia MD
Resident in Trauma and
Orthopaedic Surgery
Department of Orthopaedic and Trauma Surgery
Campus Bio-Medico University of Rome
Rome
Italy

Uma Srikumaran MD
Assistant Professor
Division of Shoulder and Sports Medicine
Department of Orthopaedic Surgery
The Johns Hopkins School of Medicine
Baltimore, MD
USA

Sebastiano Vasta MD
Orthopaedic Surgeon
Department of Orthopaedic and Trauma Surgery
Campus Bio-Medico University of Rome
Rome
Italy

Jon JP Warner MD
Chief, Harvard Shoulder Service
Professor of Orthopaedics
Harvard Shoulder Service
Department of Orthopaedics
Massachusetts General Hospital
Boston, MA
USA

Gerald R Williams, Jr MD
Professor of Orthopaedic Surgery
Chief, Shoulder and Elbow Service
Rothman Institute
Thomas Jefferson University
Philadelphia, PA
USA

Biagio Zampogna MD
Orthopaedic Surgeon
Department of Orthopaedic and Trauma Surgery
Campus Bio-Medico University of Rome
Rome
Italy

Acknowledgements

We wish to say thank you to a few people. To the talented individuals from JP Medical Publishing: Development Editors Gavin Smith and Alison Whitehouse, and Publisher Richard Furn, 'mille grazie' for the countless number of hours each of you devoted to this project. You are a talented group!

NM
JF

To the memory of my father, Giuseppe Vincenzo Maffulli: you communicated to me a love for hard work and medicine even though, when you did so, I did not realize it.

To Mamma, Dorotea Pittelli, whose unbending rules of behavior imposed on us children eventually came to fruition, at least we think.

The example that Papa and Mamma gave me remains unique, and, in retrospect, welcome.

To my beautiful wife, Gayle, who knows me and withstands my whims and peculiarities with unwavering love. And to the one whom we both love, and who never sleeps, our son Giuseppe: keep honoring the name of your nonno!

NM

To my co-editor, co-author, respected colleague, and 'caro amico'" Nicola Maffulli, a giant who is unquestionably one of the foremost experts on all things related to tendons, thank you for inviting me to participate in this worthy project. You are now my 'caro fratello'"

To my caring parents, John and Barbara Furia who continue to provide me the unconditional love, guidance and emotional support that I so need, and who continue to teach me the value of old-fashioned dedication and hard work, I thank and love you.

Finally, to my beautiful wife Elizabeth who, for years, has put up with my manuscript editing nights, busy clinical practice, hectic travel schedule, obsessive focus, and commitment to 'Getting it Right'. I thank you for your love and patience. I could not have done this without you. You are my teammate, my soul mate, and the one I want to share a cloud with for all eternity.

JF

Chapter 1 Rotator cuff: anatomy and embryology

Francisco Forriol, Umile Giuseppe Longo, Nicola Maffulli, Vincenzo Denaro

KEY FEATURES

- The rotator cuff consists of four tendons. The supraspinatus, infraspinatus, and teres minor tendons are contiguous but distinct structures, and the subscapularis tendon is separated from the other tendons by an interval containing the long head of biceps.
- All the tendons of the rotator cuff originate on the scapula and fuse to insert on both tuberosities of the proximal humerus.
- The primary function of the rotator cuff is to act as a humeral head rotator and depressor. The rotator cuff also reinforces the glenohumeral capsule, and provides stability to the glenohumeral joint.
- Functionally, the rotator cuff serves to balance the force couples around the glenohumeral joint.
- The primary aim of rotator cuff surgery is not to "cover the hole," but to balance the transverse and coronal force couples.

ANATOMY

Muscles

The rotator cuff is a group of four muscles (subscapularis, supraspinatus, infraspinatus, and teres minor) arising from the scapula; their tendons blend with the subjacent capsule of the glenohumeral joint as they attach to the tuberosities of the humerus (Minagawa et al. 1998).

Classically, the supraspinatus, infraspinatus, and teres minor tendons were considered as contiguous but distinct structures (**Fig. 1.1**), the subscapularis tendon being considered as separated from the other tendons by an interval containing the biceps tendon's long head inside the groove. Later, it was shown that all the tendons of the rotator cuff fuse to insert on both tuberosities of the proximal humerus. Fibers from teres minor (posterior) and subscapularis (anterior) interdigitate with those of supraspinatus and infraspinatus (**Fig. 1.2**). The supraspinatus and subscapularis tendons fuse to form a sheath surrounding the biceps tendon's long head at the proximal end of the groove. Fibers from the subscapularis tendon pass below the biceps tendon and join with fibers from supraspinatus to form the sheath's floor (**Fig. 1.3**), the tendinous portion of the cuff also being confluent with the glenohumeral joint capsule and the coracohumeral and glenohumeral ligaments. A thick sheet of fibrous tissue lies beneath the deep layer of the subdeltoid bursa, covering the superficial aspect of the supraspinatus and infraspinatus tendons, but not part of the bursa itself.

From a functional point of view, the rotator cuff muscles act as humeral head rotators, humeral head depressors, and humeral head steerers, actively controlling the fulcrum of the glenohumeral joint during motion (Saha 1971). These help rotations of the humerus, reinforce the glenohumeral capsule, hold the humeral head in the glenoid cavity, provide stability to the joint, and maintain a fulcrum for arm motion.

One of the most important functions of the rotator cuff is to balance the coupled forces around the glenohumeral joint. The coronal plane couple results from the balance of moments produced by the deltoid versus those produced by the inferior intact portion of the rotator cuff, including infraspinatus, teres minor, and subscapularis (Inman et al. 1996). During arm abduction, this couple will be balanced only if the line of action is below the center of rotation of the humeral head, to oppose the moment produced by the deltoid.

The transverse force couple results from the balance of moments produced by infraspinatus and teres minor posteriorly versus subscapularis anteriorly. This couple is clinically relevant in patients with massive posterior rotator cuff tears, in whom there will be superior and anterior migration of the humeral head and an inability to maintain a stable fulcrum of motion. From a surgical point of view, the primary aim of rotator cuff surgery is not to "cover the hole," but to balance the transverse and coronal force couples (Burkhart et al. 1993). The articular surface of the intact rotator cuff shows a thickening of the capsule that arches and is cable like, and surrounds a thinner crescent of tissue. The coracohumeral ligament and the posterosuperior glenohumeral ligament merge laterally with a fibrous band, which runs in a crescent shape from the middle facet of the greater tubercle, underneath the infraspinatus tendon, to the biceps groove. At this level, it merges with the transverse humeral ligament before continuing anteriorly into the fasciculus obliquus. This structure has been called a *transverse band* by Clark et al. (1990), a *rotator cable* by Burkhart et al. (1993), and *ligamentum semicirculare humeri* by Kolts et al. (2002).

Burkart introduced the suspension bridge analogy; this proposed a protective role of the cable, transferring stress along the rotator cable, and thereby shielding the thinner, avascular crescent tissue from stress, analogous to a load-bearing suspension bridge (Burkhart et al. 1993). A rotator cuff tear can be modeled on a suspension bridge, where the free margin of the tear corresponds to the supports at each end of the cable's span. This model would predict that, despite a tear in the avascular zone of the supraspinatus tendon, supraspinatus could still exert a compressive effect on the glenohumeral joint by distribution of its load along the span of the suspension bridge configuration (Burkhart et al. 1993).

Supraspinatus is responsible for approximately 50% of the torque occurring during shoulder abduction and flexion, and the deltoid is responsible for the remaining 50%.

Subscapularis

The subscapularis muscle is an internal rotator of the humerus. It arises from the subscapularis fossa, in the ventral aspect of the scapula, and inserts on the lesser tuberosity of the humerus. The upper portion of the subscapularis tendon is intra-articular, and it is the most powerful and largest muscle of the rotator cuff. A subscapular bursa, usually opening into the synovial cavity of the shoulder, is located between the muscle and the neck of the scapula. This muscle is supplied by the

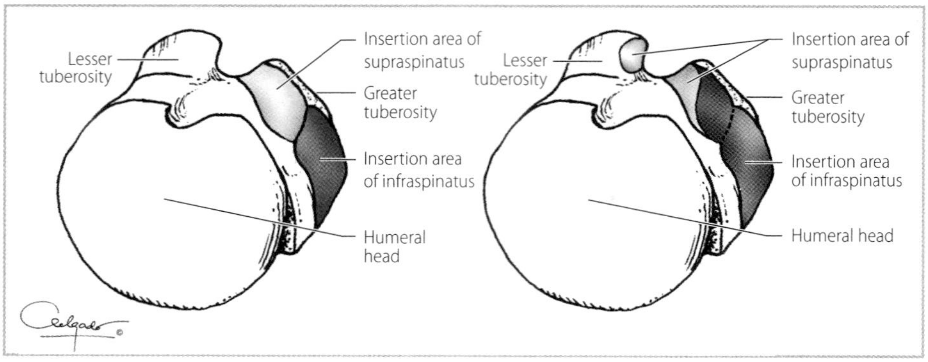

Figure 1.1 Footprint of the rotator cuff tendons.

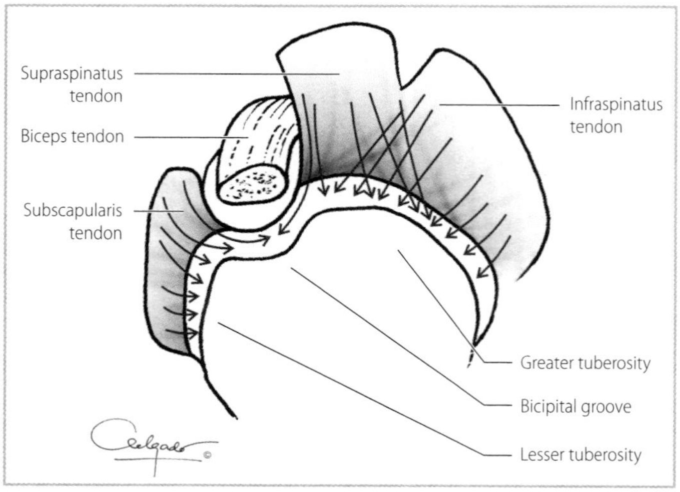

Figure 1.2 Fibers from teres minor (posterior) and subscapularis (anterior) interdigitate with those of supraspinatus and infraspinatus.

upper and lower subscapular nerves, from the posterior cord of the brachial plexus (C5 and C6 nerve roots). Subscapularis forms the most anterior part of the rotator cuff and stabilizes the shoulder, preventing anterior dislocation at 0° of abduction. Subscapularis originates from the anterior surface of the scapula, passing laterally beneath the coracoid and scapular neck and becoming tendinous at the level of the glenoid. At its insertion, the tendinous portion of subscapularis blends with fibers of the joint capsule, inserting into the lesser tuberosity. The subscapularis footprint is broad proximally and tapered distally, resulting in a comma shape (Ide 2008). It consists of a proximal tendinous part and a distal muscular part. There are marked differences between female and male specimens in the maximum longitudinal length, maximum transverse length and size of the bare area at maximum transverse distance, and distal end position (Ide et al. 2008).

The upper portion of the subscapularis tendon interdigitates with the anterior fibers of the suspraspinatus tendon, forming the rotator cuff interval, which is defined as the triangular space between the anterior aspect of the supraspinatus tendon and the superior aspect of the subscapularis tendon (Bigoni and Chung 2004). The transverse humeral ligament lies at the intertubercular sulcus, at the apex of the rotator interval for the long head of biceps (**Fig. 1.4**), the base of the rotator interval being the coracoid process. The capsular bottom of the rotator interval is made up of the coracohumeral and superior glenohumeral ligaments. The biceps pulley is a stabilizing sling of the long head of the biceps tendon against the anterior shearing stress in the rotator cuff interval (**Fig. 1.5**), and consists of four structures: the coracohumeral ligament, superior glenohumeral ligament, fibers of the supraspinatus tendon, and fibers of the subscapularis tendon.

Supraspinatus

Supraspinatus arises from the dorsal surface of the scapula in the supraspinatus fossa and the fascia covering the muscle, passing

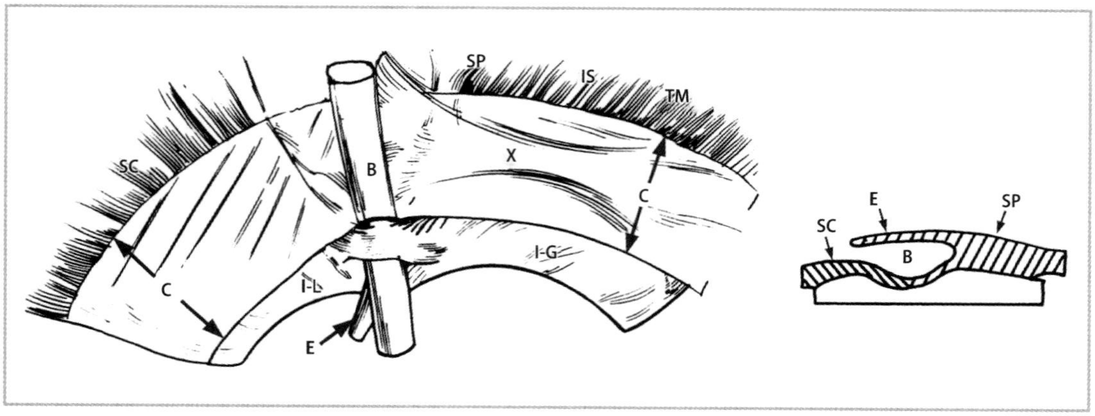

Figure 1.3 The supraspinatus and subscapularis tendons fuse to form a sheath that surrounds the long head of biceps tendon at the proximal end of the groove. Fibers from the subscapularis tendon pass below the biceps tendon and join with fibers from supraspinatus to form the floor of the sheath. B, biceps tendon; C, capsule; E, slip from supraspinatus tendon forming a roof over the biceps tendon; I-G, insertions on the greater tuberosity; I-L, insertions on the lesser tuberosity; IS, infraspinatus; SC, subscapularis; SP, supraspinatus; TM, teres minor; X, pericapsular band. (With permission from Clark JM, Harryman DT II. Tendons, ligaments, and capsule of the rotator cuff. Gross and microscopic anatomy. J Bone Joint Surg Am 1992;74:713–725).

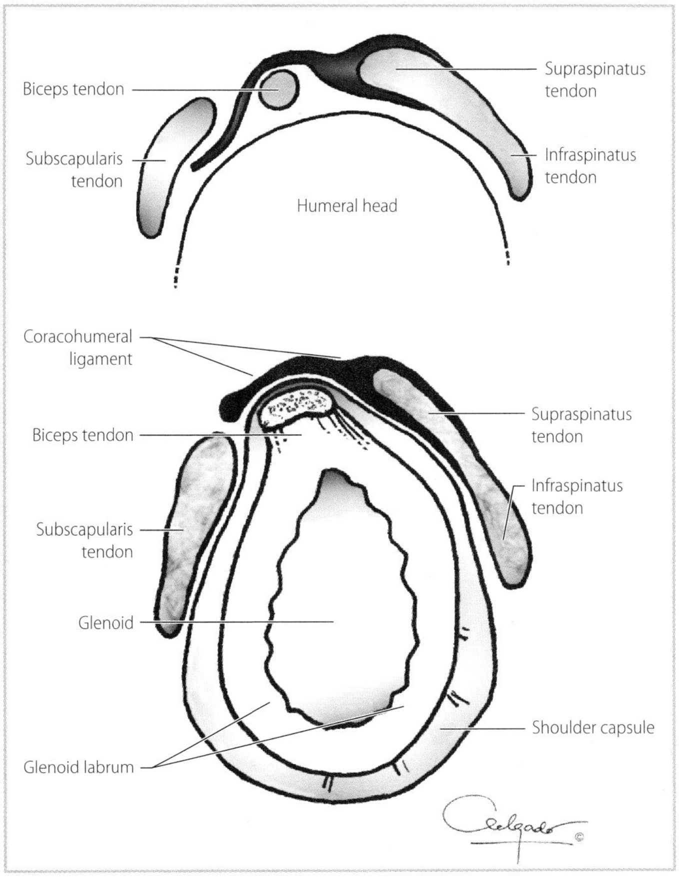

Figure 1.4 Relationships of the coracohumeral ligament (black) with the rotator cuff and scapula glenoid.

over the top of the shoulder joint to insert on the upper aspect of the greater tuberosity. It is a long thin muscle. Supraspinatus acts as an upper stabilizer of the humeral head, preventing it impinging on the undersurface of the acromion. It initiates abduction of the humerus, and is innervated by the suprascapular nerve after passing through the suprascapular notch. Supraspinatus inserts into the anteromedial area of the highest impression of the greater tuberosity. The footprint of supraspinatus is triangular, with the base lying along the articular surface. It is widest anteriorly and becomes narrow posteriorly on the greater tuberosity. The average maximum medial-to-lateral length of the footprint of supraspinatus is 6.9 mm, and that of infraspinatus is 10.2 mm (Mochizuki et al. 2008).

Most of the muscle fibers of supraspinatus, especially those of its superficial layer, run anterolaterally in front of the anterior tendinous portion, whereas the rest of the fibers from the deep layer run laterally in front of the medial margin of the highest impression on the greater tuberosity (Mochizuki et al. 2008).

A cadaveric study determined the extension of the supraspinatus tendon into subscapularis (Boon et al. 2004). Subscapularis extends over the bicipital groove, interdigitating with supraspinatus over the greater tuberosity of the humerus. The direction of subscapularis over the lesser tuberosity and that of the tendon of supraspinatus toward the bicipital groove facilitate their function in stabilizing the shoulder joint. The interdigitation area between both muscles may be disrupted as part of a rotator cuff tear (Defranco and Cole 2009).

Supraspinatus has traditionally been considered an important abductor among the rotator cuff muscles. However, infraspinatus contributes as much to abduction as supraspinatus (Hansen et al. 2008). Supraspinatus is most commonly considered an abductor of the humerus, but has also been shown to produce humeral rotation (Gates et al. 2010).

Infraspinatus

Infraspinatus arises from its covering fascia and the infraspinatus fossa; it inserts on the greater tubercle, immediately below the insertion of supraspinatus. It is a thick triangular muscle with three pennate origins.

Infraspinatus is innervated by the suprascapular nerve after it passes through the spinoglenoid notch. The supraspinatus and infraspinatus tendons join about 15 mm proximal to their insertion on the humerus.

Teres minor

Teres minor arises from the upper two-thirds of the dorsal surface of the lateral border of the scapula, and the septa between it and infraspinatus. It inserts on the greater tuberosity, below the insertion of infraspinatus.

Although there is an interval between the muscular portions of supraspinatus and teres minor, these two muscles merge just proximal to the musculotendinous junction.

Supraspinatus and infraspinatus are supplied by the suprascapular nerve (C5 and C6 nerve roots). Teres minor receives a branch from the nerve to the deltoid muscle, the axillary nerve (C5 and C6 nerve roots) [11].

Vessels

The blood flow to the shoulder muscles is supplied mainly from branches of the subclavian and axillary arteries. Vascularization of the rotator cuff muscles depends mainly on three sources: the thoracoacromial, suprahumeral, and subscapular arteries. The brachial artery is responsible for the arterial supply to both heads of biceps (Rothman and Parke 1965).

The area of supraspinatus just proximal to its insertion is markedly undervascularized compared with the remainder of the cuff (Rothman and Parke 1965). This area of poor supraspinatus blood supply is located 10–15 mm proximal to the insertion of the supraspinatus tendon, where the blood vessels travel parallel to the tendon fibers, making the tendon vulnerable to stretch and compression by the surrounding structures. The supraspinatus tendon is vulnerable in areas with poor blood supplies, the "critical or hypovascular zone."

Brooks et al. (1992) counted vessels in 5 mm^2 slices from specimens of the supraspinatus tendon taken during autopsies. They found a mean of approximately 200 microvessels at distances of 5, 10, and 15 mm from the humeral head and up to 300 at a distance of 30 mm from the tendon insertion zone. The lumen of vessels observed was reduced in the critical areas. The functional capillary density was reduced in areas adjacent to lesions of the rotator cuff (Biberthaler et al. 2003).

The vessels in the third layer of the cuff were relatively small compared with those in the more superficial layers, and the blood supply was adequate for the metabolic needs of the tissue (Clark et al. 1992). The circulation of the rotator cuff is unidirectional, with no flow crossing the tide mark at the insertion of supraspinatus. During shoulder adduction, vessels of the supraspinatus tendon are unperfused. With

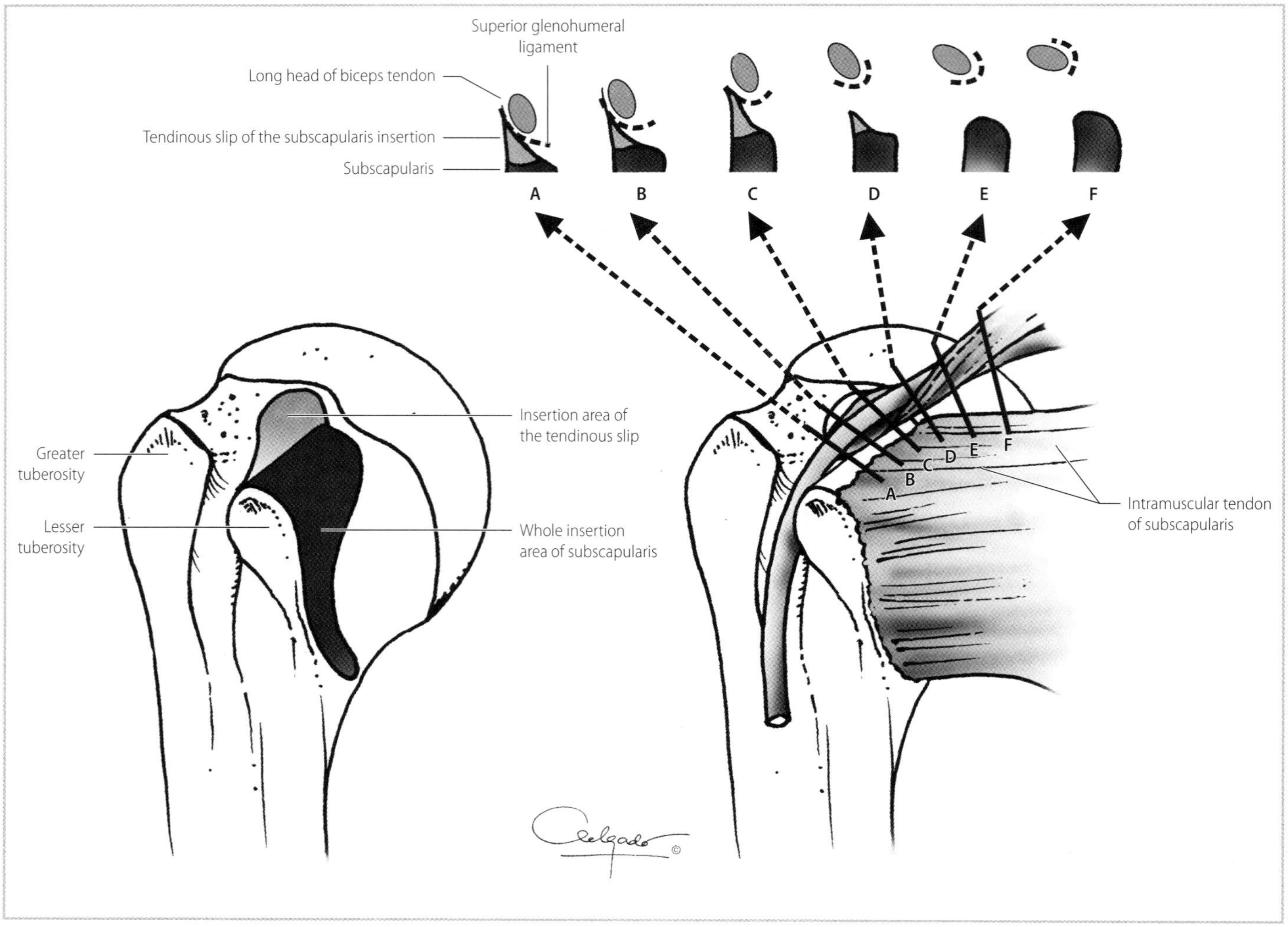

Figure 1.5 Schematic diagram. Shows the interrelationship of the coracohumeral ligament, superior glenohumeral ligament, and long biceps tendon at several planes in the rotator cuff interval.

the arm raised >30°, the intramuscular pressure of supraspinatus increases markedly.

The critical zone is probably a zone of anastomoses between the vessels supplying the bone and the tendon, and is no less vascular, except in certain positions. Although it is possible that sustained isometric contractions, prolonged adduction of the arm, or increases in subacromial pressure may reduce microcirculation, it is unlikely that frequent abduction or elevation of the arm would produce selective avascularity of the supraspinatus or biceps tendon.

Studying capillary distributions in cuff specimens, including the critical zone of supraspinatus (i.e., the anterior corner of the tendon near its insertion, which is prone to rupture and calcium deposits), Moseley and Goldie (1963) found that the critical zone was not much less vascularized than other parts of the cuff. Instead, it was rich in anastomoses between the osseous and tendinous vessels (Moseley and Goldie 1963). Both vessel diameters and lumina were approximately reduced by a third just 5 mm from the cuff edge, compared with 30 mm from the edge, but a really hypovascular area does not exist (Brooks et al. 1992). The hypovascularity could be an artifact because perfusion within the rotator cuff is a dynamic phenomenon. Reduced perfusion is obtained when the arm is in full adduction (Rathbun and Macfcnab 1970), when supraspinatus is compressed at the humeral head, the vessels are empty, and the vessel diameters dramatically decrease.

Bones and subacromial space

Three bones constitute the shoulder, namely the humerus, clavicle, and scapula. Four joints (sternoclavicular, acromioclavicular, glenohumeral joints, and the special scapulothoracic articulation) appear in the shoulder.

Scapula

The scapula is a triangular bone with three borders (superior, medial, and lateral) and three angles (superior, inferior, and lateral). The lateral angle is occupied by the smooth glenoid cavity, the articular surface receiving the head of the humerus. The glenoid cavity has a fibrocartilaginous rim around its edge, the labrum, which slightly widens and deepens the cavity.

Sixteen muscles attach to the scapula, some of which support and move the scapula, while the rest are related to the glenohumeral joint.

The anterior aspect of the scapula (subscapularis fossa) is covered by subscapularis, which also takes part in stabilizing the humeral head against the glenoid fossa. The posterior aspect of the scapula is divided by the scapular spine into two muscle compartments. The supraspinous fossa is small, and supraspinatus originates from it, whereas infraspinatus and teres minor originate from the infraspinous fossa.

The spine of the scapula provides the insertion area for the trapezius muscle. The deltoid muscle, which suspends the humerus, originates from its lower border. The spine of the scapula finishes laterally with the acromion, with the position of the acromion placing the deltoid muscle in a dominant position to provide strength during elevation of the arm.

Three types of acromion morphology have been described. Type I has a flat undersurface, type II is slightly convex, and type III is hooked. More recently, other types of acromion have been described as a type IV or convex acromion (Vanarthos et al. 1995) and an acromion with a keel (Tucker and Snyder 2004). Gagey et al. (1993) defined a new type of acromion, in which the middle third of the undersurface was convex (**Fig. 1.6**).

The angle between the scapula and the clavicle depends on function: when the shoulder is protracted, the angle is 50°, at rest it is around 60°, and with retraction the angle increases to 70°.

In the lateral corner of the scapula, where the superior and lateral borders intersect, the coracoid process projects forward like a "crow's beak." This forward location provides an efficient lever, whereby pectoralis minor, coracobrachialis, and the short head of biceps brachialis are inserted and help to stabilize the scapula.

The scapula has three ligaments of its own:

1. The coracoacromial ligament and its osseous fixations form an osteofibrous arch above the shoulder joint, which plays a role in the impingement syndrome.
2. The superior transverse scapular ligament, or its ossified arch (the scapular incisure), can cause a typical compression syndrome of the suprascapular nerve.
3. The inferior transverse scapular ligament.

Humerus

The proximal portion of the humerus is made up of the head and two tuberosities, the greater and lesser, which serve as attachments of the rotator cuff muscles. The region where the proximal extremity and the shaft of the humerus join is referred to as the surgical neck. The axillary nerve and posterior humeral circumflex artery lie together through the medial aspect of the surgical neck.

The greater tuberosity has three facets (superior, middle and inferior) for the rotator cuff tendon insertions (supraspinatus, infraspinatus, and teres minor). The lesser tuberosity serves as the attachment for subscapularis. Supraspinatus, infraspinatus, and teres minor are inserted from above to below to the greater tuberosity.

Both tuberosities are separated by the intertubercular groove, on the long head of the biceps tendon, which crosses the arm, passes through both tuberosities, reaches the humeral head, makes a right angle turn, and attaches to the superior rim of the glenoid fossa. The groove is closed by the transverse humeral ligament to restrain the tendon in the anatomical position.

Joints

Glenohumeral joint

The glenohumeral joint is characterized by its mobility and large range of motion. The normal glenohumeral joint approximates a spherical joint with a small amount of translation. Its stability is maintained by different mechanisms. Although most of these mechanisms could potentially operate throughout the entire range of motion, the relative importance of each depends on whether the shoulder is in the mid-range or end-of-range motion. The end of range is characterized by increased tensile force on the static restraints of the capsule and its ligaments. All glenohumeral motions that occur without increasing capsular tension above the baseline level are functionally in the mid-range.

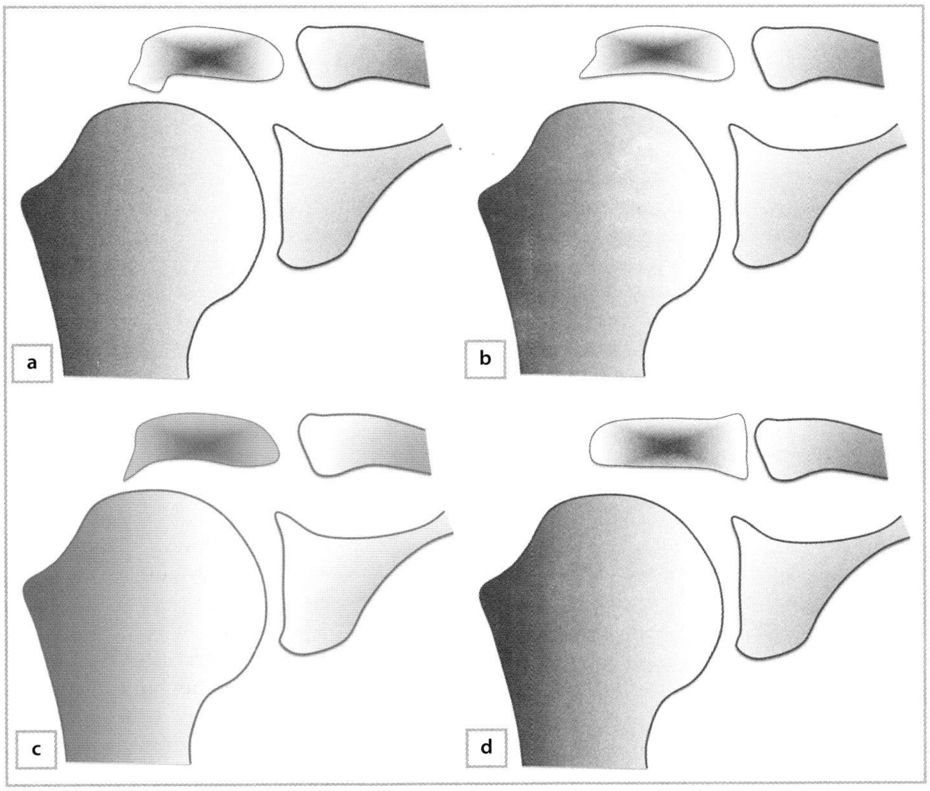

Figure 1.6 Types of spur. (a) Heel-type spur, (b) traction-type spur, (c) bird-beak spur, and (d) medial-type spur.

The glenoid labrum consists of dense connective tissue and surrounds the margin of the glenoid cavity. Two areas exhibit specialized conditions: cranially at the supraglenoid tubercle, there is an intimate relationship with the tendon of the long bicipital head and, in about 55% of cases, the labrum is stretched over the glenoid rim at the ventral side.

The glenohumeral ligament is a static stabilizer, preventing excessive translation of the humeral head, particularly in the end-of-range motion. The glenohumeral ligaments, located in the ventral articular capsule, have a stabilizing function for the ventral part of the glenoid labrum. They lift the articular lip where it crosses the glenoid notch. This "labrum-lift effect" supports the stabilizing features of the articular lip and the glenohumeral ligaments.

The coracohumeral ligament arises from the coracoid process and runs laterally, where it is split into two bands by the long head of the biceps tendon. The posterior band blends with the supraspinatus tendon to insert near the greater tuberosity, and the anterior band blends with the subscapularis tendon to insert near the lesser tuberosity. The origin of the coracohumeral ligament was thought to be the lateral aspect of the base of the coracoid process. The main insertion of the coracohumeral ligament was classically thought to be the lateral rotator interval, and some studies suggested another insertion into the supraspinatus or subscapularis tendon. Nové-Josserand et al. (2005) found that the coracohumeral ligament covers the superior glenohumeral ligament, filling the space between the supraspinatus tendon and subscapularis, uniting these tendons to complete the rotator cuff in this area.

The glenohumeral joint has a voluminous capsule that allows large amounts of motion. Medially, it is attached to the labrum and, laterally, to the anatomical neck of the humerus. The tendons of the rotator cuff reinforce the superior, posterior, and anterior aspects of the capsule. The anterior aspect is reinforced by three ligaments (Z ligaments: superior, middle, and inferior glenohumeral ligaments).

The coracoacromial arch

The coracoacromial arch is formed by the anteroinferior aspect of the acromion process, coracoacromial ligament, and inferior surface of the acromioclavicular joint. The coracoacromial ligament is often described as the roof of the shoulder. It is a thick structure that runs from the coracoid process to the anteroinferior aspect of the acromion, with some of its fibers extending to the acromioclavicular joint. The ligament is formed by two bands that join near the acromion and prevent separation of the acromioclavicular joint surfaces. Spur formation occurs preferentially in the anterolateral band. As a result, the anterolateral band is commonly involved in the impingement syndrome. The supraglenohumeral and coracohumeral ligaments were considered to be structural components of the rotator interval.

Subacromial space

The subacromial or suprahumeral space is an area located on the superior aspect of the glenohumeral joint, which is limited inferiorly by the tuberosity of the humeral head, anteromedially by the coracoid process, and superiorly by the coracoacromial arch.

The structures that are located within the suprahumeral space include, from inferior to superior, the head of the humerus, the intra-articular portion of the long head of biceps tendon, the superior aspect of the joint capsule, supraspinatus, and the upper margins of subscapularis and infraspinatus, the subdeltoid–subacromial bursae, and the inferior surface of the coracoacromial arch.

The subacromial space averages 10–11 mm in height with the arm adducted to the side. Elevating the arm decreases the distance between the acromion and the humerus to 6 mm at 90°; the space is at its narrowest point between 60° and 120° of scaption.

Acromion morphology

The mechanical effect of the acromion is the most cited predictor of rotator cuff impingement. Bigliani et al. (1991) has described three acromion shapes, and cadaveric studies have confirmed a 70% incidence of rotator cuff tears in patients with a type III acromial shape and only 3% in patients with a type I acromion. Neer (1983) concluded that 95% of all rotator cuff tears were initiated by impingement associated with the anterior third of the acromion. Bigliani et al. (1991) related the tears to the shape of the acromion and found a flat acromion or type I in 17% of the full-thickness cadaveric rotator cuff tears, a curved acromion or type II in 43%, and a hooked acromion or type III in 39%.

Enthesophytes were also significantly more common in type III acromions, and this combination was particularly associated with subacromial impingement syndrome and rotator cuff tears. In type I and IV acromions, the frequency of enthesophytes was very small (Natsis et al. 2007). Vähäkari (2010) found a greater acromial angle in patients with type III impingement syndrome than in the control group. Edelson (2006) and Nyffeler et al. (2006) suggested that acromial length or angle is more important than the acromial shape in rotator cuff tears.

Ogawa et al. (1990) classified acromial spurs according to size, and emphasized that only large spurs measuring >5 mm had diagnostic value because of the high rate of association with bursal-side tears and complete rotator cuff tears. Tucker and Snyder (2004) identified central, longitudinal, and downward-sloping spurs on the acromial undersurface, known as "acromial keel spurs," which were related to bursal-sided, partial-thickness and full-thickness rotator cuff tears. Acromial spurs are presumed to form by traction of the coracoacromial ligament (Ogata and Uhthoff 1990; Hirano et al. 2002). A relationship between acromion morphology and treatment was found. In more than 200 patients, the success of conservative management decreased with changes in acromion shapes: type I acromions responded in 89% of cases, type II in 73% of cases, and type III in 58% of cases (Wang et al. 2000).

The development of the different acromial shape is likely both congenital and acquired. With acquired causes, only age has been positively correlated to progression, from a flat to a curved or hooked acromion. Acromion shape could change with age in many cases, from type I to type III, due to traction forces (Wang et al. 2000). This implies that acromial variations and impingement are secondary to another primary intrinsic original factor. Acromial changes are also related to the fact that the disease is more symptomatic in dominant than in non-dominant arms (Yamaguchi et al. 2001). Frequency, intensity, and the nature of mechanical activities and sports may be responsible. The importance and complexity of intrinsic factors to tendon tears must also be considered (Longo et al. 2007, 2008a–c, 2009a–d, 2010a–e; Franceschi et al. 2009; Lippo et al. 2010; Longo 2010).

Coracoid process

Knowledge of the anatomy of the coracoid process and its effect on subcoracoid space is essential to understand the concept of coracoid impingement. Impingement of the rotator cuff occurs between the posterolateral coracoid and the humeral head (Franceschi et al. 2007). Changes in the coracoid process length or angulation may predispose to coracoid impingement, and place supraspinatus or subscapularis at risk of tearing (Franceschi et al. 2007).

Os acromiale and acromial spurs

Approximately 7–15% of patients have an os acromiale, and it is unlikely that this has a pathological effect on the rotator cuff. The os acromiale forms the triangular epiphysis of the scapular spine.

Bursae

The glenohumeral synovium forms variously sized bursae. Three are relevant in the clinical anatomy of the shoulder, namely the subacromial bursa, subdeltoid bursa, and subcoracoid bursa. The subcoracoid and subacromial bursae may be connected, and the subacromial bursa lies on the superior aspect of the joint. It provides two smooth serosal layers, one joined with the deltoid muscle and the other with the rotator cuff lying beneath. This bursa is also connected to the acromion, greater tuberosity, and coracoacromial ligament. As the humerus elevates, it permits the rotator cuff to slide easily beneath the deltoid muscle.

EMBRYOLOGY

Humans develop from a single cell. Through cell division, several different types of cells are produced by differentiation. The capacity of some cells to divide into cells of other types is known as pluripotency. In the earliest stages of growth, the first few generations of cells are totipotent, because each of them has the capacity to produce all the various cell types in a living person. The 9-month prenatal period begins as a few weeks of aggressive cellular differentiation, followed by an extended period (several months) of minor cellular differentiation and major multiplication, or proliferation.

Three germ layers give rise to all the tissues and organs of the body, namely the ectoderm, mesoderm, and endoderm. The ectoderm layer detects the environment. The epidermis and its appendages (mammary glands, pituitary gland, and subcutaneous glands) and the entire nervous system (central and peripheral nervous systems) derive from the ectoderm. Even the senses of smell, sight, hearing, and taste represent nothing more than neural (ectodermal) tissues that are directly exposed to specialized skin (e.g., the cornea or tympanic membrane).

The endoderm remains relatively unchanged during development, and is represented in the adult body only by thin layers of cells that line most of the internal surfaces. The endodermal tube remains open at the top (the mouth) and the bottom end (the anus). Between these two points, the entire tube of cells responsible for absorbing nutrient energy for the body remains exposed to the outside world. No endoderm is found in the limbs.

The mesoderm layer occupies every available point between the ectodermal plate and the endodermal plate, except for two places, at the cranial and caudal ends of the embryo. At these spots, the mesoderm cannot break the seal of ectoderm on endoderm. Everywhere else, there is mesoderm under the skin. The mesoderm gives rise to cartilage, bone, connective tissue, striated and smooth muscle, blood cells, kidneys, gonads, spleen, and the serous membrane lining the body cavities. Mesoderm develops into all the muscle and connective tissue (e.g., bone, ligament, tendon, and fascia) and into specialized tissues as well (e.g., blood vessels). Mesoderm develops in both rigid connective tissue (e.g., bone) and very compliant connective tissue (e.g., fascia). It gives rise to all the tissues that enable us to move.

Most studies of the developing shoulder have focused primarily on bone maturation. Analysis of soft-tissue structures of the developing shoulder, such as the rotator cuff, joint capsule, and labrum, is still incomplete.

ACKNOWLEDGMENT

Dr PJ Delgado for the drawings.

REFERENCES

Biberthaler P, Wiedemann E, Nerlich A, et al. Microcirculation associated with degenerative rotator cuff lesions. In vivo assessment with orthogonal polarization spectral imaging during arthroscopy of the shoulder. J Bone Joint Surg Am 2003;85:475–480.

Bigliani LU, Ticker JB, Flatow EL, et al. The relationship of acromial architecture to rotator cuff disease. Clin Sports Med 1991;10:823–838.

Bigoni BJ, Chung CB. MR imaging of the rotator cuff interval. Magn Reson Imaging Clin North Am 2004;12:61–73, vi.

Boon JM, de Beer MA, Botha D, Maritz NGJ, Fouche AA. The anatomy of the subscapularis tendon insertion as applied to rotator cuff repair. J Shoulder Elbow Surg 2004;13:165–169.

Brooks CH, Revell WJ, Heatley FW. A quantitative histological study of the vascularity of the rotator cuff tendon. J Bone Joint Surg Br 1992;74:151–153.

Burkhart SS, Esch JC, Jolson RS. The rotator crescent and rotator cable: an anatomic description of the shoulder's "suspension bridge." Arthroscopy 1993;9:611–616.

Clark J, Sidles JA, Matsen FA. The relationship of the glenohumeral joint capsule to the rotator cuff. Clin Orthop Relat Res 1990;254:29–34.

Clark JM, Harryman DT, II. Tendons, ligaments, and capsule of the rotator cuff. Gross and microscopic anatomy. J Bone Joint Surg Am 1992;74:713–725.

DeFranco MJ, Cole BJ. Current perspectives on rotator cuff anatomy. Arthroscopy 2009;25:305–20.

Edelson JG. The 'hooked' acromion revisited. J Bone Joint Surg Br 1995;77:284–287.

Franceschi F, Longo UG, Ruzzini L, et al. Arthroscopic management of calcific tendinitis of the subscapularis tendon. Knee Surg Sports Traumatol Arthrosc 2007;15:1482–1485.

Franceschi F, Longo UG, Ruzzini L, et al. Characteristics at haematoxylin and eosin staining of ruptures of the long head of the biceps tendon. Br J Sports Med 2009;43:603–607.

Gagey N, Ravaud E, Lassau JP. Anatomy of the acromial arch: correlation of anatomy and magnetic resonance imaging. Surg Radiol Anat 1993;15:63–70.

Gates JJ, Gilliland J, McGarry MH, et al. Influence of distinct anatomic subregions of the supraspinatus on humeral rotation. J Orthop Res 2010;28:12–17.

Gerber C, Sebesta A. Impingement of the deep surface of the subscapularis tendon and the reflection pulley on the anterosuperior glenoid rim: a preliminary report. J Shoulder Elbow Surg 2000;9:483–490.

Hansen ML, Ogtis JC, Johnson JS, et al. Biomechanics of massive rotator cuff tears: implications for treatment. J Bone Joint Surg Am 2008;90:316–325.

Hirano M, Ide J, Takagi K. Acromial shapes and extension of rotator cuff tears: magnetic resonance imaging evaluation. J Shoulder Elbow Surg 2002;11:576–578.

Ide J. An anatomic study of the subscapularis insertion to the humerus: the subscapularis footprint. Arthroscopy 2008;24:749–753.

Inman VT, Saunders JB, Abbott LC. Observations of the function of the shoulder joint. Clin Orthop Relat Res 1996;330:3–12.

Kolts I, Busch LC, Tomusk H, et al. Macroscopical anatomy of the so-called "rotator interval." A cadaver study on 19 shoulder joints. Ann Anat 2002;184:9–14.

Lippi G, Longo UG, Maffulli N. Genetics and sports. Br Med Bull 2010;93:27–47.

Longo UG. Triglycerides and total serum cholesterol in rotator cuff tears: do they matter? Br J Sports Med 2010;44:948–951.

Longo UG, Franceschi F, Ruzzini L, et al. Light microscopic histology of supraspinatus tendon ruptures. Knee Surg Sports Traumatol Arthrosc 2007;15:1390–1394.
Longo UG, Ramamurthy C, Denaro V, et al. Minimally invasive stripping for chronic Achilles tendinopathy. Disabil Rehabil 2008a;30:1709–1713.
Longo UG, Olivia F, Denaro V, et al. Oxygen species and overuse tendinopathy in athletes. Disabil Rehabil 2008b;30:1563–1571.
Longo UG, Franceschi F, Ruzzini L,et al. Histopathology of the supraspinatus tendon in rotator cuff tears. Am J Sports Med 2008c;36:533–538.
Longo UG, Ronga M, Maffulli N. Achilles tendinopathy. Sports Med Arthrosc 2009a;17:112–126.
Longo UG, Ronga M, Maffulli N. Acute ruptures of the achilles tendon. Sports Med Arthrosc 2009b;17:127–138.
Longo UG, Rittweger J, Garau G, et al. No influence of age, gender, weight, height, and impact profile in achilles tendinopathy in masters track and field athletes. Am J Sports Med 2009c;37:1400–1405.
Longo UG, Franceschi F, Ruzzini L, et al. Histopathology of the higher fasting plasma glucose levels within the normoglycaemic range and rotator cuff tears. Br J Sports Med 2009d;43:284–287.
Longo UG, Lamberti A, Maffulli N, Denaro V. Tendon augmentation grafts: a systematic review. Br Med Bull 2010a;94:165–188.
Longo UG, Lamberti A, Maffulli N, Denaro V. Tissue engineered biological augmentation for tendon healing: a systematic review. Br Med Bull 2011;98:31-59
Longo UG, Forriol F, Maffulli N, Denaro V. Evaluation of histological scoring systems for tissue-engineered, repaired and osteoarthritic cartilage. Osteoarthr Cartilage 2010c;18:1001; author reply 1002.
Longo UG, Fazio V, Poeta ML, et al. Bilateral consecutive rupture of the quadriceps tendon in a man with BstUI polymorphism of the COL5A1 gene. Knee Surg Sports Traumatol Arthrosc 2010d;18:514–518.
Longo UG, Fazio V, Poeta ML, et al. Bilateral consecutive rupture of the quadriceps tendon in a man with BstUI polymorphism of the COL5A1 gene. Knee Surg Sports Traumatol Arthrosc 2010e;18:514–518.
Minagawa H, Itoi E, Konno N, et al. Humeral attachment of the supraspinatus and infraspinatus tendons: an anatomic study. Arthroscopy 1998;14:302–306.
Mochizuki T, Sugaya H, Uomizu M, et al. Humeral insertion of the supraspinatus and infraspinatus. New anatomical findings regarding the footprint of the rotator cuff. J Bone Joint Surg Am 2008;90:962–969.
Moseley HF, Goldie I. The arterial pattern of the rotator cuff of the shoulder. J Bone Joint Surg Br 1963;45:780–789.
Natsis K, Tsikaras P, Totlis T, et al. Correlation between the four types of acromion and the existence of enthesophytes: a study on 423 dried scapulas and review of the literature. Clin Anat 2007;20:267–272.
Neer CS, 2nd. Impingement lesions. Clin Orthop Relat Res 1983;173:70–77.
Nové-Josserand L, Edwards TB, O´Connor DP, Walch G. The acromiohumeral and coracohumeral intervals are abnormal in rotator cuff tears with muscular fatty degeneration. Clin Orthop Rel Res 2005; 433:90–98.
Nyffeler RW, Werner CM, Sukthankar A, Schmid MR, Gerber C. Association of a large lateral extension of the acromion with rotator cuff tears. J Bone Joint Surg Am 2006;88:800–805.
Ogata S, Uhthoff HK. Acromial enthesopathy and rotator cuff tear. A radiologic and histologic postmortem investigation of the coracoacromial arch. Clin Orthop Relat Res 1990;254:39–48.
Ogawa K, Inokuchi W, Naniwa T. Subacromial impingement associated with deltoid contracture. A report of two cases. J Bone Joint Surg Am 1999;81:1744–1746.
Rathbun JB, Macnab I. The microvascular pattern of the rotator cuff. J Bone Joint Surg Br 1970;52:540–553.
Rothman RH, Parke WW. The vascular anatomy of the rotator cuff. Clin Orthop Relat Res 1965;41:176–186.
Saha AK. Dynamic stability of the glenohumeral joint. Acta Orthop Scand 1971;42:491–505.
Tucker TJ, Snyder SJ. The keeled acromion: an aggressive acromial variant – a series of 20 patients with associated rotator cuff tears. Arthroscopy 2004;20:744–753.
Vähäkari M. Acromial shape in asymptomatic subjects: a study of 305 shoulders in different age groups. Acta Radiol 2010;51:202–206.
Vanarthos WJ, Monu JU. Type 4 acromion: a new classification. Contemp Orthop 1995;30:227–229.
Wang JC, Horner G, Brown ED, et al. The relationship between acromial morphology and conservative treatment of patients with impingement syndrome. Orthopedics 2000;23:557–559.
Yamaguchi, K, Ball CM, Galatz LM. Arthroscopic rotator cuff repair: transition from mini-open to all-arthroscopic. Clin Orthop Relat Res 2001;390:83–94.

Chapter 2 Surgical anatomy and rotator cuff tear pattern

Francesco Franceschi, Angelo Del Buono, Rocco Papalia, Nicola Maffulli, Vincenzo Denaro

KEY FEATURES

- Rotator cuff tears can be classified by shape, the number of tendons involved, and the size of the tear, including its anteroposterior and medial lateral dimensions.
- Partial-thickness rotator cuff tears are either interstitial, indicating a defect entirely within the substance of the cuff, or communicating, denoting disruption of the tendon fibrils on the underside of the cuff, with free communication between the joint space and the defect.
- The coracoacromial arch marks the superior boundary of the subacromial space and protects the rotator cuff from external trauma inflicted on the top of the shoulder.
- Knowledge of the three-dimensional tear pattern is a critical initial step in achieving a quality repair.

Many factors influence the management of rotator cuff tears, including knowledge of rotator cuff anatomy and tear pattern. Tear pattern recognition is critical to ensure an accu rate anatomical rotator cuff repair (Codman 1934) and to appropriately reproduce the normal action of the fibers (Wolfgang 1974, Patte 1990, McLaughlin 1944). This chapter explains how rotator cuff anatomy and tear pattern influence decision-making in the management of rotator cuff disease.

ROTATOR CUFF ANATOMY

The rotator cuff is a group of four muscles (subscapularis, supraspinatus, infraspinatus, and teres minor) that function as dynamic stabilizers of the spherical humeral head in the shallow glenoid fossa **(Table 2.1)** (Codman 1934). Their short, flat, broad tendons fuse intimately with the fibrous capsule, which in turn is enveloped and circumferentially strengthened by the rotator cuff, except where the rotator interval is located.

Table 2.1 Physiology of the shoulder muscles

Shoulder muscles
Superficial
Deltoid: main abductor, especially in the range 90–180°
Teres major: adduction and internal rotation
Deep
Supraspinatus: abduction (0–90°) and external rotation
Infraspinatus: external rotation
Teres minor: external rotation
Subscapularis: adduction and internal rotation
Long head of biceps: humeral head depressor

The rotator interval

This is a triangular anatomical area in the anterosuperior aspect of the shoulder, which is defined by the coracoid process at its base, the anterior margin of the supraspinatus tendon superiorly, and the superior margin of the subscapularis tendon inferiorly. The rotator interval is reinforced externally by the coracohumeral ligament (CHL) and internally by the superior glenohumeral ligament (SGHL); it is traversed by the intra-articular biceps tendon. This anatomical complex plays an important role in the normal function of the shoulder joint. The imaging assessment can be difficult, but arthroscopic evaluation of this area is often required to confirm suspected pathology (De Palma 2008)

Subscapularis

Subscapularis is a large, flat muscle that fills the entire subscapular fossa and comprises the anterior portion of the rotator cuff. Subscapularis is covered by a thick fibrous aponeurosis, and is innervated by the upper and lower subscapular nerves. Almost all tendon fibers blend with the anterior capsule just lateral to the glenoid rim, and extend laterally to subcapsularis's insertion on the lesser tuberosity. A large subscapular bursa is located between the muscle and the joint capsule, and communicates with the cavity of the joint capsule. The axillary nerve runs along the inferior scapular border and is, therefore, susceptible to injury after an anterior dislocation. It acts as an internal rotator, especially in maximum internal rotation, opposing the volume and power of infraspinatus and teres minor posteriorly (De Palma 2008).

Infraspinatus

Infraspinatus originates from the infraspinous fossa on the posterior aspect of the scapula and extends laterally in very close proximity to the posterior fibrous capsule. The tendon insertion is fixed to the middle aspect of the greater tuberosity. It is covered by a thick fascia, which is fixed to the scapular spine and inserted into the lateral margin of the scapula up to the proximal portion of the humerus. The muscle is intimately associated with teres minor, divided by a clearly visible intermuscular septum. Innervation is from the suprascapular nerve. Along with teres minor, infraspinatus serves as the primary external rotator of the shoulder (Soslowsky et al. 1997).

Teres minor

Teres minor is a narrow muscle originating from the mid to upper axillary border of the scapula and the lower portion of the intermuscular septum. After extending laterally and superiorly, together with the capsule, its fairly thick tendon inserts to the inferior facet of the greater tubercle. This muscle is innervated by a branch of the axillary nerve. Together with infraspinatus, it acts as an external rotator and glenohumeral stabilizer (Terry and Chopp 2000).

Supraspinatus

Originating from the supraspinous fossa, suprapinatus extends anterioraly and laterally, and inserts on the superior aspect of the greater tuberosity, just posterior to the bicipital groove. The tendon extends to the joint capsule and runs under the coracoacromial ligament, above the infraspinatus tendon. The muscle is covered by a thick fascia fixed to the superior scapular margin and the medial scapular margin, and by a thick aponeurosis to the spine of the scapula up to the acromion. The tendon is wrapped in a synovial sheath, which merges into the capsule of the shoulder joint, together with superficial muscle bundles of the articular muscles. Innervation is from the suprascapular nerve. Along with deltoid, it initiates forward elevation of the arm and functions as a glenohumeral stabilizer.

At the insertion point, supraspinatus, infraspinatus, and teres minor cannot be distinguished into anatomical units. The coracohumeral ligament passes along the interval placed between supraspinatus and subscapularis, where the biceps tendon and its synovial covering pass through the joint capsule (Ward et al. 2006).

Long head of biceps

The long head of biceps acts together with the rotator cuff as a humeral head depressor. The biceps tendon originates from the supraglenoid tubercle, leaves the joint through an exit between the superior capsule and the head of the humerus, and continues in the bicipital groove. The intracapsular tendon is located under the coracohumeral ligament, between supraspinatus and subscapularis. It continues into the bicipital groove, enveloped in a synovial covering deriving from the joint synovial membrane.

ANATOMY OF THE CORACOACROMIAL ARCH AND THE STRUCTURES IN THE SUBACROMIAL REGION

The coracoacromial arch marks the superior boundary of the subacromial space. It is formed by the acromion, coracoacromial ligament, and coracoid process. Anatomically, the arch protects the rotator cuff from external trauma inflicted on the top of the shoulder. However, the arch can also be a cause of injury, particularly when the shoulder is positioned in abduction and forward elevation. Indeed, mechanical loads acting on the arch have been shown to be involved in the development of rotator cuff disease. Together with the humerus, rotator cuff, and subacromial bursa, the arch is frequently referred to as the superior humeral articulation. The rotator cuff muscles are close to the undersurface of the coracoacromial ligament, acromion, and acromioclavicular joint, whereas the subacromial bursa lies between the rotator cuff and arch.

Acromion

The shape of the acromion shows considerable interindividual variation. In a cadaveric study on 140 shoulders Bigliani et al. (1986) found three types of acromion: flat (type I), curved (type II), and hooked (type III) (see **Fig. 5.11**). Relationships between acromial morphology and extent of rotator cuff tearing have been found. In fact, types II and III acromion may lead to rotator cuff extrinsic mechanical compression, shown to be responsible for degenerative changes of cuff tendons. In addition, an anatomical investigation has demonstrated how acromial length, height, and inclination are associated with rotator cuff degeneration.

The coracoacromial ligament

This is a strong triangular structure that stretches from the outer edge of the coracoid and inserts into the inner border of the acromion, just in front of the acromioclavicular joint. It has been hypothesized that its thickening may result in predisposition to shoulder impingement and rotator cuff degeneration. The ligament functions as a dynamic stabilizer, which is able to protect the acromion and coracoid from surrounding muscular loadings.

With regard to the *subacromial bursa*, it may be a single structure extending as far as the base of the coracoid or this portion may be a separate bursa often referred to as the subcoracoid bursa. Hypertrophic alterations in the bursa may be the cause of bursal impingement against the arch, interfering with the smooth rhythmical elevation and descent of the arm (DeFranco and Cole 2009).

ROTATOR CUFF TEARS

The histopathological changes involved in cuff tendon rupture mostly occur gradually and progressively, except in the rare cases of acute traumatic avulsion through normal tissue. Partial tears are either interstitial, indicating a defect entirely within the substance of the cuff, or communicating, denoting disruption of the tendon fibrils on the underside of the cuff with free communication between the joint space and the defect (Wolfgang 1974).

As reported by Codman (1934), the partial-thickness tears are referred to as either articular-side or bursal-side lesions, developed respectively on the undersurface of or over supraspinatus, and interstitial tears.

Ellman (1990) classified partial-thickness rotator cuff tears into three grades according to their depth: grade 1 tears involve <3 mm, grade 2 tears involve 3–6 mm, and grade 3 tears are >6 mm, or 50% of tendon thickness (**Table 2.2**).

Complete tears by definition allow free communication between the joint space and the subacromial bursa, and may be categorized by use of different classification systems (Codman 1934; McLaughlin 1944; Wolfgang 1974; Patte 1990; Ellman 1993).

As McLaughlin described in 1944, rotator cuff tears were classified as (1) transverse ruptures, (2) vertical splits, and (3) retracted tears. Later cuff tear classifications often described the one-dimensional length of a tendon tear or the number of tendons torn. To obtain three-dimensional information on indicated surgical options, such as end-to-bone repair, side-to-side repair, or interval slides, the tear configuration has been assessed by use of preoperative magnetic resonance imaging (MRI) or at arthroscopy.

As De Orio and Cofield described in 1984, the tear was categorized as small, medium, large, or massive, based on the length of the greatest diameter of the tear. However, a one-dimensional description

Table 2.2 Classification of partial-thickness tears

Location	Grade : Depth
Articular surface	1: <3 mm
Bursal surface	2: 3–6 mm
Interstitial	3: >6 mm

Based on Ellman H. Diagnosis and treatment of incomplete rotator cuff tears. Clin Orthop Relat Res 1990;254:64–74.

of a tear can be misleading because a cuff tear described as massive, difficult to repair, and characterized by unfavorable prognosis may in fact be easily repaired with a positive outcome. Harryman et al. (1991) assessed the tear status on the number of tendons torn. These systems do not differentiate specific tear pattern or method of repair.

In summary, characteristics of each rotator cuff tear at surgery may be recorded as follows: (1) classification of the tear by shape as either a crescent-shaped tear or a U-shaped tear (Burkhart 2000); (2) the number of tendons involved; and (3) by the size of the tear, including its anteroposterior and medial lateral dimensions in centimeters.

Tear shape

As Burkhart (Davidson and Burkhart 2010) noted, the cuff tear pattern is much more accurately assessed by arthroscopic inspection than through an open view: arthroscopic visualization provides a much more accurate three-dimensional assessment of tear configuration compared with findings detected by open means. Based on the shape, rotator cuff tears can be classified as crescent-shaped or U-shaped tears. Crescent-shaped tears, including large tears, are not far retracted and can usually be pulled away from the bone **(Fig. 2.1)**. They are typically repaired directly to the bone with no or minimal tension.

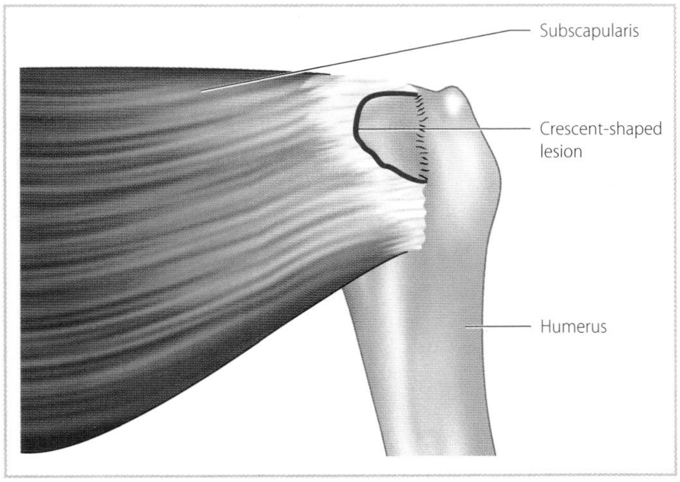

Figure 2.1 Crescent-shaped lesion.

In contrast, U-shaped tears generally extend much farther medially, to the glenoid, or even medial to the glenoid **(Fig. 2.2)**. The medial extension of the tear is not considered as a retraction, but represents the configuration that an L-shaped tear assumes under action of its muscle tendon components. To repair such a tear, the surgeon must reconstitute the two limbs of the "L," without trying to sufficiently mobilize the medial margin of the tear from the glenoid and scapular neck over to the humeral bone bed. The large tensile loads could result in repair failure.

Tendon involvement

Harryman et al. (1991) characterized the cuff status in terms of the integrity of the different tendons: type 0 refers to an intact cuff; type lA to the mildest identifiable pattern of tear, considered as thinning or a partial-thickness defect of the supraspinatus tendon; type lB tear is a full-thickness defect of the supraspinatus tendon; type II is a full-thickness defect involving the supraspinatus and infraspinatus tendons; and type III is a full-thickness defect involving the supraspinatus, infraspinatus, and subscapularis tendons.

Tear size

Tear size measures may be made in centimeters, including the total linear extent of the tear. As reported by De Orio and Cofield (1984), the length of the greatest diameter of the tear has been used to devise four categories of tear. Small tears measure ≤1 cm, medium tears <3 cm, large tears measure from 3 cm to 5 cm, and massive tears are >5 cm **(Fig. 2.3)**. The retraction is measured in centimeters from the greater tuberosity footprint to the leading edge of the tendon, with reference to a calibrated probe for arthroscopic cases and using a ruler in open cases, accounting for the original tear pattern that is presumed to have retracted and remodeled over time (**Table 2.3**).

Tear mobility

Before and after the release of soft-tissue contractures, mobility is subjectively assessed as excellent, moderate, or poor, on the basis of excursion and elasticity of the tendon complex. The tears with no adhesions are referred to as excellent; in these the muscle tendon unit may be easily inserted into the anatomical footprint. When inherent mild stiffness and minimal adhesions allow muscle tendon units to

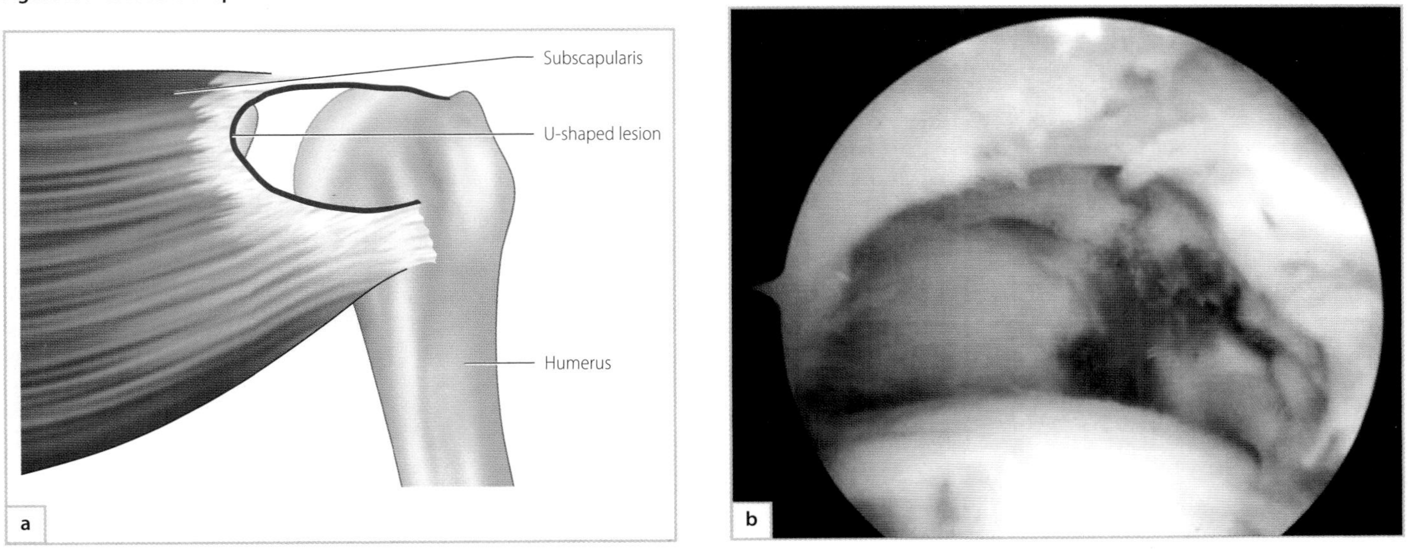

Figure 2.2 Different shapes: (a) U-shaped lesion; (b) arthroscopic finding of U-shaped tear.

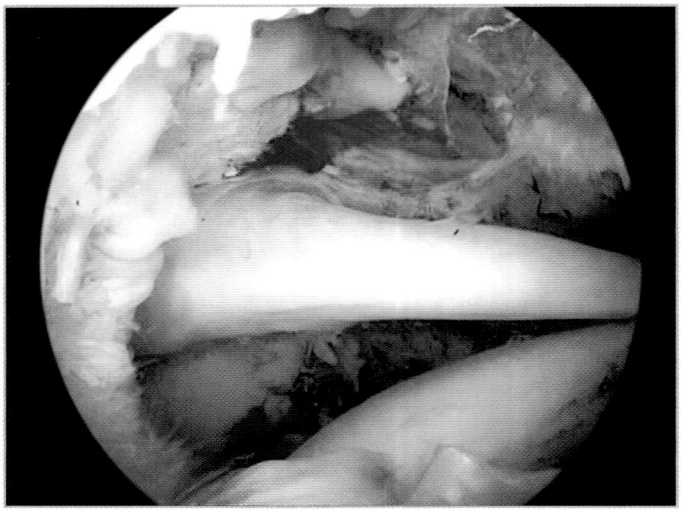

Figure 2.3 **Massive rotator cuff tear.**

Table 2.3 Classification of full-thickness tears

Lesion	Size (cm)	Involved tendons
Small	<1	<1
Medium	1–3	1
Large	3–5	2
Massive	>5	>2

be pulled to the footprint with tension, this is referred to as moderate. Finally, significant intrinsic stiffness, global adhesions, and the inability to perform anatomical repair are characteristics of poor mobility. These tears are unrepairable or can be pulled only to the medial footprint (Sallay et al. 2007).

Tissue quality

Tendon thickness and suture-holding properties determine the tissue quality. Excellent quality refers to normal tendon thickness, with no signs of remodeling, which easily holds suture. Moderate quality refers to tendon tissue exhibiting thinning and remodeling, but which still holds sutures. Poor quality is characteristic of thin and attritional tendons which hold sutures poorly or not at all.

Chronicity

Acute tears are classified as those that occur in the 6 weeks before surgery, presenting hypervascularity and fresh tear edges at surgical evaluation. Chronic rotator cuff tears are characterized by insidious onset of symptoms or a history of injury longer than 6 weeks. The intraoperative assessment shows signs of healing and remodeling at the tear edge.

If a recent injury or exacerbation occurs in the setting of an already existing chronic rotator cuff tear, the tears are considered as acute on chronic. At surgery, there is often evidence of recent injury, usually manifested by synovitis and acute reactive tissue.

Tear extension

McLaughlin (1944) and Wolfgang (1974) subdivided the complete tears into small transverse tears and larger triangular or crescentic ones. The transverse tears are located in the critical area in the superior portion of the cuff and run perpendicular to the cuff fibers. If there is retraction, they enlarge and assume a triangular or crescentic configuration. Massive complete tears result from either progressive cuff retraction, as a smaller tear enlargement, or severe trauma which avulsed a large portion of the insertion of the cuff. In some instances, a large area of the humeral head has been completely uncovered by such a tear.

Sallay et al. (2007) categorized the tear patterns by using a morphological classification system.

Transverse tear

The tendon was detached only from the greater tuberosity without evidence of involvement of the tendon or the rotator interval. Ellman's linear tears and crescent-shaped tears are included in the subgroup.

Anterior L tears

The detachment from the greater tuberosity with anterior extension into or near the rotator interval is termed anterior L tears (Ellman's reverse L tear).

Posterior L tears

The tendon is detached from the greater tuberosity which extends to posterior supraspinatus or into the substance of the infraspinatus tendon (Ellman's L tear).

Tongue-shaped tears

A posterior L tear extends into the rotator interval.

Shaped tears

V-shaped tears

It is avulsed from the greater tuberosity with a central longitudinal split component; the apex of the tear is centered relative to the base of the tear.

U-shaped tears

This is a large retracted tear with a falciform edge and with no specific pattern on initial inspection.

Complex tears

This is poor tissue quality or extensive delamination that did not fit any of the previously mentioned patterns and was not classified.

Boileau et al. (2005) determined the extent of the tear intraoperatively, under direct arthroscopic visualization, with the arthroscope in the lateral portal after debridement of the degenerated tendon edges. To evaluate associated tendon delamination, the assessment was performed in both the coronal and sagittal planes, according to a system that was an evolution of Thomazeau's classification (Thomazeau et al. 1997). Tendon retraction in the coronal plane is classified according to the position of the tear medial edge in reference to the surrounding anatomy **(Fig. 2.4)**.

If the tear edge is lying over the greater tuberosity, the tear retraction is classified as a stage I tear. These tears are usually <1 cm in greatest diameter. A stage II tear involves exposure of the humeral head, but the glenoid is still covered. These tears measure >1 cm and <3 cm in greatest diameter. A stage III tear is the glenoid exposure. These tears are severely retracted and measure between 3 and 5 cm in greatest diameter. A stage IV tear is medially retracted to the glenoid and measures >5 cm in greatest diameter. To assess the extent of the tear in the sagittal plane, the cuff is divided into six sectors (A, B, C, D, E, or F) **(Fig. 2.5)**. The most frequent tear pattern is the stage D and DE tears. The stage D tear is strictly limited to the supraspinatus

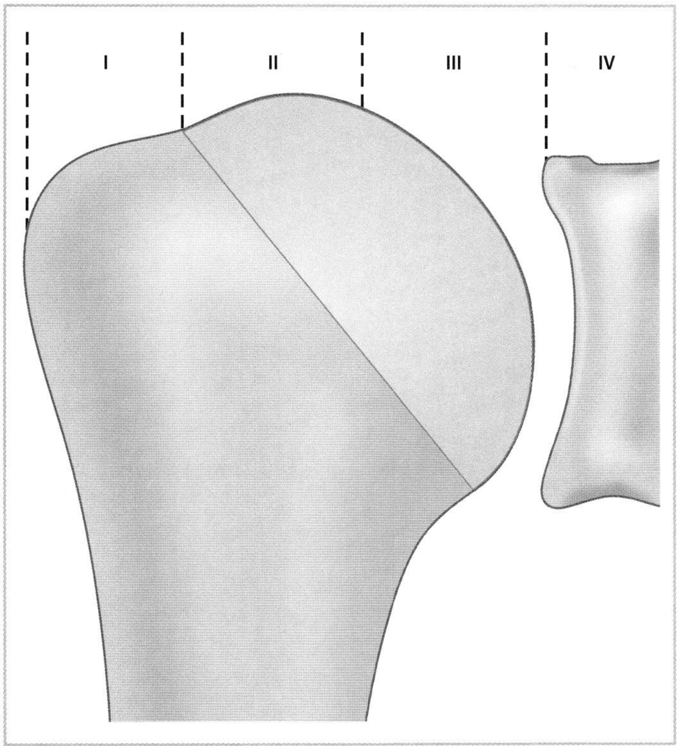

Figure 2.4 Classification of the extent of complex rotator cuff tears based on Thomazeau's classification for the coronal plane.

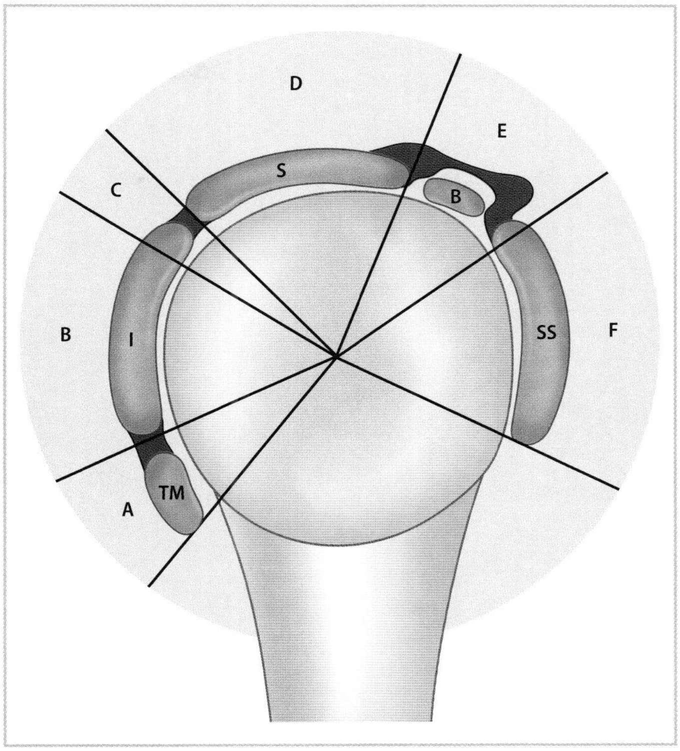

Figure 2.5 Classification of the extent of complex rotator cuff tears based on Thomazeau's classification for the sagittal plane. B, biceps; I, infraspinatus; S, supraspinatus; SS, subscapularis; TM, teres minor.

tendon, whereas the stage DE tear refers to the supraspinatus tear extended anteriorly to the rotator interval, with the long head of biceps uncovered, and/or associated subscapularis delamination or fraying. The stage CD tear is the supraspinatus tear associated with infraspinatus delamination. The stage CDE tear is the supraspinatus tear associated with anterior and posterior delamination or cleavage.

The delamination (or cleavage) is different from a partial-thickness tear. The former refers to tendon degenerative changes and fibrillation with no insertion disruption, the latter to a partial disruption of the tendon insertion from its footprint. This is an arthroscopic diagnosis.

CONCLUSION

The quality and mobility of rotator cuff tissue can be correlated with tear pattern, size, retraction, and chronicity. Tear type is correlated with tendon retraction, tear size, cuff mobility, and tissue quality. On the basis of this information, the surgeon can anticipate tear patterns that may improve pattern recognition and facilitate anatomical repair. Awareness of these three-dimensional tear patterns and their orientation is especially important during arthroscopic repair.

REFERENCES

Bigliani L, Morrison D, April E. The morphology of the acromion and it relationship to rotator cuff tears. Orthopaed Transact 1986;10:228.

Boileau P, Brassart N, Watkinson DJ, et al. Arthroscopic repair of full-thickness tears of the supraspinatus: does the tendon really heal? J Bone Joint Surg Am 2005;87:1229–1240.

Burkhart SS. A stepwise approach to arthroscopic rotator cuff repair based on biomechanical principles. Arthroscopy 2000;16:82–90.

Codman EA. Operative treatment of shoulder lesions. In: The Shoulder: Rupture of the supraspinatus tendon and other lesions in or about the subacromial bursa. Boston: Thomas Todd, 1934: 225–261.

Davidson J, Burkhart SS. The geometric classification of rotator cuff tears: a system linking tear pattern to treatment and prognosis. Arthroscopy 2010;26:417–424.

De Franco MJ, Cole BJ. Current perspectives on rotator cuff anatomy. Arthroscopy 2009;25:305–320.

De Orio JK, Cofield RH. Results of a second attempt at surgical repair of a failed initial rotator cuff repair. J Bone Joint Surg Am 1984;66:563–567.

De Palma AF. The classic. Surgical anatomy of the rotator cuff and the natural history of degenerative periarthritis. Surg Clin North Am 1963;43:1507–1520.

Ellman H. Diagnosis and treatment of incomplete rotator cuff tears. Clin Orthop Relat Res 1990;254:64–74.

Ellman H. Rotator cuff disorders. In: Ellman H, Gartsman GM (eds), Arthroscopic Shoulder Surgery and Related Disorders. Philadelphia, PA: Lea & Febiger, 1993: 98–119.

Harryman DT, Mack LA, Wang KY, et al. Repairs of the rotator cuff. Correlation of functional results with integrity of the cuff. J Bone Joint Surg Am 1991;73:982–989.

Inman VT, Saunders JB, Abbott LC. Observations on the function of the shoulder joint. J Bone Joint Surg Am 1944;26:1–30.

McLaughlin H. Lesions of the musculotendinous cuff of the shoulder. J Bone Joint Surg Am 1944;26:31–51.

Patte D. Classification of rotator cuff lesions. Clin Orthop Relat Res 1990;254: 81–86.

Rodosky MW, Harner CD, Fu FH. The role of the long head of the biceps muscle and superior glenoid labrum in anterior stability of the shoulder. Am J Sports Med 1994;22:121–130.

Sallay PI, Hunker PJ, Lim JK. Frequency of various tear patterns in full-thickness tears of the rotator cuff. Arthroscopy 2007;23:1052–1059.

Soslowsky LJ, Carpenter JE, Bucchieri JS, Flatow EL. Biomechanics of the rotator cuff. Orthop Clin North Am 1997;28:17–30.

Terry GC, Chopp TM. Functional anatomy of the shoulder. J Athl Train 2000;35:248–255.

Thomazeau H, Boukobza E, Morcet N, et al. Prediction of rotator cuff repair results by magnetic resonance imaging. Clin Orthop Relat Res 1997;344: 275–83.

Ward SR, Hentzen ER, Smallwood LH, et al. Rotator cuff muscle architecture: implications for glenohumeral stability. Clin Orthop Relat Res 2006;448: 157–63.

Wolfgang GL. Surgical repair of tears of the rotator cuff of the shoulder. Factors influencing the result. J Bone Joint Surg Am 1974;56:14–26.

Chapter 3 Why does the rotator cuff fail? The pathophysiology of rotator cuff disease

Gerald R. Williams, Robert J. Gillespie

KEY FEATURES

- There are three broad categories of partial-thickness rotator cuff tears: bursal sided, articular sided, and intratendinous.
- Partial-thickness rotator cuff tears increase the strain on the cuff, change the biomechanical characteristics of the surrounding rotator cuff, and may progress from partial- to full-thickness rotator cuff tears.
- Rotator cuff failure is a multifactorial process.
- Recent research points to various intrinsic factors as being major causes of rotator cuff failure.

INTRODUCTION AND HISTORICAL REVIEW

Failure of the rotator cuff is a condition that prevents it from fulfilling its physiological role, whether for activities of daily living or for competitive athletics. The pathophysiology of rotator cuff failure has been a subject of controversy. It is unclear when the first description of the rotator cuff and its failure appeared.

In 1834, JG Smith wrote that shoulder pain was caused by a rupture of the tendons in the rotator cuff. In 1934, Codman and Akerson argued that the articular side of the tendon is where most tears occur. Many authors have agreed with this theory because it has been supported by cadavers, surgery, and magnetic resonance imaging (MRI) studies (Clark et al. 1990, Wolff et al. 2006, Löhr and Uhthoff 2007, Gerber 2010).

Mclaughlin also wrote on lesions of the rotator cuff approximately 10 years after Codman's work. McLaughlin classified tears as being either complete or incomplete, with incomplete tears receiving the designation of bursal sided, intratendinous, and articular sided (Harrison and McLaughlin 1944). Similar to Codman's early work, Mclaughlin reported that the articular-sided tear of the rotator cuff was more common than the others.

However, in 1972, Charles Neer proposed that impingement syndrome was where the rough surface of the anterior acromion was striking against and damaging the rotator cuff. He suggested that there was a continuum from bursitis to partial-thickness rotator cuff to complete tears. Neer (1972) believed that 95% of rotator cuff tears started with impingement wear, rather than trauma or circulatory impairment.

It is clear from these classic works, and the multitude of studies that have followed, that there is no single cause of failure of the rotator cuff. Tendon degeneration, vascular factors, trauma, impingement, instability, scapulothoracic dysfunction, and congenital abnormalities have all been implicated and shown to have some role in the failure of the rotator cuff (**Table 3.1**). These etiologies can be categorized into two broad categories of rotator cuff failure as originally described by Codman and Neer: extrinsic and intrinsic.

The focus of this chapter starts with a brief anatomy review and biomechanical overview of the rotator cuff because a basic understanding of both of these concepts is key to understanding the causes of rotator cuff failure. The role of partial-thickness rotator cuff tears, and what influence these injuries have in the pathophysiology of full-thickness rotator cuff disease, are discussed. Finally the most recent theories and causes of rotator cuff failure since the early works of Codman and Neer are reviewed, separated broadly into intrinsic and extrinsic causes.

Anatomy of the rotator cuff

The anatomy of the rotator cuff is discussed in more detail in Chapter 1; however, a brief review is indicated here in order to fully understand the pathophysiology of rotator cuff failure. The normal anatomy of the rotator cuff is made up of four muscle–tendon units: supraspinatus, infraspinatus, teres minor, and subscapularis. All four of these muscles have their origin on the body of the scapula, and they envelope the humeral head as they insert on to their respective tuberosities on the proximal humerus (**Fig. 3.1**) (Clark and Harryman 1992, Cooper et al. 1993). The rotator cuff adheres to the glenohumeral capsule, except at the rotator interval and axillary recess, in order to provide circumferential reinforcement. Clark and Harryman (1992) performed gross and microscopic studies examining the rotator cuff and surrounding tissue. In normal healthy tissue, the tendon is very strong, with a transition of tendon to fibrocartilage to bone, forming a common insertion on the tuberosities of the humerus (Clark and Harryman 1992).

Both subscapularis and infraspinatus fibers interdigitate and fuse with anterior and posterior fibers of supraspinatus, converging as they insert on the humerus (**Fig. 3.1**). In addition, they found that the rotator cuff tendons and surrounding ligaments and capsule were made up of five layers: the first (bursal side) is a thin layer made up mostly of the coracohumeral ligament; the second is thicker and made up of parallel tendon fibers; the third is slightly thinner than the second and is made up of tendinous structures without the uniform orientation seen in the second layer; the fourth is composed of thick bands

Table 3.1 Etiology of rotator cuff disease

Intrinsic	Extrinsic
Avascularity	Subacromial Impingement
Smoking	Coracoid Impingement
Cholesterol	Trauma
Aging/Degeneration	Os acromiale
	Overuse

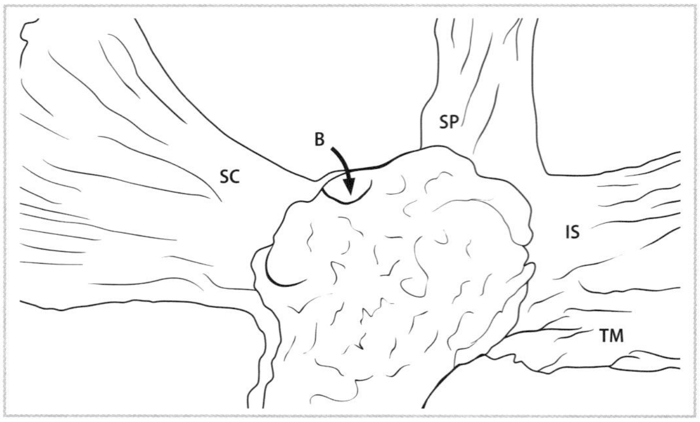

Figure 3.1 The bony and soft-tissue anatomy of the rotator cuff complex, showing the interdigitation of the rotator cuff tendons with common insertion sites. B, bicipital groove; IS, infraspinatus; SC, subscapularis; SP, supraspinatus; TM, teres minor. (From Clark JM, Harryman DT. Tendons, ligaments, and capsule of the rotator cuff. Gross and microscopic anatomy. J Bone Joint Surg Am 1992;74:713– 725.)

of collagen amid loose connective tissue; and the fifth and deepest layer (articular side), which is considered the capsule, is a continuous sheet of interwoven collagen fibrils, approximately 1.5–2.0 mm thick (**Fig. 3.2**) (Clark and Harryman 1992).

Subscapularis is the largest and most powerful muscle of the rotator cuff. It has dual innervations from the upper and lower subscapular nerves, which arise from the posterior cord of the brachial plexus. Internal rotation of the shoulder is the main mechanism of action of subscapularis, but it also contributes to arm abduction and humeral head depression (Otis et al. 1994).

Teres minor and infraspinatus make up the posterior portion of the rotator cuff. The suprascapular nerve innervates infraspinatus and the axillary nerve contributes to the innervation of teres minor. Their main action is external rotation of the humerus and stabilization of the glenohumeral joint with the other rotator cuff muscles.

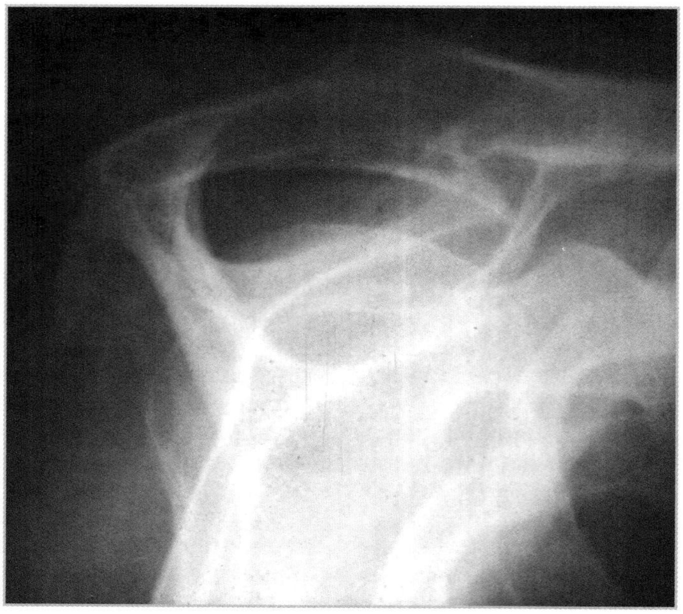

Figure 3.2 Scapular outlet view showing evidence of a type III acromion, as described by Bigliani and coworkers (1986).

Supraspinatus also receives its innervations from the suprascapular nerve. It contributes to humeral head compression as well as assisting the deltoid muscle with humeral abduction (Howell et al. 1986). Supraspinatus is situated between the humeral articular surface and the acromial arch, where it is protected by a synovial cavity on both sides (Glaser et al. 2007).

The deltoid muscle is superficial to the rotator cuff's musculotendinous unit and receives its innervations from the axillary nerve. It has three heads, anterior, middle, and posterior, which all vary in structure and function. All three heads exhibit differences in activity depending on the position of the arm; a description of this is beyond the scope of this chapter.

The long head of the biceps tendon has been considered by some to be a functional part of the rotator cuff because it receives its origin from the supraglenoid tubercle and travels between supraspinatus and subscapularis, attaching to its muscle in the distal part of the arm. The biceps tendon may assist in compressing the humeral head as well as guiding the humerus during elevation (Clark et al. 1990).

The acromion is a scapular process that has three separate centers of ossification, the pre-acromion, mesoacromion, and a meta-acromion. When these centers fail to fuse (usually by age 22), it is referred to as an os acromiale. Some have found an association between os acromiale and rotator cuff degeneration and impingement (Bigliani et al. 1986) but recent studies have shown a prevalence of rotator cuff tears that is comparable to that in patients with os acromiale and a standard population with an unknown status of rotator cuff tears (Boehm et al. 2005). The variability of the shape of the acromion between individuals in the sagittal plane has also been studied by Bigliani and coworkers (1986) in a cadaveric study. Three predominant types were identified: type I acromion had a flat undersurface and was present in 17%, type II (curved undersurface) in 43%, and type III (hooked undersurface) in 40% (**Fig. 3.2**). The role that the shape of the acromion plays in rotator cuff disease remains controversial. The coracoacromial arch consists of the anterior undersurface of the acromion and the coracoacromial ligament. This concave surface provides a smooth surface for gliding of the cuff musculature during shoulder movements. This space is normally lubricated by the subacromial and subdeltoid bursae (**Fig. 3.3**).

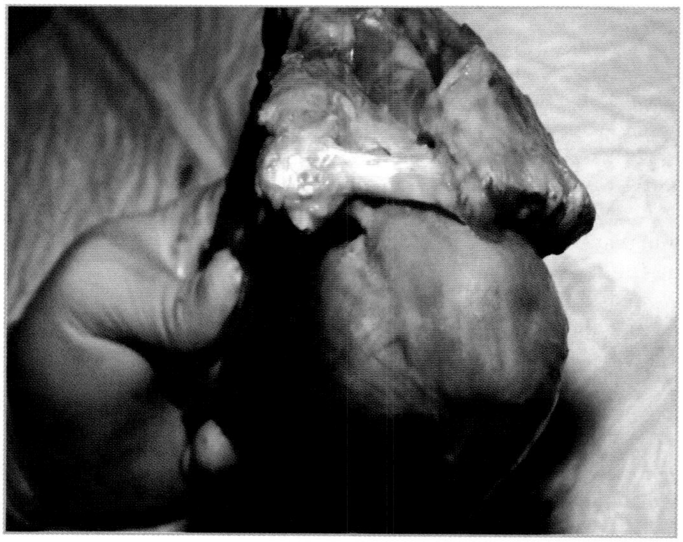

Figure 3.3 Cadaveric dissection of the coracoacromial arch with the deltoid musculature removed, showing the contour of the undersurface of the acromion and coracoacromial ligament.

Multiple vessels contribute to the vascularity of the rotator cuff. The anterior and posterior humeral circumflex vessels supply the superior as well as the anterior and posterior portions of the cuff, respectively. Most patients will have a branch of the thoracoacromial artery which provides nutrients to supraspinatus, as well as the suprascapular artery which supplies the superior cuff. Other contributions may include the suprahumeral branches of the axillary artery and branches of the subscapular artery. Finally, osseous vessels coming from the tuberosities of the proximal humerus have also been included in the vascular supply to the rotator cuff (Brooks et al. 1992). Areas of avascularity around the rotator cuff have been controversial in the literature and are discussed in more detail later in the chapter.

BIOMECHANICS OF THE ROTATOR CUFF

Function of the rotator cuff

The four muscles of the rotator cuff have three main functions: to rotate the humerus, compress the humeral head into the glenoid fossa (not necessarily depress), and provide muscular balance to the other shoulder musculature and surrounding soft tissue. This last function was clearly elucidated by Matsen and coworkers in the following example: use of the anterior deltoid in forward elevation without rotation needs to have the cross-body and internal rotation forces of the anterior deltoid neutralized by other muscles of the shoulder girdle, such as infraspinatus and posterior deltoid (Clark et al. 1990, Sharkey et al. 1994, Halder et al. 2002). Loss of these balancing muscles can lead to uncoordinated movements of the proximal humerus in unwanted directions. Clearly, the rotator cuff plays an integral role in the balanced and coordinated movement of the humerus. Compression of the humeral head into the glenoid also helps the dynamic stability of the shoulder through multiple force couples (Inman et al. 1944).

In normal activities, the force that the rotator cuff transmits ranges from 140 N to 200 N. In the sixth or seventh decade of life, the ultimate tensile strength of the rotator cuff has been measured as between 600 and 800 N (Itoi et al. 1995). Tendon fibers fail when the applied load exceeds their strength, which in turn leads to the following four detrimental effects: it increases the load on the neighboring unruptured cuff fibers; it detaches muscles fibers from bone, decreasing the maximum force that can be delivered by the cuff muscles; it distorts the normal cuff anatomy, which potentially compromises the blood supply to the rotator cuff, in turn potentially leading to ischemic events; and it exposes the rotator cuff to joint fluid that contains lytic enzymes, which could inhibit tendon healing (Andarawis-Puri et al. 2010). This same group has performed elegant studies examining the effect of a rotator cuff tendon tear on the neighboring tendons in a rat model, showing increased cross-sectional area in the intact tendons as well as decreased mechanical properties (Perry et al. 2009).

The biomechanical relationship between cuff muscles, as well as the strength and mechanism of force couples, continue to give us a better understanding of why and how failure occurs in the rotator cuff. In the following sections, the role of intrinsic and extrinsic causes of rotator cuff failure are outlined, as well as their effect on the force–tension relationship of the cuff.

PATHOPHYSIOLOGY OF PARTIAL TEARS OF THE ROTATOR CUFF

The controversy surrounding the exact etiology of rotator cuff failure is largely dependent on the etiology and prevalence of different types of partial-thickness rotator cuff tears. There are three broad types of partial rotator cuff tears that can be classified according to Ellman (1990): bursal side, articular side, and intratendinous. The average thickness of the rotator cuff tendon is 10–12 mm and each of these types of partial-thickness tears can be graded based on the thickness of the tear (Ruotolo et al. 2004) (see **Table 2.2**). One reason to discuss partial-thickness tears in this chapter is the different etiologies and pathology that have been implicated for each subtype. As natural history studies of partial-thickness rotator cuff tears have shown propagation to full-thickness tears, many conclusions can be made on the failure of the rotator cuff to convert to full-thickness tears (**Fig. 3.4**).

Nakajima and coworkers (1994) studied 60 supraspinatus tendons from cadavers and found that the histological and biomechanical properties of the bursal- and joint-side tendon layers were different. The bursal layers are composed primarily of tendon bundles, which may elongate with a tensile load and are resistant to rupture, whereas the joint-side layers, a complex of tendons, ligaments, and joint capsule, do not stretch and tear easily. They suggested that intratendinous lamination is caused by differential shear stress within the supraspinatus tendon (Nakajima et al. 1994). This supports the theory that the rotator cuff has multiple mechanisms of failure, at both the macroscopic and the microscopic levels. Although there are very few data available on the natural history of partial-thickness rotator cuff tears, there is a substantial body of evidence to suggest that most partial tears do not heal on their own (Ellman 1990, Hamada et al. 1997, Wolff et al. 2006, Gerber 2010). Patients may have intermittent symptoms, but the biomechanical and biologic data suggest that most of these tears progress to become larger rather than smaller with time, in addition to progressing to full-thickness tears.

Interestingly, Kim and coworkers (2010) recently looked at the location of partial-thickness and full-thickness rotator cuff tears and found that they were in a similar location, with 93% and 89% of full-thickness

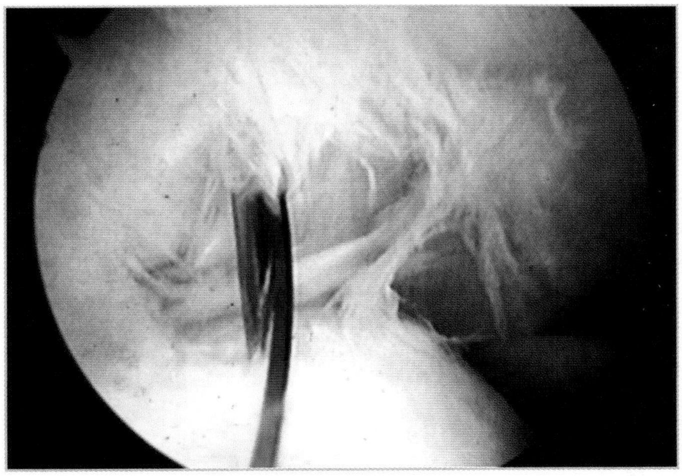

Figure 3.4 Arthroscopic view of an articular-sided, partial-thickness rotator cuff tear.

and partial-thickness tears located 13–17 mm posterior to the biceps tendon, respectively. This further supports the theory that partial-thickness rotator cuff tears are a likely precursor to full-thickness tears, and probably progress as a result of a continued insult to the tendon integrity. Studies such as this emphasize the importance of understanding the pathophysiology of partial-thickness tears because this could give us a better understanding of full-thickness rotator cuff disease.

Throughout the clinical orthopedic literature, articular-sided tears are about two to three times more common than their bursal-sided counterparts, with intratendinous tears having inconsistent prevalence (Ellman 1990, Gerber 2010). However, some have reported a smaller difference in the ratio of partial-thickness rotator cuff tears because Fukuda and coworkers (1994) reported a prevalence of 13% for partial-thickness rotator cuff tears in 200 cadaveric specimens. Of these, 18% were bursal sided, 27% articular sided, and 55% intratendinous. As a result of the inherent differences between the various partial-thickness tears, a brief overview of each type of partial tear is presented below, as well as their potential role in the overall pathophysiology of rotator cuff failure.

Bursal-sided rotator cuff tears

When Neer originally described subacromial impingement in 1970, he felt that 95% of rotator cuff tears were a result of extrinsic causes, most being from subacromial impingement (Neer 1970). In addition Hijioka and coworkers (1993) performed a cadaveric study that found a significant correlation between the severity of the undersurface of the acromion and the changes in the rotator cuff. Their results suggested that the degeneration of the rotator cuff is aggravated by friction and rubbing against the undersurface of the acromion, and can lead to a complete tear (Hijioka et al. 1993). However, others have shown that changes on the undersurface of the acromion are the result, and not the cause, of changes to the rotator cuff. The impingement observed in patients with bursal-sided cuff injuries may still be due to a primarily intrinsic etiology that produces weakness of the rotator cuff. This weakness, in turn, may lead to superior migration of the humerus which causes increased subacromial impingement, initiating a "vicious cycle" as described by Ozaki and coworkers (1988). Recent anatomical and clinical studies have shown that articular-sided tears are more common, making it less likely that subacromial impingement is the sole cause of all rotator cuff disease as originally described by Neer.

Articular-sided, partial-thickness, rotator cuff tears

Articular partial-thickness tears go back to the work of Codman and his early descriptions of rotator cuff disease (Codman and Akeron 1931). Yamanaka and coworkers (1994) performed a study observing the natural history of partial-thickness rotator cuff tears and were one of the first to document progression of joint-sided, partial-thickness tears to full-thickness tears, supporting the theory that most full-thickness tears are a result of partial rotator cuff tear progression. Internal impingement, as first described by Walch and coworkers (1992) as well as Jobe and coworkers (Paley et al. 2000), is another cause of articular-sided tears. Both groups showed that repetitive overhead athletes could have a "kissing" lesion of the posterosuperior glenoid and the undersurface of the rotator cuff, leading to partial-thickness rotator cuff tears. Currently, most studies in the English literature believe that articular-sided tears are two to three times more common than bursal-sided tears and, left untreated, have a risk of propagation to full-thickness rotator cuff tears (**Fig. 3.5**).

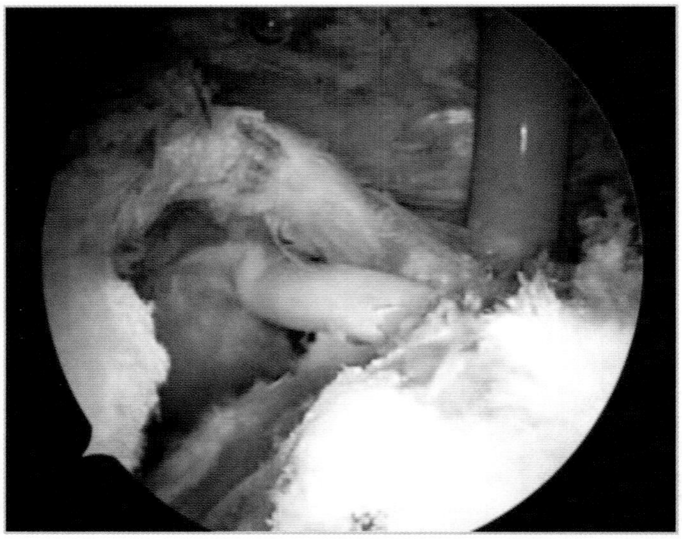

Figure 3.5 Arthroscopic view from the subacromial space of a massive full-thickness rotator cuff tear.

Intratendinous partial-thickness rotator cuff tears

Intratendinous partial-thickness tears of the rotator cuff are less well described in the English literature than their articular-sided and bursal-sided counterparts. This is due to the difficulty in diagnosing them both with radiological and arthroscopic findings. They likely occur more often than originally thought, with some reports having the incidence higher than articular- or bursal-sided tears, but they often occur at the same time as bursal-sided and articular-sided tears as well as with subacromial bursitis (Fukuda et al. 1994). Fukuda and coworkers also noted that trauma always seemed to be associated with intratendinous tears, and others have confirmed this finding with almost 85% of their intrasubstance tears having an association with trauma (Uchiyama et al. 2010). It is possible that partial-thickness intratendinous tears of the rotator cuff may be a precursor to full-thickness tears in some individuals. The causes of these tears could be multifactorial, but at this time are more likely to be a result of intrinsic etiologies that contribute to the overall health of the individual and tendon, and less likely to be a result of extrinsic causes of rotator cuff failure.

Partial-thickness rotator cuff tears have been shown to increase the strain and change the biomechanical characteristics of the surrounding rotator cuff (Soslowsky et al. 2000). These biomechanical studies support the progression of partial-thickness to full-thickness rotator cuff tears because changes in mechanics of the surrounding tissue would make these tendons more susceptible to further injury and/or progression of the tear. Knowing that partial-thickness tears are a likely precursor for most patients with full-thickness tears is crucial to our understanding of the overall failure of the rotator cuff. The three broad categories of partial-thickness rotator cuff tears discussed earlier (bursal, articular, and intratendinous) all have different and highly variable etiologies. As we examine the intrinsic and extrinsic causes of rotator cuff failure in the following sections, it is important to remember the different types of partial-thickness tears and where their causes fall in the spectrum of rotator cuff disease.

INTRINSIC CAUSES OF ROTATOR CUFF FAILURE

Avascularity

The relationship between the vascular blood supply to the rotator cuff and its role in the failure of these muscles continues to be controversial. Although a compromised vascular supply has been suggested as a cause of rotator cuff disease, no study has been able to fully validate this claim. Codman originally suggested that a critical portion existed in the distal tendon predisposing it to calcification and degeneration. He believed that a vascular mechanism, in conjunction with trauma, led to tearing of the rotator cuff. Other studies have supported these early findings in cadaveric studies showing zones of hypovascularity near the insertion of the tendon (Rothman and Parke 1965). In addition, Rudzki et al. (2008) examined age-related dynamic changes in the vascularity in the rotator cuff in vivo, and found that there was a significant decrease in blood flow to the supraspinatus tendon in patients over the age of 40 compared with patients younger than 40. They further suggested that this was consistent with the increased prevalence of rotator cuff pathology in older age groups because the decreased blood supply may predispose a patient to tendinopathy and possible attrition or failure.

By contrast, other studies have failed to show decreases in the vascular supply to critical portions of the rotator cuff (anterosuperior corner of supraspinatus). Moseley and Goldie (1963) performed microinjection studies on cadaveric shoulders and found a watershed area that corresponded to the critical zone of the tendon (that was most susceptible to tears), but that this area was not necessarily less vascularized than other portions of the cuff. However, Rathbun and Macnab (1970) noted that avascular areas existed within the supraspinatus tendon, especially in the adducted position. In addition they did note that the zones of relative avascularity would precede cuff degeneration. When tendon degeneration did occur, secondary vascular changes could be seen.

In 1990, a study by Lohr and Ulthoff showed that the bursal side of the cuff was well vascularized whereas the articular side had a sparse vascular supply. They concluded that this may predispose the articular side of the rotator cuff to failure. Intraoperative laser Doppler flowmetry has also been used to assess cuff vascularity. The aim of the study by Swiontowski and coworkers (1990) was to clarify the discrepancy between the prior cadaveric studies that showed hypovascular zones within the supraspinatus tendon and surgical findings of increased vascularity in patients with impingement syndrome. Intact tendons and those with tendinitis demonstrated increased zones of vascularity where the greatest mechanical impingement occurred. Partial tears also exhibited increased vascularity at this critical zone; however, patients with complete tears had variable vascularity. They concluded that impingement causes a hypervascular response resulting in resorption of injured tendon fibers and mediates the progression of rotator cuff disease (Swiontowski et al. 1990). Finally, Funakoshi and coworkers (2010) did an elegant in vivo study showing that there was a significant decrease in blood flow in the intratendinous region in elderly people compared with young people, but age had no effect on blood flow in bursal tissue. They also noted that rupture of the tendon did not seem to affect the blood supply to the tendon, which is contrary to what had been found in previous studies.

Many of the discussed studies have inherent shortcomings, whether they are cadaveric, postmortem, or microinjection studies. Further study should focus on in vivo methods as well as microscopic tissue evaluation to help answer some of the unanswered and controversial questions, about the vascular supply of the cuff tendons and its role in the ultimate failure of the rotator cuff. Regardless, the ability to heal an injury of any type in the human body requires adequate blood supply, so the question in future studies will not be so much if vascularity plays a role in full-thickness rotator cuff tears but rather how much of the injury seen in rotator cuff tears is due to a vascular etiology alone.

Smoking

Recently, more attention has been placed on intrinsic causes of rotator cuff failure including environmental factors such as smoking. We believe that smoking should be discussed as an adjunct to the role of vascularity in rotator cuff disease. As has been previously discussed, a zone of relative avascularity in the area proximal to supraspinatus and infraspinatus insertion at the greater tuberosity may be a factor in rotator cuff disease. As tobacco and nicotine use are known contributors to microvascular disease and soft-tissue healing, it may compromise the precarious blood supply to the supraspinatus/infraspinatus tendon, thus increasing the incidence of tendinous pathology with a decreased chance of healing in the rotator cuff. Kane and coworkers (2006) evaluated the rotator cuff of 72 shoulders in 36 cadavers and compared the incidence of macroscopic and microscopic disease within the rotator cuff tendon. History of smoking was also documented. Of the 36 shoulders that exhibited macroscopic rotator cuff tears, 23 were from cadavers with a history of smoking compared with only 13 from cadavers with no history of smoking. Furthermore, the presence of advanced microscopic rotator cuff pathology (grade 3 or 4 fibrous degeneration) was more than twice as likely in the cadavers with a history of smoking (22/32) compared with only 10 of 32 shoulders from cadavers with no history of smoking. None of the data in this study were statistically significant (Kane et al. 2006). However, Baumgarten and coworkers (2010) performed a retrospective review of patients who had diagnostic ultrasonography for atraumatic shoulder pain. History of smoking, mean duration of smoking (23.4 versus 20.2 years), mean packs per day of smoking, and mean pack-years of smoking were all correlated with an increased risk for rotator cuff tear. In addition, they observed a dose-dependent and time-dependent relationship between smoking and rotator cuff tears Baumgarten et al. 2010). As more studies are performed with regard to the history of rotator cuff failure, evidence will come to the forefront that activities such as smoking contribute to the degeneration of the rotator cuff (**Table 3.2**).

Table 3.2 Risk factors associated with an increased incidence of rotator cuff tears

Risk factor	Rotator cuff tears		P
	Present	Absent	
Age (years)	63	49	<0.001
Ever smoked (%)	62	48	0.002
Smoked within 10 years of presentation (%)	35	30	0.0006
Mean no. of packs smoked per day	1.25	1.1	0.004
Mean years smoking	23	20	0.05
Mean pack years	30	22	0.002

Data from Baumgarten KM, Gerlach D, Galatz LM, et al. Cigarette smoking increases the risk for rotator cuff tears. Clin Orthop Relat Res 2010;468:1534–1541.

Cholesterol

Recently, Abboud and coworkers (2010) delineated a relationship of hypercholesterolemia to rotator cuff disease. They found that total cholesterol, triglycerides, and low-density lipoprotein (LDL) were all higher in patients with rotator cuff disease and that there was a trend toward a lower high-density lipoprotein (HDL) in these patients versus the control group. Whether this represents a true independent risk factor for rotator cuff disease or is part of the overall continuum of aging and its effect on rotator cuff disease remains unclear. More work is currently being performed to determine the exact role of cholesterol in rotator cuff disease. Similar to cigarette smoking, intrinsic factors such as cholesterol, which contribute to the overall health of a patient, undoubtedly contribute to the health of the rotator cuff tendons.

Aging/Degeneration

The effect of aging is that of progressive degeneration of all elements of the rotator cuff. Since Codman and Akerson (1931) noted that tendinous defects in supraspinatus were typically found 1 cm medial to the insertion, and that this finding had an increased frequency with increasing age, many studies have been performed showing that age has a direct effect on the failure of the rotator cuff. DePalma et al. (1949) also noted that partial-thickness tears typically begin to occur in patients aged >40 and increase in frequency with age. Hashimoto and coworkers (2003) did an elegant study showing degenerative change, myxoid degeneration, and loss of collagen orientation in full-thickness tears. They concluded that, in the setting of microtrauma, degeneration from aging appears to be the main cause of rotator cuff tears. Rudzki and coworkers (2008) examined dynamic changes and found that vascularity to the cuff decreased significantly in the over 40 group versus the under 40 group, giving a cause for the age-related degeneration of the rotator cuff. In addition to these studies that examined the pathology and vascularity of the rotator cuff as it related to aging, others have performed radiological studies in an attempt to stratify increasing age and its effect on the integrity of the rotator cuff. Sher et al. (1995) lent support to the theory that degeneration and aging were one of the main causes of rotator cuff failure, together with an MRI study in asymptomatic volunteers, the findings of which showed that 54% of patients aged >60 years had a partial- or full-thickness rotator cuff tear, and those individuals between the age of 40 and 60 had a prevalence of 28% whereas those under 40 had an incidence of 4%, all of which were partial-thickness tears (see **Fig. 3.4**).

In addition, Milgrom and coworkers (1995) also found an increased incidence of rotator cuff tears in asymptomatic individuals using ultrasonography, in which 50% of individuals in the seventh decade had a tear and 80% of those aged >80 years had either a partial-thickness or a full-thickness tear. More recently, Yamaguchi et al. (2006) performed a retrospective study and found that there was approximately a 10-year difference in the average age of patients with no rotator cuff tear (48.7 years), a partial-thickness rotator cuff tear (58.7 years), and a full-thickness rotator cuff tear (67.8 years). In addition, they found that 35.5% of patients with symptomatic full-thickness tears had one on their asymptomatic side and patients with a symptomatic shoulder with no rotator cuff tear had an almost 98% chance of having no rotator cuff tear on their asymptomatic side. Why some patients develop symptoms from a rotator cuff tear and others do not remains a large area of interest in the orthopedic literature but is outside the scope of this chapter.

As these studies demonstrate, when a patient ages, the risk of having a rotator cuff tear increases. What has not yet been fully delineated in the literature is how aging causes rotator cuff failure. It is likely that, as we age, the blood supply to the rotator cuff is compromised and other factors such as overuse, high cholesterol, and smoking all contribute to the degeneration of the rotator cuff, ultimately leading to a full-thickness failure.

EXTRINSIC CAUSES OF ROTATOR CUFF FAILURE

Subacromial impingement

In 1972, Neer published a landmark paper examining the role of the acromion in rotator cuff disease. His observations from surgery and cadaveric dissections highlighted the role of the excrescences and bony spurs from the anterior third of the acromion and coracoacromial ligament as a source of impingement. This was in contrast to the widely held belief at that time that the lateral acromion was the major source of pathology. He believed that up to 95% of rotator cuff tears were due to impingement of the acromion on the rotator cuff. Bigliani and coworkers (1986) further subcategorized the acromion into a classification system that is still used today (see **Fig. 3.2**). A follow-up study by the same group then confirmed the association of rotator cuff tears and the hooked (type III) acromion (see **Fig. 3.2**) (Morrison and Bigliani 1987). A simplified two-dimensional finite element model was used by Luo et al. (1998) to investigate the stress environment in the supraspinatus tendon, specifically on the bursal side of the rotator cuff. The results demonstrated that subacromial impingement generated high stress concentrations in and around the critical zone of the rotator cuff which were high enough to initiate a tear. This further supported extrinsic causes of rotator cuff failure. Interestingly, they found that potential tears could occur on the bursal side, the articular side, or within the tendon, which is different from previously held views that subacromial impingement caused bursal-sided tears (Luo et al. 1998).

In addition, Gerber and coworkers (Schneeberger et al. 1998) showed that bursal-sided cuff tears could be caused after creating subacromial impingement in a rat model. Subacromial impingement of the infraspinatus tendon was experimentally created in 28 young adult rats. All rats with experimental subacromial impingement showed an infraspinatus tear on the bursal side of the tendon. An isolated tear on the articular side or within the tendon was not seen. Experimental subacromial impingement in the rat caused bursal-sided rotator cuff tears. The type of partial tears that are most frequently observed in clinical practice, i.e., intratendinous and articular-sided tears, were not seen in this experimental model (Schneeberger et al. 1998). Flatow and coworkers (1994) examined fresh frozen, human cadaveric shoulders using stereophotogrammetry to determine possible regions of subacromial contact with the rotator cuff. They found that the acromial undersurface and rotator cuff tendons were in closest proximity between 60° and 120° of elevation. Contact was consistently more pronounced for type III acromions and was usually centered on the supraspinatus insertion. As a result of this, the authors believed that anterior acromioplasty may be indicated in patients with symptomatic type III acromions (Flatow et al. 1994).

However, other studies have not corroborated the findings of the previous studies, showing that subacromial impingement can lead to failure of the rotator cuff. Oh et al. (1999) classified the characteristics of the acromion using MR or CT arthrography. The presence of spurs and characteristics was noted and correlated with the incidence of rotator cuff tears. They did not find a major difference between acromial shape and cuff tear. They did, however, note an increased incidence of acromial spurs as the patient population changed Oh et al. 1999). Nicholson et al. (1996) also found spur formation on the anterior acromion to be an age-dependent process. This anatomical study found the morphological condition of the acromion to be an age-independent factor. Their data suggested that the variations seen in acromial morphological conditions are not acquired from age-related changes and spur formation, and thus contribute to impingement disease independent of and in addition to age-related processes (Nicholson et al. 1996).

Ozaki and coworkers (1988) also looked at the relationship between anatomical changes of the undersurface of the acromion and the pathological findings of the rotator cuff. Their cadaveric study of 200 shoulders demonstrated an association between bursal-sided, partial-thickness rotator cuff tears and abnormalities on the undersurface of the acromion. Acromial abnormalities were also seen in full-thickness tears of the rotator cuff. The prevalence of acromial changes did correlate with age. Of particular interest was that, in specimens with articular-sided tears, the undersurface of the acromion was almost always intact. Their data further support the contention, originally proposed by Codman, that rotator cuff tears represent a degenerative process, and that acromial abnormalities are secondary changes as a result of a tear on the bursal side of the cuff (Ozaki and coworkers 1988).

Whether the overlying coracoacromial arch or the age-related degenerative properties mediate the process seen in rotator cuff disease, it seems plausible that many of the intrinsic and extrinsic factors discussed thus far may all have a contributory role in rotator cuff failure.

Overuse

In an active individual, the loads that the rotator cuff fibers have to withstand can be considerable when the humerus is actively moving in the direction of action of the rotator cuff. In addition, the glenoid rim can often abut the rotator cuff in extremes of motion, predisposing the cuff tendon to injury. Walch et al. (1992) and Jobe (Paley et al. 2000) initially described impingement in the throwing athlete that led to partial-thickness rotator cuff tears. In the study performed by Walch and coworkers (1992), 17 patients who did not have evidence of anterior instability or superior labral pathology were found to have impingement of the posterosuperior glenoid and rotator cuff in the throwing position (see **Fig. 5.15**). They believed that this was likely physiological, but that if repeated thousands of times, such as in a throwing athlete, it could lead to a rotator cuff injury and shoulder pain. Paley and coworkers (2000) confirmed these findings in a study on professional overhead throwing athletes, 93% of whom exhibited undersurface fraying of the rotator cuff. However, others have proposed that the pathological condition in the rotator cuff was not an abrasive phenomenon, but rather a result of a hypertwist mechanism with large shear stresses, leading to a fatigue failure of both the rotator cuff and the biceps tendon insertion point of the labrum.

Burkhart and coworkers (2003) went on to assert that internal impingement is not a pathological condition, but rather a natural restraint to hyperexternal rotation. Despite this, in a patient who exposes the shoulder to significant overuse, there are good basic science data to support repetitive motion as being an etiological factor in rotator cuff disease: Soslowsky and coworkers (2000) performed an excellent basic science study looking at overuse in a rat model, examining both the mechanical and the histological changes associated with overuse of the rotator cuff. They found that there was an increase in cellularity, loss of normal collagen alignment, and an increase in the cross-sectional area of the tendon with a loss of some its biomechanical properties. It is clear from these clinical and basic science studies that overuse and, more specifically, internal impingement can have a role in the failure of the rotator cuff (Drakos et al. 2009). It is likely that rotator cuff tears that occur from overuse and internal impingement occur in small select populations and do not have as large a role in most rotator cuff tears seen every day in the outpatient setting.

Coracoid impingement

Gerber and coworkers (1985) recognized, in 1985, that the subcoracoid space (region between the coracoid process and the lesser tuberosity or head of the humerus) was a potential source for shoulder pain. This space must accommodate subscapularis, capsule, and articular cartilage, and still leave room for the soft tissues to glide between the coracoid process and the humerus. Minor variations in the surrounding anatomy can result in a much greater chance of impingement, especially with the shoulder elevated, medially rotated, and adducted. Intraoperative findings in patients diagnosed with this relatively rare entity showed anything from superficial erosions to complete cuff destruction. Many of the patients had these symptoms as a result of iatrogenic changes (Trillat's procedure or posterior glenoid osteotomy), although it was also seen in patients with no history of trauma or prior surgical procedure. Others have described this syndrome of pain and impingement in an entirely idiopathic patient population but no evidence of rotator cuff tears was seen (Dines et al. 1990). This is a rare condition that will cause rotator cuff tears intermittently and must be kept in the differential diagnosis in the pathophysiology of rotator cuff tears.

Os acromiale

Congenital abnormalities such as os acromiale and an association with rotator cuff tears have been described (Mudge et al. 1984, Boehm et al. 2005). The acromion is made up of three centers of ossification that typically unite with the scapula and themselves by age 15–18 years. The incidence of os acromiale is anywhere from 1% to 15% in the literature, and Boehm and coworkers (2005) published their study on rotator cuff tears associated with an os acromiale. They treated 33 patients surgically with repair of the rotator cuff and various treatments of os acromiale, ranging from excision to fusion. The authors believed that it remained controversial whether os acromiale was a pathological condition leading to rotator cuff tears (Boehm et al. 2005) (**Fig. 3.6**). Similar to coracoid impingement, it is unlikely that an os acromiale is a significant contributor to the development of rotator cuff disease in all individuals, but maintaining it in the differential diagnosis will decrease the likelihood of missing this extrinsic cause of rotator cuff disease in a patient presenting with a history of shoulder pain and dysfunction.

Trauma

The incidence of rotator cuff tears in patients who are over 40 and sustain a shoulder dislocation are well known and can occur from 14% to 80% of the time, with the incidence increasing as patients age (Stayner et al. 2000, Glaser et al. 2007). In the older patient, the poste-

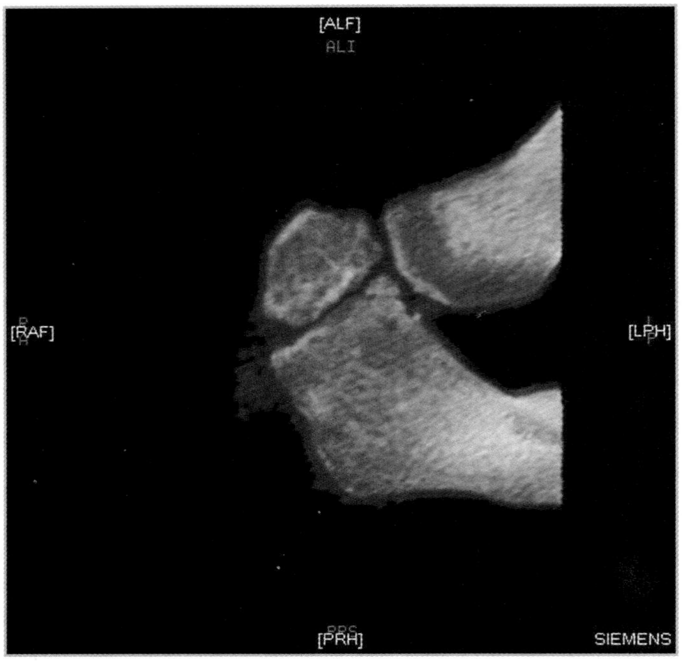

Figure 3.6 MRI axillary view, showing the presence of an os acromiale in a symptomatic patient.

rior structures – the rotator cuff and greater tuberosity complex – are weaker by attrition and tend to disrupt, usually leaving the anterior capsuloligamentous complex intact. After trauma most symptomatic rotator cuff tears occur as a result of an event or injury in the setting of rotator cuff disease (**Fig. 3.7**). The ability to determine whether pre-existing disease was present before the event is largely based on history of pain or disability. Neviaser et al. (1988) reported on a series of patients who had concurrent rupture of the rotator cuff with an anterior dislocation of the shoulder joint. All patients in this series were older than 40, all having supraspinatus torn and some with injury to infraspinatus occurring to a variable degree. Patients who had recurrent instability had a subscapularis tear. These patients were all treated with a primary repair of the rotator cuff. Posterior dislocations can also result in a tear of the rotator cuff. Schoenfield and Lippitt (1998) reported on a 22 year old with an isolated rotator cuff tear after a posterior dislocation. Fractures of the greater tuberosity can also result in rotator cuff tears. Neer (1970) reported that a greater tuberosity fracture results in an obligate tear at the region of the rotator interval. The diagnosis of rotator cuff tears after a traumatic injury is beyond the scope of this chapter but should remain in the differential for all patients aged >35 years who have difficulty raising their arm after treatment for shoulder dislocations, because cuff tears and brachial plexus injuries can be difficult to differentiate and can occur together.

Other forms of traumatic cuff tears can occur as partial-thickness tears in throwing or overhead athletes. One proposed mechanism

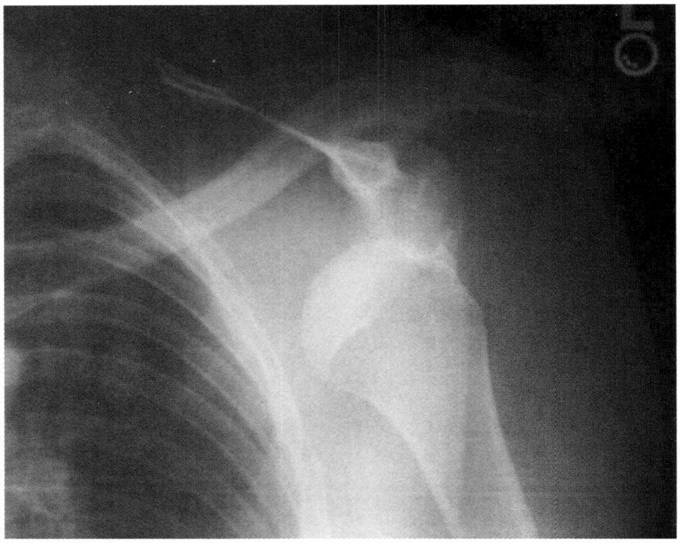

Figure 3.7 Anteroposterior radiograph of anteroinferior shoulder dislocation.

for this is fatigue of the scapular stabilizers from repeated overhead motions. This then causes the humeral head and rotator cuff to abut against the acromion during overhead activities, causing fraying and eventual tears of the rotator cuff. A similar mechanism with traumatic disruption of the shoulder suspensory complex, through the acromioclavicular or coracoclavicular ligaments, could also result in similar rotator cuff abnormalities (Glaser et al. 2007).

CONCLUSION

Rotator cuff failure is likely a result of multiple etiologies, with no single cause being the sole reason for failure. The pendulum currently has swung back to the days of Codman, with basic science and clinical research pointing to intrinsic factors as being the major causes of failure in the rotator cuff. There is no question that trauma will continue to play a large role in the development of rotator cuff tears, but it appears that it may be a separate entity from the rotator cuff tear with no evidence of trauma (Kim et al. 2010). In summary, with the exception of traumatic tear of the rotator cuff, it is likely that, as a patient ages, multiple etiologic factors contribute to the degeneration and, ultimately, failure of the rotator cuff. It is unlikely that any patient has one single cause of failure except in the unique situation of a young patient with a traumatic event to the shoulder. As research in this expanding field continues, it will be important to study the exact contributions that factors such as smoking, hypercholesterolemia, and vascular insult have on the failure of the rotator cuff. It is our hope that prevention and treatment of rotator cuff failure can be optimized in the future with new pharmaceutical interventions or changes in our non-surgical and surgical management, based on the research that is currently ongoing in the field of rotator cuff disease.

REFERENCES

Abboud JA, Kim JS.The effect of hypercholesterolemia on rotator cuff disease. Clin Orthop Relat Res. 2010;468:1493–1497.

Andarawis-Puri N, Kuntz AF, Kim SY. Effect of anterior supraspinatus tendon partial-thickness tears on infraspinatus tendon strain through a range of joint rotation angles. J Shoulder Elbow Surg 2010;19:617–623.

Baumgarten KM, Gerlach D, Galatz LM, et al. Cigarette smoking increases the risk for rotator cuff tears. Clin Orthop Relat Res 2010;468:1534–1541.

Bigliani LU, Morrison DS, April EW. The morphology of the acromion and rotator cuff impingement. Orthop Trans 1986;10:288.

Boehm TD, Rolf O, Martetschlaeger F, Kenn F, Gohlke W. Rotator cuff tears associated with os acromiale. Acta Orthop 2005;76:241–244.
Brooks CH, Revell WJ, Heatley FW. A quantitative histological study of the vascularity of the rotator cuff tendon. J Bone Joint Surg Br 992;74:151–153.
Burkhart SS, Morgan CD, Kibler WB. The disabled throwing shoulder: spectrum of pathology part I: pathoanatomy and biomechanics. Arthroscopy 2003;19:404–420.
Clark JM, Sidles JA Matsen FA III. The relationship of the glenohumeral joint capsule to the rotator cuff. Clin Orthop Rel Res 1990;254:29–34.
Clark JM, Harryman DT. Tendons, ligaments, and capsule of the rotator cuff. Gross and microscopic anatomy. J. Bone Joint Surg Am 1992;74:713–725
Codman EA, Akerson TB. The pathology associated with rupture of the supraspinatus tendon. Ann Surg 1931;93:348–359.
Cooper DE, O'Brien SJ, Warren RF. Supporting layers of the glenohumeral joint: An anatomic Study. Clin Orthop 1993;289:144–155.
DePalma AF, Callery G, Bennett GA. Variational Anatomy and Degenerative Lesions of the Shoulder Joint. Instructional Course Lectures, vol. 6. American Academy of Orthopaedic Surgeons, 1949: 255–281.
Dines DM, Warren RF, Inglis AE, Pavlov H. The coracoid impingement syndrome. J Bone Joint Surg Br 1990;72:314–316.
Drakos MC, Rudzki JR, Allen AA, Potter HG, Altchek DW. Internal impingement of the shoulder in the overhead athlete J Bone Joint Surg Am 2009;91:2719–2728.
Ellman H. Diagnosis and treatment of incomplete rotator cuff tears. Clin Orthop Relat Res 1990;254:64–74.
Flatow EL, Soslowsky LJ, Ticker JB, et al. Excursion of the rotator cuff under the acromion. Patterns of subacromial contact. Am J Sports Med 1994;22:779–788.
Funakoshi T, Iwasaki N, Kamishima T, et al. In vivo visualization of vascular patterns of rotator cuff tears using contrast-enhanced ultrasound. Am J Sports Med 201038:2464–2471.
Fukuda H, Hamada K, Nakajima T, Tomonaga A. Pathology and pathogenesis of the intratendinous tearing of the rotator cuff viewed from en bloc histologic sections. Clin Orthop Relat Res 1994;304:60–67.
Gerber C, Terrier F, Ganz R. The role of the coracoid process in the chronic impingement syndrome. J Bone Joint Surg Br 1985;67:703–708.
Gerber C. Partial rotator cuff tears. International Guest Speaker presentation at the 29th Annual Meeting of the Arthroscopy Association of North America. May 20–23, 2010, Hollywood, CA.
Glaser DL, Sher JS, Ricchetti ET, Williams GR, Soslowsky LJ. Anatomy, biomechanics, and pathophysiology of rotator cuff disease. In: Williams GR & Iannotti J (eds), Disorders of the Shoulder, vol 1, 2nd edn. Philadelphia, PA: Lippincott Williams & Wilkins, 2007: 3–38.
Halder AM, O'Driscoll SW, Heers G, et al. Biomechanical comparison of effects of supraspinatus tendon detachments, tendon defects, and muscle retractions. J. Bone Joint Surg Am 2002;84:780–785
Hamada K, Tomonaga A, Gotoh M, Yamakawa H, Fukuda H. Intrinsic healing capacity and tearing process of torn supraspinatus tendons: In situ hybridization study of α1(I) procollagen mRNA. J Orthop Res 1997;15:24–32.
Harrison L, McLaughlin ?. Lesions of the musculotendinous cuff of the shoulder: I. The exposure and treatment of tears with retraction J. Bone Joint Surg Am 1944;26:31–51
Hashimoto T, Nobuhara K, Hamada T. Pathologic evidence of degeneration as a primary cause of rotator cuff tear.Clin Orthop Relat Res 2003;415:111–120.
Hijioka A, Suzuki K, Nakamura T, Hojo T. Degenerative change and rotator cuff tears. An anatomical study in 160 shoulders of 80 cadavers.Arch Orthop Trauma Surg 1993;112:61–64.
Howell SM, Imobersteg AM, Seger DH, Marone PJ. Clarification of the role of the supraspinatus muscle in shoulder function. J. Bone Joint Surg Am 1986;68:398–404.
Inman VT, Saunders JB, Abbott LC. Observations on the function of the shoulder joint. J Bone Joint Surg Am 1944;26:1–30.
Itoi E, Berglund LJ, Grabowski KK, et al. Tensile properties of the supraspinatus tendon. J Orthop Res 1995;13:578–584.
Kane SM, Dave A, Haque A, Langston K. The incidence of rotator cuff disease in smoking and non-smoking patients: a cadaveric study. Orthopedics 2006;29:363–366.
Kim HM, Dahiya N, Teefey SA, et al. Location and initiation of degenerative rotator cuff tears: an analysis of three hundred and sixty shoulders. J Bone Joint Surg Am 2010;92:1088–1096.
Lohr JF, Uhthoff HK. The microvascular pattern of the supraspinatus tendon. Clin Orthop 1990;254:35–38.
Löhr JF, Uhthoff HK [Epidemiology and pathophysiology of rotator cuff tears] [Article in German]. Orthopade 2007;36:788–795.
Luo ZP, Hsu HC, Grabowski JJ, Morrey BF, An KN Mechanical environment associated with rotator cuff tears. J Shoulder Elbow Surg 1998;7:616–620.
Milgrom C, Schaffler M, Gilbert S, van Holsbeeck M. Rotator-cuff changes in asymptomatic adults. The effect of age, hand dominance and gender. J Bone Joint Surg Br 1995;77:296–298.
Morrison DS, Bigliani LU. The clinical significance of variations in acromial morphology. Orthop Trans 1987;11:234.
Moseley HF, Goldie I. The arterial pattern of the rotator cuff of the shoulder. J Bone Joint Surg Br 1963;45:780–789.
Mudge MK, Wood VE, Frykman G. Rotator cuff tears associated with os acromiale. J. Bone Joint Surg Am 1984;66:427–429.
Nakajima T, Rokuuma N, Hamada K, Tomatsu T, Fukuda H. Histologic and biomechanical characteristics of the supraspinatus tendon: Reference to rotator cuff tearing. J Shoulder Elbow Surg 1994;3:79–87.
Neer CS II. Displaced proximal humeral fractures: Part I. Classification and evaluation. J Bone Joint Surg Am 1970;52:1077–1089.
Neer CS II. Anterior acromioplasty for the chronic impingement syndrome in the shoulder: a preliminary report. J Bone Joint Surg Am 1972;54:41–50.
Neviaser RJ, Neviaser TJ, Neviaser JS. Concurrent rupture of the rotator cuff and anterior dislocation of the shoulder in the older patient. J Bone Joint Surg Am 1988;70:1308–1311.
Nicholson GP, Goodman DA, Flatow EL, Bigliani LU. The acromion: Morphologic condition and age-related changes. A study of 420 scapulas. J Shoulder Elbow Surg 1996;5:1–11.
Oh JH, Kim JY, Lee HK, Choi JA. Classification and clinical significance of acromial spur in rotator cuff tear: heel-type spur and rotator cuff tear. Clin Orthop Relat Res 2010;468:1542–50.
Otis JC, Jiang CC, Wickiewicz TL, et al. Changes of the moment arms of the rotator cuff and deltoid muscles with abduction and rotation. J Bone Joint Surg Am 1994;76:667–676.
Ozaki J, Fujimoto S, Nakagawa Y, Masuhara K, Tamai S. Tears of the rotator cuff of the shoulder associated with pathological changes in the acromion. A study in cadavera. J Bone Joint Surg Am 1988;70:1224–1230.
Paley KJ, Jobe FW, Pink MM, Kvitne RS, ElAttrache NS. Arthroscopic findings in the overhand throwing athlete: evidence for posterior internal impingement of the rotator cuff. Arthroscopy 2000;16:35–40.
Perry SM, Getz CL, Soslowsky LJ. After rotator cuff tears, the remaining (intact) tendons are mechanically altered. J Shoulder Elbow Surg 2009;18:52–57.
Rathbun JB, Macnab I. The microvascular pattern of the rotator cuff. J Bone Joint Surg Br 1970;52:540–553.
Rothman RH, Parke WW. The vascular anatomy of the rotator cuff. Clin Orthop 1965;41:176–186.
Rudzki JR, Adler RS, Warren RF, et al. Contrast-enhanced ultrasound characterization of the vascularity of the rotator cuff tendon: age- and activity-related changes in the intact asymptomatic rotator cuff. J Shoulder Elbow Surg 2008;17(1 suppl):96S–100S.
Ruotolo C, Fow JE, Nottage WM. The supraspinatus footprint: an anatomic study of the supraspinatus insertion. Arthroscopy 2004;20:246–249.
Schneeberger AG, Nyffeler R, Gerber C. Structural changes of the rotator cuff caused by experimental subacromial impingement in the rat. J Shoulder Elbow Surg 1998;7:375–380.
Schoenfeld AJ, Lippitt SB. Rotator cuff tear associated with a posterior dislocation of the shoulder in a young adult: a case report and literature review. J Orthop Trauma 2007;21:150–152.
Sharkey NA, Marder RA, Hanson PB. The entire rotator cuff contributes to elevation of the arm. J Orthop Res 1994;12:699–708.
Sher JS, Uribe JW, Posada A, Murphy BJ, Zlatkin MB. Abnormal findings on magnetic resonance images of asymptomatic shoulders. J. Bone Joint Surg Am 1995;77:10–15.
Smith JG. Pathological appearances of seven cases of injury of the shoulder joint with remarks. London Med Gazette 1834;14:280.
Soslowsky LJ, Thomopoulos S, Tun S, et al. Neer Award 1999. Overuse activity injures the supraspinatus tendon in an animal model: a histologic and biomechanical study. J Shoulder Elbow Surg 2000;9:79–84.
Stayner LR, Cummings J, Andersen J, Jobe CM. Shoulder dislocations in patients older than 40 years of age.Orthop Clin North Am 2000;31:231–239.
Swiontowski MF, Iannotti JP, Boulas HJ, et al. Intraoperative assessment of rotator cuff vascularity using laser Doppler flowtometry. In Post M, Morrey

BF, Hawkins RJ (eds), Surgery of the Shoulder. St Louis, MO: Mosby-Year Book, 1990: 208–212.

Uchiyama Y, Hamada K, Khruekarnchana P, et al. Surgical treatment of confirmed intratendinous rotator cuff tears: retrospective analysis after an average of eight years of follow-up. J Shoulder Elbow Surg. 2010;19:837–846.

Walch G, Boileau P, Noel E, Donell ST. Impingement of the deep surface of the supraspinatus tendon on the posterosuperior glenoid rim: An arthroscopic study. J Shoulder Elbow Surg 1992;1:238–245.

Wolff AB, Sethi P, Sutton KM, et al. Partial-thickness rotator cuff tears. J Am Acad Orthop Surg 2006;14:715–725.

Yamaguchi K, Ditsios K, Middleton WD, et al. The demographic and morphological features of rotator cuff disease. A comparison of asymptomatic and symptomatic shoulders. J Bone Joint Surg Am 2006;88:1699–1704

Yamanaka K, Matsumoto T. The joint side tear of the rotator cuff. A followup study by arthrography . Clin Orthop Relat Res 1994;304:68–73.

Chapter 4 Epidemiology and genetic basis of rotator cuff pathology

Umile Giuseppe Longo, Alessandra Berton, Filippo Spiezia, Nicola Maffulli, John Furia, Vincenzo Denaro

KEY FEATURES

- The incidence of cuff tears has been reported to range from 5 to 39%.
- Partial-thickness tears are more common than full-thickness defects.
- The etiology of rotator cuff disease is multifactorial. Studies have suggested that genetic factors contribute to the pathogenesis of rotator cuff tears, but knowledge is still incomplete.
- Tobacco smoking and diabetes mellitus are well-defined risk factors for rotator cuff lesions.
- Genetics may predispose to the production of a failed healing response and/or tear progression.

EPIDEMIOLOGY

Diseases of the rotator cuff are common. The incidence of cuff tears has been reported to range from 5% (Neer 1983) to 39%. However, prevalence rates and epidemiological variables of rotator cuff disease vary across studies. This lack of uniformity is, in part, the cause of this phenomenon, and the differences between cadaveric studies and population studies are also a factor.

Results from cadaver dissection studies (Meyer 1924; Codman and Akerson 1931; Keyes 1933, 1935; Wilson and Duff 1943; Grant and Smith 1948; DePalma et al. 1949, 1950; Cotton and Rideout 1964; Neer 1983; Yamanaka et al. 1983; Fukuda et al. 1987, 1990; Uhthoff et al. 1991; Lehman et al. 1995; Quiniann et al. 2011) have helped clarify this issue. Keyes, in 1933, found full-thickness tears of the supraspinatus tendon in 13.4% of shoulders of 73 unselected cadavers. Wilson and Duff (1943) found full-thickness tears of supraspinatus in 11% and partial-thickness tears in 10% of the shoulders of a series of 108 cadavers, while DePalma and co-workers (1949) noted an even higher (39%) rate of tears of the rotator cuff in 100 cadaver specimens.

Advanced age is a risk factor for rotator cuff lesions (Meyer 1924; Codman aand Akerson 1931; Keyes 1933, 1935; Grant and Smith 1948; DePalma et al. 1949, 1950; Fukuda et al. 1990, 1987; Lehman et al. 1995; Quiniann et al. 2011). Approximately 30% of the elderly population have full-thickness rotator cuff tears (Quiniann et al. 2011). Keyes (1933) reported no full-thickness tears below the age of 50. In contrast, there was a 31% prevalence of rotator cuff tears in specimens from people aged >50. Yamanaka and coworkers (Fukuda et al. 1990; Yamanaka and Matsumoto 1994) found similar results. Fukuda et al. (1987) reported no tears below age 40 and a 30% prevalence of tears in those over 40. Lehman et al. (1995) noted that the prevalence of full-thickness tears in those aged <60 and >60 years was 6% and 30%, respectively.

Studies that record the incidence of partial-thickness tears reveal that they are more common than full-thickness defects, with a prevalence of 13% versus 7%, respectively (Fukuda et al. 1987). Others have reported a prevalence ranging from 20% to 37%. In living individuals, it is difficult to report the true incidence of rotator cuff tears because not all are symptomatic (DePalma et al. 1949). Thus, studies on asymptomatic individuals are essential to obtain a correct view of the magnitude of the problem of rotator cuff pathology.

The best methods to investigate asymptomatic individuals are arthrography, magnetic resonance imaging (MRI), and ultrasonography. Petersson (1984) showed the presence of tears in apparently healthy shoulders arthrographically, more frequently observed in individuals aged between 70 and 75 years.

Using MRI, Sher et al. (1995) reported a high prevalence of rotator cuff tears in a cohort of asymptomatic individuals: 25 (54%) of the 46 individuals aged >60 years had a tear of the rotator cuff. Partial-thickness tears were more common than full-thickness tears, and the incidence of tears increased with age.

Using ultrasonography, Milgrom et al. (1995) studied 90 asymptomatic adults, and reported that rotator cuff tears were present in 15 (65%) of 23 adults aged >70. These results were consistent with those of Keyes (1933), who reported a progressive increase of rotator cuff lesions after the fifth decade of life, with no correlation with hand dominance, exertional shoulder activities, and gender. The prevalence of stage 3 impingement lesions was 5–11% in the fourth and fifth decades of life, 50% in the seventh decade, and 80% in the ninth and tenth decades. They concluded that rotator cuff lesions were regarded as a natural correlate of aging, often occurring without symptoms.

The relevance of the asymptomatic condition has recently been considered (Yamaguchi et al. 2001; Yamaguchi and Lashgari 2002). Investigations into the natural history of cuff tears, monitoring their size and pain progression, help in understanding factors that may influence symptom presentation and whether a secondary prevention intervention is necessary. Many initially asymptomatic tears induce pain and decrease the ability to perform activities of daily living (Yamaguchi et al. 2001, 2006). This trend has been correlated with progression in tear size (Yamaguchi et al. 2006).

Patients frequently have bilateral disease but unilateral shoulder pain. Larger rotator cuff tears have been observed more commonly in painful shoulders than in non-painful shoulders. Non-painful shoulders become symptomatic over a mean of 2.8 years (Yamaguchi et al. 2001). Thus, the development of new symptoms may indicate enlargement of the tear.

Arthrographic progression of partial-thickness tears with increasing age is relatively common (Yamanaka and Matsumoto 1994). At 1-year follow-up, 4 of 40 tears showed apparent resolution, 4 reduced in size, 21 enlarged, and 11 progressed to a full-thickness tear.

Shoulder disease ranks among the most common musculoskeletal disorders, being the third cause of musculoskeletal disease (16%), after the back (23%) and knee (19%) (Urwin et al. 1998). In the USA, 17 million individuals are at risk for shoulder disability (Milgrom et al. 1995; Sher et al. 1995). Many patients with shoulder problems do not require medical consultations and treatment.

Community survey, hospital-based studies, and surveillance systems of work-related disorders help to characterize the epidemiology of symptomatic rotator cuff tears.

A large survey in the Netherlands reported that 21% of surveyed individuals were referred to a specialist for the evaluation of shoulder pain (Bonger 2001). A survey of the British population recorded shoulder tendinopathy in 6.1% of women and 4.5% of men (Walker-Bone et al. 2004).

Shoulder disorders are particularly common in the working population. In epidemiological surveillance systems of work-related, upper-limb musculoskeletal disorders in France's Pays de la Loire region, rotator cuff syndrome was the most frequent disorder (Roquelaure et al. 2006). Men were less commonly affected (6.8% of cases) than women (9% of cases), unilateral pathology occurred in 52% of patients, and bilateral presentation occurred in 16% of shoulders. In about 4% of cases, rotator cuff syndrome was newly diagnosed and presented with high pain intensity (4.8 of 10).

Pain was manifested during active shoulder elevation (50% of cases), by resisted abduction, internal and external rotation (15% of cases), or both (26% of cases). Pain was sometimes elicited during the resisted elbow flexion test. The prevalence rate of rotator cuff syndrome reported in other studies on French workers exposed to repetitive work is even higher, ranging between 29% in highly exposed workers and 16% in weakly exposed workers (Leclerc et al. 1998).

The possible association between mechanical overuse and cuff tearing has been well investigated. Symptomatic disease is more often localized to the dominant arm, but 36% of cases also have a full-thickness tear on the non-dominant side (Yamaguchi et al. 2006). Moreover, 28% of symptomatic patients had full-thickness tears on the non-dominant shoulder only, and 70% of patients with full-thickness tears undertake light work only (Harryman et al. 2003).

An infraspinatus tendon tear together with a supraspinatus tendon tear causes greater difficulty in overhead movements than a supraspinatus tear alone (Harryman et al. 2003). In some cases, onset of symptoms coincides with sports activities such as throwing, tennis, skiing, and swimming. In one study, 42% of 137 swimmers in the USA showed shoulder problems related to subluxation and cuff disease (Richardson et al. 1980). The problems were attributed to errors in technique (Neer and Welsh 1977; Albright et al. 1978; Penny and Smith 1980). Elderly athletes more frequently present with rotator cuff injuries (18%) than younger athletes (Jarvinen 1992).

Epidemiological studies have helped identify several risk factors for rotator cuff disorders. Tobacco smoking and diabetes mellitus have been well defined as risk factors for rotator cuff lesions. Smoking has been associated with musculoskeletal pain and dysfunction (Leino-Arjas 1999), rotator cuff tendinopathy (Stenlund et al. 1993), and shoulder pain (Leino-Arjas 1999; Hellsing and Bryngelsson 2000; Kaergaard and Andersen 2000). Tendon healing is negatively influenced by both tobacco smoking and diabetes mellitus (Chen et al. 2003; Mallon et al. 2004; Galatz et al. 2006). In middle-aged to slightly elderly populations, increasing body mass index is associated with rotator cuff tendinopathy and rotator cuff-related surgery. However, additional research is required to better demonstrate this association (Wendelboe et al. 2004).

Epidemiological information describes well the relevance of rotator cuff problems. Its high prevalence rate causes high direct and indirect costs in industrialized countries. It is responsible for high healthcare costs in western industrialized countries (Meislin et al. 2005) and relevant costs for workers' compensation systems (Hegmann and Moore 1998). Moreover, it is troublesome because of the poor medical and social prognosis (Roquelaure et al. 2004).

GENETICS

The etiology of rotator cuff disease is multifactorial, and involves both biological and mechanical factors. Extrinsic and intrinsic theories are well described. All of these factors may be responsible for the development of the pathology, but any single factor is not sufficient to determine the disease on its own.

Genetics may also be an important aspect of rotator cuff pathology (Lippi et al. 2010; Longo et al. 2010a, 2010b, 2010c). Studies have suggested that genetic factors contribute to the pathogenesis of rotator cuff tears, but knowledge is still incomplete.

Preliminary studies report familiar predisposition towards rotator cuff disease (Harvie et al. 2004; Yamaguchi et al. 2006; September et al. 2007; Gwilym et al. 2009). Yamaguchi et al. (2006) described a definite correlation between family history and risk of rotator cuff tear (10.9% compared with 6.9%; $p = 0.06$) in 586 patients who underwent diagnostic shoulder ultrasonography for shoulder pain.

Harvie et al., in 2004, carried out a retrospective cohort study on 205 patients diagnosed with full-thickness tears of the rotator cuff. Siblings and spouses were compared. It demonstrated the genetic susceptibility to the development of full-thickness tears. Siblings had a relative risk of full-thickness tears of 2.42, and a risk of experiencing symptoms of 4.65 compared with controls.

Genetics may be expressed via tendon ultrastructure through apoptosis and regenerative capacity (Gwilym et al. 2009). The degeneration that is commonly associated with aging may present only in those patients who have a genetic predisposition. Rotator cuff tears have a different prevalence in patients stratified by family history and matched for age, gender, and environmental conditions (Gwilym et al. 2009). Moreover, considering only patients under the age of 40, the risk of rotator cuff disease is significantly elevated for their relatives to a genetic distance of third cousins (Tashjian et al. 2009). These data are derived from a population-based, multigenerational study of familial clustering of rotator cuff disease which, according with previous observations, showed an elevated risks for first- and second-degree relatives, and indicated young patients as being the best group in whom to study genetic predisposition (Tashjian et al. 2009).

Evidence suggests that genetics may influence symptom presentation (Buskila 2007; Foulkes and Wood 2008). Symptoms may present at any point of the sensorineural pathway of the cuff (Harvie et al. 2004). Heritable components of pain have been demonstrated by the evidence of relative risk of painful tear of 1.44 in siblings of symptomatic patients, compared with 1 in control individuals (Gwilym et al. 2009). Pain presentation seems to be influenced by the same genetic factors that predispose to rotator cuff tears and tear progression.

In siblings of patients, tear size has a higher tendency to progress. Increased tear size was observed in 16.1% of siblings, compared with 1.5% of the control group over a period of 5 years (Gwilym et al. 2009).

The precise gene abnormalities that contribute to rotator cuff pathology are unknown. It is difficult to select single genes involved in rotator cuff pathology, because it is a multifactorial condition in which different gene products and environments interact.

Most information about a genetic role in tendinopathies concerns the Achilles tendon. The correlation between ABO blood group system and Achilles tendon ruptures has been previously described (Jozsa et al. 1989; Kujala et al. 1992; Kannus and Natri 1997), and explained by the presence of two structural genes, tenascin C (*TNC*) and collagen type Va1 (*COL5A1*), on the same region of chromosome 9. Polymorphisms of these tendon components have been associated with Achilles tendon injuries (Mokone et al. 2005, 2006). Similar mechanisms may help elucidate the pathogenesis of rotator cuff disease

Knowledge of a genetic role in the pathogenesis of rotator cuff tears will help to identify individuals at risk and to develop biological augmentations for prevention and treatment of rotator cuff tears. Studies are still in their infancy. Predisposing genes need to be identified, and their relationship with environmental factors described. The study of the molecular biology of gene products should integrate anatomical and physiological assumptions to apply scientific findings in clinical setting.

REFERENCES

Albright JA, Jokl P, Shaw R, Albright JP. Clinical study of baseball pitchers: correlation of injury to the throwing arm with method of delivery. Am J Sports Med 1978;6:15–621.

Bonger PM. Leader. BMJ 2001;322:64–65.

Buskila D. Genetics of chronic pain states. Best Pract Res 2007;21:535–547.

Chen AL, Shapiro JA, Ahn AK, Zuckerman JD, Cuomo F. Rotator cuff repair in patients with type I diabetes mellitus. J Shoulder Elbow Surg 2003;12:416–421.

Codman EA, Akerson IB. The pathology associated with rupture of the supraspinatus tendon. Ann Surg 1931;93:348–359.

Cotton RE, Rideout DF. Tears of the humeral rotator cuff: a radiological and pathological necropsy survey. J Bone Joint Surg Br 1964;46:314–328.

Denaro V, Ruzzini L, Barnaba SA, et al. Effect of pulsed electromagnetic fields on human tenocyte cultures from supraspinatus and quadriceps tendons. Am J Phys Med Rehabil 2011;90:119–127.

Denaro V, Ruzzini L, Longo UG, et al. Effect of dihydrotestosterone on cultured human tenocytes from intact supraspinatus tendon. Knee Surg Sports Traumatol Arthrosc 2010;18:971–976.

DePalma A, Callery G, Bennett G. Variational anatomy in degenerative lesions of the shoulder joint. Instr Course Lect 1949;6:255–281.

DePalma A, White J, Callery G. Degenerative lesions of the shoulder joint at various age groups which are compatible with good function. Instr Course Lect 1950;7:168–180.

Foulkes T, Wood JN. Pain genes. PLoS Genetics 2008;4:e1000086.

Fukuda H, Mikasa M, Yamanaka K. Incomplete thickness rotator cuff tears diagnosed by subacromial bursography. Clin Orthop Relat Res 1987;223:51–58.

Fukuda H, Hamada K, Yamanaka K. Pathology and pathogenesis of bursal-side rotator cuff tears viewed from en bloc histologic sections. Clin Orthop Relat Res 1990;254:75–80.

Galatz L, Silva M, Rothermich S, et al. Nicotine delays tendon-to-bone healing in a rat shoulder model. J Bone Joint Surg Am 2006;88:2027–2034.

Grant J, Smith G. Age incidence of rupture of the supraspinatus tendon. Anat Rec 1948;100:666.

Gwilym SE, Watkins B, Cooper CD, et al. Genetic influences in the progression of tears of the rotator cuff. J Bone Joint Surg Br 2009;91:915–917.

Harryman DT 2nd, Hettrich CM, Smith KL, et al. A prospective multipractice investigation of patients with full-thickness rotator cuff tears: the importance of comorbidities, practice, and other covariables on self-assessed shoulder function and health status. J Bone Joint Surg Am 2003;85:690–696.

Harvie P, Ostlere SJ, Teh J, et al. Genetic influences in the aetiology of tears of the rotator cuff. Sibling risk of a full-thickness tear. J Bone Joint Surg Br 2004;86:696–700.

Hegmann K, Moore J. Common neuromusculoskeletal disorders. In: King PM (ed.), Sourcebook of Occupational Rehabilitation. New York: Plenum Press, 1998: 30–32.

Hellsing A, Bryngelsson I. Predictors of musculoskeletal pain in men: a twenty-year follow-up from examination at enlistment. Spine 2000;25:3080–3086.

Jarvinen M. Epidemiology of tendon injuries in sports. Clinics Sports Med 1992;11:493– 504.

Jozsa L, Balint JB, Kannus P, Reffy A, Barzo M. Distribution of blood groups in patients with tendon rupture. An analysis of 832 cases. J Bone Joint Surg Br 1989;71:272–274.

Kaergaard A, Andersen J. Musculoskeletal disorders of the neck and shoulders in female sewing machine operators: prevalence, incidence, and prognosis. Occup Environ Med 2000;57:528–534.

Kannus P, Natri A. Etiology and pathophysiology of tendon ruptures in sports. Scand J Med Sci Sports 1997;7:107–112.

Keyes EL. Observations on rupture of the supraspinatus tendon: based upon a study of seventy-three cadavers. Ann Surg 1933;97:849–856.

Keyes E. Anatomic observations on senile changes in the shoulder. J Bone Joint Surg Am 1935;17:953–960.

Kujala UM, Jarvinen M, Natri A, et al. ABO blood groups and musculoskeletal injuries. Injury 1992;23:131–133.

Leclerc A, Franchi P, Cristofari MF, et al. Carpal tunnel syndrome and work organisation in repetitive work: a cross sectional study in France. Study Group on Repetitive Work. Occup Environ Med 1998;55:180–187.

Lehman C, Cuomo F, Kummer FJ, Zuckerman JD. The incidence of full thickness rotator cuff tears in a large cadaveric population. Bull Hosp Joint Dis 1995;54:30–31.

Leino-Arjas P. Smoking and musculoskeletal disorders in the metal industry: a prospective study. Occup Environ Med 1999;55:828–833.

Lippi G, Longo UG, Maffulli N. Genetics and sports. Br Med Bull 2010;93:27–47.

Longo UG, Fazio V, Poeta ML, et al. Bilateral consecutive rupture of the quadriceps tendon in a man with BstUI polymorphism of the ***COL5A1*** gene. Knee Surg Sports Traumatol Arthrosc 2010a;18:514–518.

Longo UG, Lamberti A, Maffulli N, Denaro V. Tendon augmentation grafts: a systematic review. Br Med Bull 2010b;94:165–188.

Longo UG, Lamberti A, Maffulli N, Denaro V. Tissue engineered biological augmentation for tendon healing: a systematic review. Br Med Bull 2010c;95:63–77.

Mallon WJ, Misamore G, Snead DS, Denton P. The impact of preoperative smoking habits on the results of rotator cuff repair. J Shoulder Elbow Surg 2004;13:129–132.

Meislin RJ, Sperling JW, Stitik TP. Persistent shoulder pain: epidemiology, pathophysiology, and diagnosis. Am J Orthop 2005;34:5–9.

Meyer A. Further evidences of attrition in the human body. Am J Anat 1924;34:241–267.

Milgrom C, Schaffler M, Gilbert S, Van Holsbeeck M. Rotator cuff changes in asymptomatic adults. The effect of age, hand dominance and gender. J Bone Joint Surg Br 1995;77:296–298.

Mokone GG, Gajjar M, September AV, et al. The guanine-thymine dinucleotide repeat polymorphism within the tenascin-C gene is associated with achilles tendon injuries. Am J Sports Med 2005;33:1016–1021.

Mokone GG, Schwellnus MP, Noakes TD, Collins M. The ***COL5A1*** gene and Achilles tendon pathology. Scand J Med Sci Sports 2006;16:19–26.

Neer CS, 2nd. Impingement lesions. Clinical Orthop Relat Res 1983;70–77.

Neer CS, 2nd, Welsh RP. The shoulder in sports. Orthop Clinics North Am 1977;8:583–591.

Penny JN, Smith C. The prevention and treatment of swimmer's shoulder. Can J Appl Sport Sci 1980;5:195–202.

Petersson CJ. Ruptures of the supraspinatus tendon. Cadaver dissection. Acta Orthop Scand 1984;55:52–56.

Quiniann E, Sinert R. Rotator cuff injury. Available at: www.emadicine.com/emerg/tople512.htm (accessed 21 August 2011).

Richardson AB, Jobe FW, Collins HR. The shoulder in competitive swimming. Am J Sports Med 1980;8:159–163.

Roquelaure Y, Cren S, Rousseau F, et al. Work status after workers' compensation claims for upper limb musculoskeletal disorders. Occup Environ Med 2004;61:79–81.

Roquelaure Y, Ha C, Leclerc A, et al. Epidemiologic surveillance of upper-extremity musculoskeletal disorders in the working population. Arthr Rheum 2006;55:765–778.

September AV, Schwellnus MP, Collins M. Tendon and ligament injuries: the genetic component. Br J Sports Med 2007;41:241–246; discussion 246.

Sher JS, Uribe JW, Posada A, Murphy BJ, Zlatkin MB. Abnormal findings on magnetic resonance images of asymptomatic shoulders. J Bone Joint Surg Am 1995;77:10–15.
Stenlund B, Goldie I, Hagberg M, Hogstedt C. Shoulder tendinitis and its relation to heavy manual work and exposure to vibration. Scand J Work Environ Health 1993;19:43–49.
Tashjian RZ, Farnham JM, Albright FS, Teerlink CC, Cannon-Albright LA. Evidence for an inherited predisposition contributing to the risk for rotator cuff disease. J Bone Joint Surg Am 2009;91:1136–1142.
Uhthoff HK, Sarkar K. Surgical repair of rotator cuff ruptures. The importance of the subacromial bursa. . J Bone Joint Surg Am 1991;73:399–401.
Urwin M, Symmons D, Allison T. Estimating the burden of musculoskeletal disease in the community. Ann Rheum Dis 1998;57:649–655.
Walker-Bone K, Palmer K, Reading I, Coggon D, Cooper C. Prevalence and impact of musculoskeletal disorders of the upper limb in the general population. Arthr Rheum 2004;51:642–651.
Wendelboe AM, Hegmann KT, Gren LH, et al. Associations between body-mass index and surgery for rotator cuff tendinitis. J Bone Joint Surg Am 2004;86:743–747.
Wilson C, Duff G. Pathologic study of degeneration and rupture of the supraspinatus. Arch Surg 1943;47:121–135.
Wilson PW. Established risk factors and coronary artery disease: the Framingham Study. Am J Hypertens 1994;7:7S–12S.
Yamaguchi K, Lashgari C. Natural history of rotator cuff disorders and non surgical treatment. In: Norris TR (ed.), Orthopaedic Knowledge Update. Shoulder and Elbow 2. 2nd edn. Rosemont, IL: American Academy of Orthopaedic Surgeons, 2002: 155–162.
Yamaguchi K, Tetro A, Blam O, et al. Natural history of asymptomatic rotator cuff tears: a longitudinal analysis of asymptomatic tears detected sonographically. J Shoulder Elbow Surg 2001;10:199–203.
Yamaguchi K, Ditsios K, Middleton W, et al. The demographic and morphological features of rotator cuff disease. a comparison of asymptomatic and symptomatic shoulders. J Bone Joint Surg Am 2006;88:1699–1704.
Yamanaka K., Fukuda, H, Hamada K, Mikasa M. Incomplete thickness tears of the rotator cuff. Orthop Surg Traumatol (Tokyo) 1983;26:7–13.
Yamanaka K, Matsumoto T. The joint side tear of the rotator cuff. A followup study by arthrography. Clin Orthop Relat Res 1994;68–73.

Chapter 5 Rotator cuff biomechanics

Giuseppe Porcellini, Eugenio Cesari, Fabrizio Campi, Paolo Paladini

KEY FEATURES

- The rotator cuff tendons act as a combined and integrated structure.
- Both the bone and soft-tissue structures of the shoulder have a marked impact on the function of the rotator cuff.
- The rotator cuff muscles are the primary dynamic stabilizers of the glenohumeral joint.
- The deltoid muscle acts as a shoulder elevator when supraspinatus is torn or dysfunctional.
- The fibers on the articular side of the rotator cuff are more likely to experience greater tensile loads than those on the bursal side.
- There are two main theories for the cause of rotator cuff tears: extrinsic impingement and intrinsic degeneration.

Although many factors influence the management of rotator cuff disease, understanding the anatomy of the rotator cuff and how it relates to function in tears of the rotator cuff is of fundamental importance. Both the bony and the soft-tissue structures have a marked impact on rotator cuff function. Recent research has expanded our knowledge about the rotator cuff, as well as about the coracoacromial arch, bursae, and neurovascular structures; several controversies have arisen as a result, including: the influence of the morphology of the acromion, coracoacromial ligament, and coracoid process on the development of rotator cuff tears; the role of the subacromial bursa as a source of pain or an essential contributor to a fibrovascular response for rotator cuff healing; the anatomical definition of the rotator cuff footprint; and the anatomical location of the neurovascular structures surrounding the rotator cuff.

ROTATOR CUFF MUSCLES

The shoulder complex comprises 30 muscles. These muscles both move the shoulder and stabilize it – some are "movers," others are "shakers." The rotator cuff muscles predominantly stabilize the glenohumeral joint, an inherently unstable joint, and contribute to movement.
The rotator cuff muscles are:

- supraspinatus
- infraspinatus
- teres minor
- subscapularis.

The tendons of these muscles coalesce to form the rotator cuff (**Figs 5.1** and **5.2**). The muscles merge at the level of the rotator cuff, except for the tendon of subscapularis, which is separate and joins the rest of the cuff via the rotator interval (**Figs 5.3** and **5.4**). They perform multiple functions during shoulder movement, including glenohumeral abduction, external rotation (ER), internal rotation (IR), and control of translation of the humeral head. Infraspinatus and subscapularis have significant roles in scapular plane abduction (scaption), producing forces that are two to three times greater than the force of supraspinatus. However, supraspinatus still remains a more effective shoulder abductor because of its more effective moment arm. Both deltoids and rotator cuff provide significant abduction torque, with an estimated contribution of up to 35–65% by middle deltoid, 30% by subscapularis, 25% by supraspinatus, 10% by infraspinatus, and 2% by anterior deltoid.

During abduction, the force of the middle deltoid has been estimated to be 434 N, followed by 323 N from anterior deltoid, 283 N from subscapularis, 205 N from infraspinatus, and 117 N from supraspinatus. These forces not only abduct the shoulder, but also stabilize the joint and neutralize the antagonistic effects of undesirable actions.

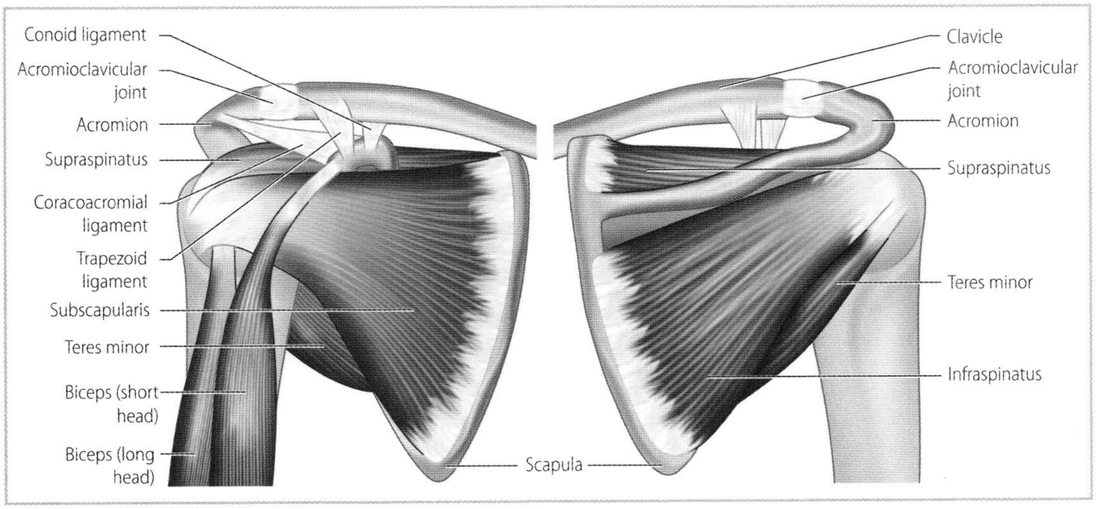

Figure 5.1 Anatomy of the RTC tendons – right shoulder (anterior view, left and posterior view, right)

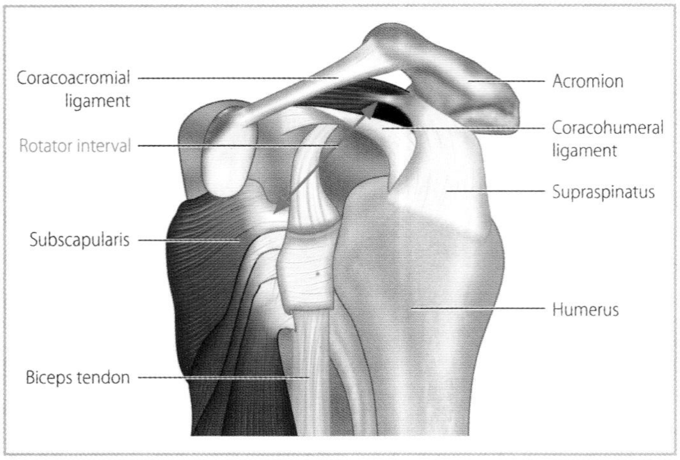

Figure 5.2 Rotator cuff interval and shoulder girdle anatomy – left shoulder. (From Lennard Funk 2005).

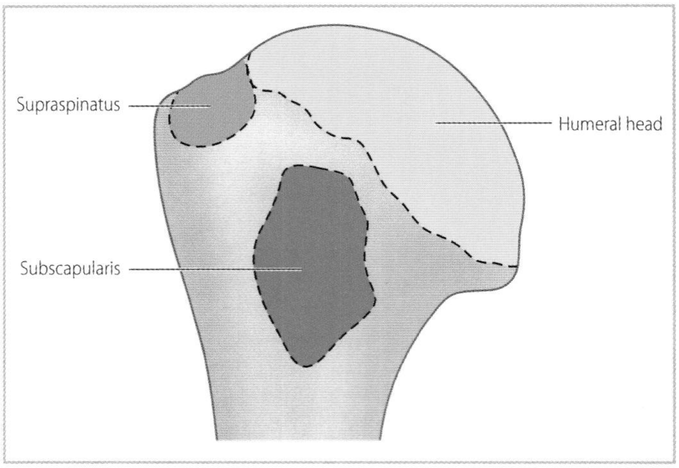

Figure 5.4 Right shoulder showing the footprint of the subscapularis tendon (blue) and the supraspinatus tendon (green). Yellow indicates the humeral head.

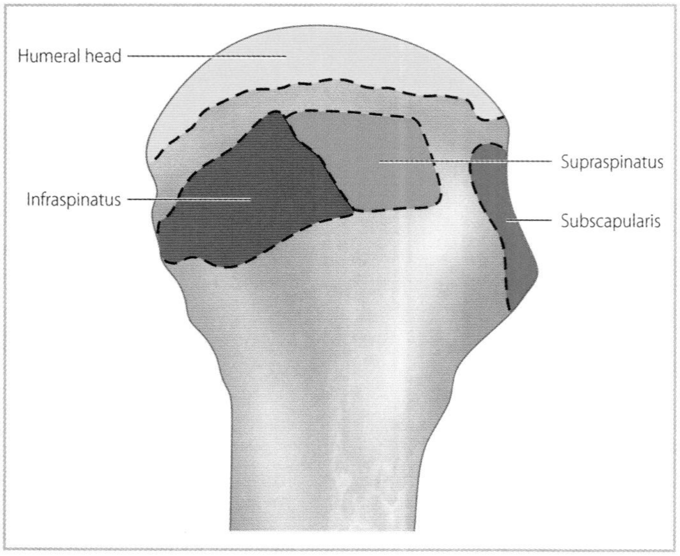

Figure 5.3 Right shoulder showing the footprint of the supraspinatus tendon (green), infraspinatus tendon (red), and subscapularis tendon (blue) anterior to biceps groove. The humeral head is also indicated in yellow.

A relatively high force from the rotator cuff not only helps abduct the shoulder but also neutralizes the superior directed force produced by the various components of deltoid at lower abduction angles. Even though the force produced by anterior deltoid is relatively high, its ability to abduct the shoulder is low, given its very small moment arm, especially at low abduction angles.

Deltoid is a more effective abductor at higher abduction angles, whereas the rotator cuff muscles are more effective abductors at lower abduction angles. During maximum humeral elevation, the scapula normally rotates upward 45–55°, tilts posteriorly 20–40°, and rotates externally 15–35°. The scapular muscles are important during humeral elevation because they cause these motions, especially serratus anterior, which contributes to scapular upward rotation, posterior tilt, and external rotation. Serratus anterior also helps stabilize the medial border and inferior angle of the scapula, preventing scapular internal rotation (winging) and anterior tilt. If the normal scapular movements are disrupted by abnormal scapular muscle firing patterns, weakness, fatigue, or injury, the shoulder complex functions less efficiently with increased risk of injury. Scapula position and humeral rotation can affect injury risk during humeral elevation. Compared with scapular protraction, scapular retraction both increases subacromial space width and enhances supraspinatus force production during humeral elevation. Moreover, scapular internal rotation and scapular anterior tilt, both of which decrease subacromial space width and increase impingement risk, are greater when performing scaption with internal rotation ("empty can") compared with scaption with external rotation ("full can").

The activity of supraspinatus is similar between "empty can" and "full can" movements, although the "full can" results in lesser risk of subacromial impingement. Infraspinatus and subscapularis activity have generally been reported to be higher in the "full can" compared with the "empty can," whereas posterior deltoid activity has been reported to be higher in the "empty can" than the "full can" position (**Figs 5.5** and **5.6**).

The progression of a rotator cuff tear or dysfunction leads to superior subluxation of the humeral head, with consequent dysfunction of the shoulder. The rotator cuff stabilizes the glenohumeral joint through force couples in both the coronal and transverse planes. Deltoid and supraspinatus both contribute to abduction equally. As the arm is abducted, the resultant joint reaction force is directed toward the glenoid. This "compresses" the humeral head against the glenoid, and improves the stability of the joint when the arm is abducted and overhead (Parsons et al. 2002). Throughout the range of motion, the compressive resultant joint reaction force in the transverse plane contributes to joint stability. This is the predominant mechanism resisting superior humeral head displacement with cuff tears. As long as the force couple between subscapularis and infraspinatus remains balanced, the joint remains centered (Parsons et al. 2002; Escamilla et al. 2009).

Supraspinatus

Supraspinatus not only is an initiator of abduction, but also acts throughout the range of abduction of the shoulder. It has equal abduction power to deltoid and lies in the scapular plane, i.e., 30° to the coronal plane.

The function of supraspinatus is complex. In addition to initiating shoulder abduction and stabilizing the glenohumeral joint, it contributes to humeral rotation. From three-dimensional shoulder

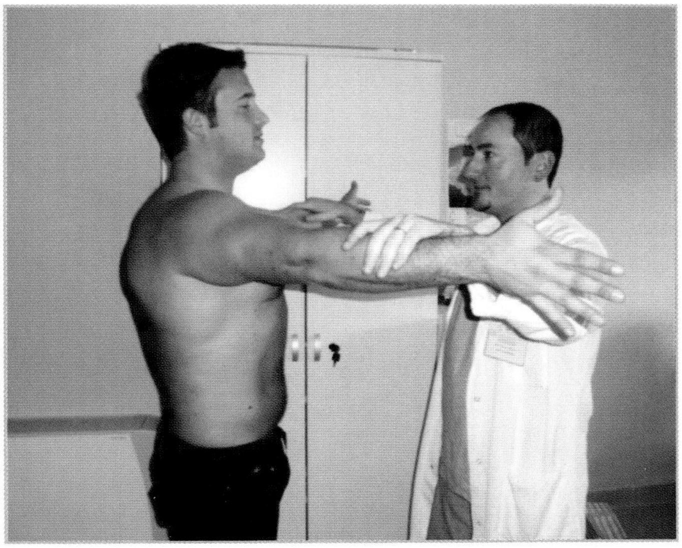

Figure 5.5 The "full can" exercise. The patient elevates the upper extremity at approximately 30° horizontal abduction in the plane of the scapula and full glenohumeral external rotation

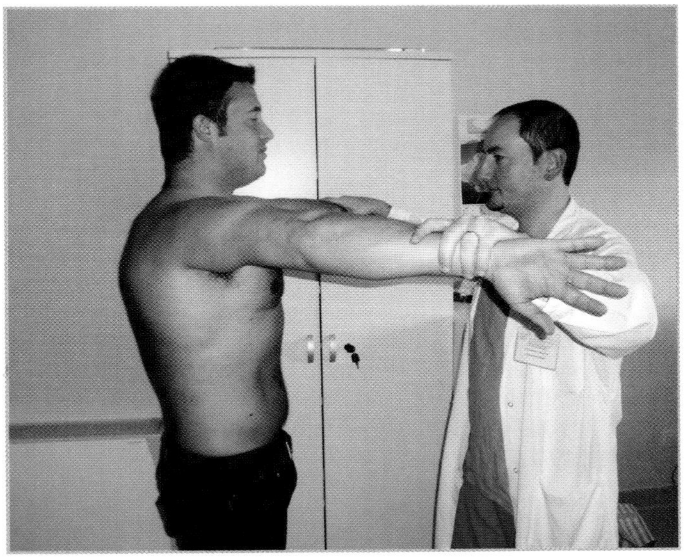

Figure 5.6 The "empty can" exercise. The patient elevates the upper extremity at approximately 30° horizontal abduction in the plane of the scapula and full glenohumeral internal rotation.

models, the predicted supraspinatus force during maximum effort isometric scapular plane abduction (scaption) at the 90° position was 117 N (Escamilla et al. 2009). In addition, supraspinatus activity increases as resistance increases during scaption movements, peaking at 30–60° for any given resistance. At lower scaption angles, the activity of supraspinatus increases to provide additional humeral head compression within the glenoid fossa to counter the humeral head superior translation from deltoids. Given the decreasing moment arm with abduction, supraspinatus is more effective during scaption at smaller abduction angles, but it still produces abductor torque (a function of both moment arm and muscle force) at larger abduction angles. The abduction moment arm for supraspinatus peaks at approximately 3 cm close to 30° abduction, but maintains an abduction moment arm of >2 cm throughout the shoulder abduction range of movement. Its ability to produce abduction torque during scaption appears to be greatest with the shoulder in neutral rotation or in slight internal or external rotation (Escamilla et al. 2009).

The external rotation lag sign (ERLS) is a test designed to assess the integrity of the supraspinatus and infraspinatus tendons. Blonna et al. (2010) determined the electromyographic (EMG) pattern of shoulder girdle muscles during a series of external rotation tasks conducted at full adduction and 20° to assess the final contribution of supraspinatus to the ERLS by measuring the amount of lag after a supraspinatus block induced by botulinum toxin. They demonstrated that supraspinatus contributed 20% of the electrical activities during the ERLS, significantly greater than the contributions of the other shoulder girdle muscles, except for infraspinatus. The selective block of supraspinatus caused a lag of 4° in all 10 shoulders at 20° but no increase in lag at 0° of elevation. The ERLS is potentially able to detect an isolated supraspinatus tear if the test is performed correctly (20° of abduction). The deltoid and biceps muscles are almost silent during the test, limiting confounding factors (Blonna et al. 2010).

Supraspinatus is composed of distinct anterior and posterior regions. Anatomical dissections (Volk and Vangsness 2001), magnetic resonance (MR) images of healthy volunteers (Vahlensieck et al. 1994) and a detailed study by Roh et al. (2000) described the specific structural differences between the two subregions while estimating the muscle forces that each could produce.

The distinct anatomy can be summarized as follows:

- The anterior subregion has a larger muscle that produces 71% of the total force. That force is transmitted through a thicker, more tubular tendon which accounts for 47% of the total tendon cross-sectional area.
- The posterior subregion has a smaller muscle that produces 29% of the total force that is transmitted through a wider, thinner tendon which accounts for 53% of the total tendon cross-sectional area.

The anterior subregion induces either internal or external rotation depending on the initial position of the humerus, whereas the posterior subregion does not produce internal rotation and instead induces either no rotation or external rotation. These results can be partly explained by the findings of Ihashi et al. (1998), who, investigating the relationship between the "leading edge" of the supraspinatus tendon and the center of rotation of the humeral head, found that the position of the long axis of the supraspinatus tendon varied with respect to the center of rotation of the humeral head, depending on the initial position of the humerus. At 30° and 60° of internal rotation, the long axis was anterior to the center of the head, at neutral rotation, it was near the center of rotation, and, at 30° of external rotation, supraspinatus was posterior to the head. Thus, supraspinatus can function as either an internal or an external rotator depending on the position. **Figure 5.7** shows how the positions of the anterior and posterior subregions of supraspinatus may vary with humeral rotation, and demonstrates why the anterior subregion was found to both internally and externally rotate the humerus.

Further evidence that supraspinatus can function as either an internal or an external rotator of the humerus is provided by the biomechanical studies of supraspinatus moment arms. In particular, Langenderfer et al. (2006) divided supraspinatus into three equal subregions, and calculated the moment arms at different positions of abduction. Overall, the anterior third was an internal rotator at positions of internal rotation, and an external rotator at positions of external rotation. To our knowledge, no biomechanical studies account for the difference in muscle force production between the anterior and posterior subregions when testing supraspinatus repair constructs, confirming that, at nearly all starting positions of the humerus, loading

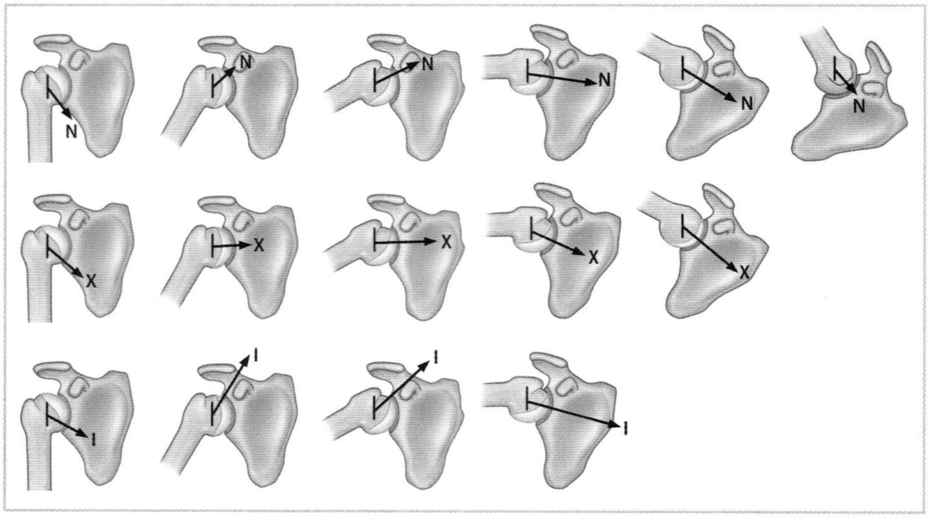

Figure 5.7 The resultant force vectors of the shoulder during arm elevation with the arm in neutral (N), external rotation similar to the "full can" exercise (X) and internal rotation similar to the "empty can" exercise (I). Note the superiorly oriented force vector with internal rotation at 30° and 60° elevation. (Adapted from Poppen NK, Walker PS. Forces at the glenohumeral joint in abduction. Clin Orthop Relat Res 1978;135:165–170.)

supraspinatus physiologically did not lead to a functional difference when compared with loading the muscle non-physiologically. The one condition where there was a difference (30° of humeral abduction and neutral rotation) is frequently used in biomechanical studies. It is uncertain whether this finding would lead to different conclusions in studies that do not allow for humeral rotation during testing.

Similarly, recent biomechanical studies using humeral rotational models did not account for the difference in subregional muscle force. Park and Phelps (1994) and Ahmad et al. (2008) studied gap formation in supraspinatus repairs with dynamic humeral external rotation and variable static humeral rotation positions, respectively. Park and Phelps (1994) found a regional difference in gap formation and tendon strain, with the anterior tendon demonstrating greater values of each. Ahmad et al. (2008) found that gap formation was different depending on which static humeral rotation position was used for testing. Both studies loaded supraspinatus as a whole. Had they accounted for the difference in force production between the two subregions, their results may have changed, with larger gap formations or tendon strains, depending on the position tested. These findings may explain a frequently encountered clinical problem as well.

Patients often have tears of supraspinatus on MRI without much clinical weakness (so-called functional tears) given the minimal contribution (29%) of the posterior part of the muscle to the whole force of supraspinatus. Specifically, the intact anterior subregion may compensate for the loss in abduction force, and an intact infraspinatus, which shares some of its footprint with posterior supraspinatus, may compensate for loss in external rotation force (Gates et al. 2010). Recently, Su et al. (2009) investigated the biomechanical effects of the size of anterosuperior rotator cuff tears on superior and anterosuperior translation, including tears interrupting the anterior cable attachment and the anterior force couple. Five cadaveric shoulders were subjected to different loading conditions in both the superior and the anterosuperior directions in the intact state, with supraspinatus completely cut and with sequentially larger anterosuperior rotator cuff tears. They found that isolated tears of supraspinatus had no significant biomechanical consequences under any condition tested. Anterosuperior translation was greater than superior translation in the intact specimen, and for every combination of anterosuperior rotator cuff defect. With supraspinatus and the superior half of subscapularis (i.e., the anterior cable attachment) released, there was no significant increase in anterosuperior or superior glenohumeral translation in response to lower loading conditions (10–20 N). At higher loading conditions (40–50 N), tears of supraspinatus and the superior half of subscapularis led to significantly increased translation in both directions. They concluded that simulated anterosuperior rotator cuff tears involving the superior half of subscapularis significantly alter shoulder biomechanics and lead to increased anterosuperior and superior glenohumeral translation under higher loads.

The anterior attachment of the rotator cuff cable is an important determinant of the biomechanics of anterosuperior rotator cuff tears at higher loads but not at lower loads. Preserving the inferior half of subscapularis was sufficient to maintain relatively normal shoulder kinematics under lower loading conditions. Tears of the entire subscapularis altered glenohumeral kinematics at essentially all loads. Su et al. (2010), in a cadaver study, investigated the biomechanical effects of posterosuperior rotator cuff tear size and loading the long head of biceps tendon in the presence of tears of the rotator cuff of various sizes, demonstrating that, as long as inferior infraspinatus remained intact, there was no significant differences in glenohumeral translation for any different load studied. Once supraspinatus and the entire infraspinatus were released, 50 N of load led to significantly increased translation in both superior and anterosuperior directions. For the intact specimens and for all sizes of rotator cuff tears, biceps loading led to a significant decrease in glenohumeral translation.

Partial repair of massive rotator cuff tears may improve the biomechanics of the shoulder, re-establishing the shoulder's essential force couples, thus converting a "dysfunctional symptomatic" rotator cuff tear into a "functional tear." Accordingly, the restoration of the force couple of the remaining anterior and posterior parts of the rotator cuff re-establish the muscle biomechanics ratio between internal and external humeral head rotators, leading to better function of the glenohumeral joint (Burkhart 2001). These biomechanical data can justify the preventive role of partial repair on computed tomography arthrography (CTA) development, in cases of easy repair of the infraspinatus tendon on Burkhart's original footprint, as recently demonstrated by Mochizuki et al. (2008). Specifically, they found that the footprint of supraspinatus was much smaller than previously reported and that the infraspinatus footprint covers a substantial amount of the entire greater tuberosity (Mochizuki et al. 2008). Muscle transfers of latissimus dorsi and pectoralis major have also been described to improve pain and function, usually in younger patients with irreparable rotator cuff tears. The transferred latissimus dorsi was recently supposed to act as an effective depressor in restricting cranial migration of the humeral head. However, postoperative radiographs showed minimal or no depression, especially in the neutral or externally rotated position. With internal rotation, 9 of the 14 patients treated showed slightly improved positioning of the humeral head in relation to the glenoid (Weening and Willems 2010).

Infraspinatus and teres minor

Infraspinatus and teres minor comprise the posterior cuff, which provides glenohumeral compression, and external rotation and abduction, and resists superior and anterior humeral head translation by exerting a posteroinferior force on the humeral head. The external rotation provided from the posterior cuff helps clear the greater tuberosity from under the coracoacromial arch during overhead movements, minimizing subacromial impingement. These two muscles lie below the scapular spine, and are external rotators of the shoulder. Infraspinatus primarily acts with the arm in neutral, and teres minor is more active with external rotation in 90° abduction. From three-dimensional biomechanical models, the maximum predicted isometric infraspinatus force was 723 N for external rotation at 90° abduction and 909 N for external rotation at 0° abduction. The maximum predicted teres minor force was much less than infraspinatus during maximum external rotation – both 90° abduction (111 N) and 0° abduction (159 N).

The effectiveness of the posterior cuff to laterally rotate depends on glenohumeral position. For infraspinatus, its superior, middle, and inferior heads all produce its largest external rotation torque at 0° abduction, primarily because its moment arm is greatest at 0° abduction (approximately 2.2 cm). As the abduction angle increases, the moment arms of the inferior and middle heads decrease slightly but stay relatively constant, whereas the moment arm of the superior head progressively decreases until it is about 1.3 cm at 60° adduction. These data imply that infraspinatus is a more effective external rotator at lower abduction angles compared with higher abduction angles. Although infraspinatus activity during external rotation is similar at 0°, 45°, and 90° abduction, external rotation at 0° abduction has been shown to be the optimal position to isolate infraspinatus, and there is a trend towards greater infraspinatus activity during external rotation at lower abduction angles compared with higher abduction angles.

Teres minor produces a relatively constant external rotation torque (relatively constant moment arm of 2.1 cm) throughout arm abduction, which implies that the abduction angle does not affect the effectiveness of teres minor to produce external rotation torque. Teres minor activity during external rotation is similar at 0°, 45°, and 90° abduction. In addition, both infraspinatus and teres minor activities are similar during external rotation movements regardless of abduction position. What is not readily apparent is the significance of infraspinatus as a shoulder abductor in the scapular plane. From three-dimensional biomechanical shoulder models, predicted infraspinatus force during maximum isometric effort scaption (90° position) is 205 N, nearly twice the predicted force from supraspinatus in this position. Liu et al. (1997) reported that, in scaption with neutral rotation, infraspinatus had an abductor moment arm that was small at 0° abduction but increased to 1 cm at 15° abduction and remained fairly constant throughout increasing abduction angles. Moreover, infraspinatus activity increases, peaking at 30–60° for any given resistance.

As resistance increases, infraspinatus activity increases to produce a higher torque in scaption, and infraspinatus activity at lower scaption angles increases to resist superior humeral head translation from the increased activity of deltoid. Also, the abductor moment arm of infraspinatus generally increased as abduction with internal rotation increased, such as performing the "empty can" exercise. In contrast, the abductor moment arm of infraspinatus generally decreased as abduction with external rotation increased, similar to performing the "full can" exercise. These data imply that infraspinatus may be more effective in producing abduction torque during the "empty can" compared with the "full can." Moreover, MRI data demonstrate similar infraspinatus activity during abduction with internal rotation and abduction with external rotation.

In contrast to infraspinatus, teres minor produces a weak shoulder adductor torque, given its lower attachments to the scapula and humerus. It is a weak adductor of the humerus regardless of its rotational position. In addition, because of its posterior shoulder position, it also helps to generate a weak horizontal abduction torque. Although its activity is similar to infraspinatus during external rotation, EMG and MRI demonstrated that the activity of teres minor during flexion, abduction, and scaption is less than infraspinatus activity. Even though teres minor produces an adduction torque, it is active during humeral head elevation movements because it contracts to enhance joint stability by resisting superior humeral head translation and providing humeral head compression within the glenoid fossa. This is especially true at lower abduction angles and when abduction and scaption movements encounter greater resistance. In contrast to arm abduction, scaption, and flexion, teres minor activity is much higher during prone horizontal abduction at 100° abduction with external rotation, exhibiting activity similar to infraspinatus. Teres minor activity is also high during standing high, mid, and low scapular rowing, and standing forward scapular punch, and even during internal rotation exercises to stabilize the glenohumeral joint (Escamilla et al. 2009).

Subscapularis

Subscapularis is the main internal rotator of the shoulder. It is the largest and strongest cuff muscle, providing 53% of the total cuff strength. The upper 60% of the insertion is tendinous and the lower 40% is muscle. It is a passive restraint in neutral, but not abduction. It provides glenohumeral compression stability, internal rotation, and abduction. From three-dimensional biomechanical shoulder models, predicted subscapularis force during maximum effort internal rotation was 1725 N at 90° abduction and 1297 N at 0° abduction. Its superior, middle, and inferior heads produce its largest internal rotation torque at 0° abduction, with a peak moment arm of approximately 2.5 cm. As the abduction angle increases, the moment arms of the inferior and middle heads stay relatively constant, whereas the moment arm of the superior head progressively decreases until it is about 1.3 cm at 60° abduction. These data imply that the upper portion of subscapularis (innervated by the upper part of the subscapular nerve) is a more effective internal rotator at lower abduction angles compared with higher abduction angles.

However, there is no significant difference in upper subscapular activity among internal rotation exercises at 0°, 45°, and 90° abduction. Abduction angle does not appear to affect the ability of lower subscapularis (innervated by the lower subscapular nerve) to produce internal rotation torque. Lower subscapularis muscle activity is affected by abduction angle. One study reported significantly greater lower subscapularis activity with internal rotation at 0° abduction compared with internal rotation at 90° abduction, whereas another reported greater lower subscapularis activity with internal rotation at 90° abduction compared with internal rotation at 0° abduction. Performing internal rotation at 0° abduction produces similar amounts of upper and lower subscapularis activity. The movement most optimal to isolation and activation of subscapularis is the Gerber lift-off against resistance, which is performed by lifting the dorsum of the hand off the mid-lumbar spine (against resistance) and simultaneously extending and internally rotating the shoulder. Performing the Gerber test produces similar amounts of upper and lower subscapularis activity. Subscapularis produces significant abduction torque during humeral elevation. Its force during maximum effort scaption (90° isometric position) is about 283 N, approximately 2.5 times the predicted force from supraspinatus in this position.

Liu et al. (1997) reported that, in the scapular plane, abduction with neutral rotation of subscapularis produced a peak abductor moment arm of 1 cm at 0° abduction and then slowly decreased to 0 cm at 60° abduction. Moreover, the abductor moment arm of subscapularis generally decreased as abduction with internal rotation increased, such as performing the "empty can" exercise. In contrast, the abductor moment arm of subscapularis generally increased as abduction with external rotation increased, such as performing the "full can" exercise. Otis et al. (1994) reported that the superior, middle, and inferior heads of subscapularis had abductor moment arms (greatest in the superior head and lowest in the inferior head) that vary as a function of humeral rotation. These moment arm lengths for the three muscle heads are approximately 0.4–2.2 cm at 45° of external rotation, 0.4–1.4 cm at neutral rotation, and 0.4–0.5 cm at 45° of internal rotation. This implies that subscapularis is more effective in scaption with external rotation compared with scaption with internal rotation. The simultaneous activation of subscapularis and infraspinatus during humeral elevation not only produces both abductor moments and inferior directed force to the humeral head to resist superior humeral head translation, but also neutralizes the internal rotation and external rotation torques that the muscles produce, further enhancing joint stability (Escamilla et al. 2009).

Deltoid

The deltoid muscle is the only shoulder elevator if supraspinatus is torn and dysfunctional. Therefore, most rehabilitation is directed toward this muscle. It comprises anterior, middle, and posterior portions that are more active depending on the direction of arm elevation.

The abductor moment arms during scaption at 0° abduction with neutral rotation are approximately 0 cm for anterior deltoid and 1.4 cm for middle deltoid, and progressively increase with increasing abduction. By 60° abduction the moment arms increase to approximately 1.5–2.0 cm for anterior deltoid and 2.7–3.2 cm for middle deltoid. From 0° to 40° abduction the moment arms for anterior and middle deltoids are less than the moment arms for supraspinatus, subscapularis, and infraspinatus. This implies that anterior and middle deltoids are not effective abductors at low abduction angles (especially anterior deltoids), whereas supraspinatus, infraspinatus, and subscapularis are more effective abductors at low abduction angles. These data are supported by an EMG Study (Park et al. 2007) in which anterior and middle deltoid activity generally peaks between 60° and 90° of scaption, whereas supraspinatus, infraspinatus, and subscapularis activity generally peaks between 30° and 60° of scaption. The abductor moment arm for anterior deltoid changes considerably with humeral rotation, increasing with external rotation and decreasing with internal rotation.

At 60° external rotation and 0° abduction, a position similar to the beginning of the "full can," the anterior deltoid moment arm was 1.5 cm (compared with 0 cm in neutral rotation), which makes the anterior deltoid an effective abductor even at small abduction angles. By 60° abduction with external rotation, its moment arm increases to approximately 2.5 cm (compared with 1.5–2.0 cm in neutral rotation). In contrast, at 60° internal rotation and 0° abduction, a position similar to the beginning of the "empty can" exercise, its moment arm was 0 cm, which implies that anterior deltoid is not an effective abductor with humeral internal rotation. By 60° abduction and internal rotation, its moment arm increased to only about 0.5 cm. Although the abductor moment arms for middle and posterior deltoids did change significantly with humeral rotation, the magnitude of these changes was too small to be clinically relevant.

From EMG and MRI data, both anterior and middle deltoids exhibit similar activity between the "empty can" and "full can." Posterior deltoid does not effectively contribute to the scapular plane abductor from 0° to 90°, but more effectively functions as a scapular plane adductor due to an adductor moment arm. As its adductor moment arm decreases with increase in abduction, this muscle becomes less effective as a scapular plane adductor at higher abduction angles, and may change to a scapular plane abductor beyond 110° abduction. These biomechanical data are consistent with EMG and MRI data, in which posterior deltoid activity is low not only during scaption but also during flexion and abduction. However, high to very high posterior deltoid activity has been reported in the "empty can" exercise when compared with the "full can" exercise, which implies that internal rotation during scaption increases posterior deltoid activity. Posterior and middle deltoid activity remain similar between internal rotation and external rotation positions while performing prone horizontal abduction at 100° abduction.

Peak isometric abduction torque has been reported to be 25 N/m at 0° abduction and neutral rotation. Up to 35–65% of this torque is produced by middle deltoid, up to 30% by subscapularis, up to 10% by infraspinatus, up to 2% by anterior deltoid, and 0% by posterior deltoid. This implies that both deltoids and the rotator cuff provide significant abduction torque. The ineffectiveness of anterior and posterior deltoids in producing abduction torque may appear surprising, but the low abduction torque for anterior deltoid does not mean that this muscle is only minimally active. In fact, as anterior deltoid has an abductor moment arm near 0 cm, at 0° abduction, the muscle could be very active and generating very high force, but very little torque, because of the small moment arm. At 0° abduction, the force produce by deltoid attempts to translate the humeral head superiorly, which is resisted largely by the rotator cuff. Therefore, highly active deltoids may also result in a highly active rotator cuff, especially at low abduction angles during humeral elevation.

The torque data are supported by muscle force data from deltoids and the rotator cuff during maximum effort abduction with the arm 90° abducted and in neutral rotation. The forces produced by posterior deltoid and teres minor were only 2 N and 0 N, respectively, which further demonstrates the ineffectiveness of these muscles as shoulder abductors. In contrast, the force produced by middle deltoid was the highest, at 434 N, which supports the high activity in this muscle during abduction. Anterior deltoid produced the second highest force of 323 N, which may appear surprising given the low abductor torque for this muscle at 0° abduction. However, force and torque are not the same. It is important to remember that the moment arm of anterior deltoid progressively increases as abduction increases, and that muscle force is produced not only to produce joint torque, but also to provide joint stabilization (Escamilla et al. 2009).

STATIC AND DYNAMIC RESTRAINTS

In addition to the dynamic stabilizers mentioned above, there are important secondary restraints to superior displacement of the humeral head with cuff tears.

Coracoacromial arch

The coracoacromial arch is the combination of the coracoid, coracoacromial ligament, and acromion. These form an arch above the rotator cuff and humeral head. The morphology of the acromion is relevant to the surgical management of rotator cuff disease for several reasons. First, abnormalities in the development of the acromion may lead to the formation of an os acromiale, with approximately 8% of patients having one. In 33% of patients, an os acromiale occurs bilaterally. Recent studies suggest an association between os acromiale and rotator cuff tears, but this relationship is not well defined (Park and Phelps 1994; Boehm et al. 2005). In fact, on the basis of the data in the literature, it is unlikely that the os acromiale has a pathological effect on the rotator cuff (Boehm et al. 2003). The presence of an os acromiale also does not influence the number of tendons involved in the rotator cuff tear. These findings are important considerations in the preoperative planning for rotator cuff repairs. Boehm et al. (2005) retrospectively reviewed the surgical management of 33 patients who undergone treatment for a rotator cuff tear and an os acromiale. They concluded that, at the time of rotator cuff repair, resection is appropriate for a small, symptomatic os acromiale. A large and symptomatic os acromiale can be fused to the acromion. However, fusion of the os acromiale after rotator cuff repair does not result in a better clinical outcome compared with acromioplasty or unsuccessful fusion (Boehm et al. 2003).

Furthermore, acromioplasty as a treatment for os acromiale should be used with caution because it may destabilize the acromion. The morphology of the acromion and its relationship to impingement as a cause of rotator cuff disease are controversial. As a result, the debate continues over whether rotator cuff tears are caused by degenerative changes in the cuff tendons or by extrinsic mechanical compression resulting from a hooked acromion.

Neer (1972) developed the concept that rotator cuff tears result from subacromial impingement. Subsequently, the technique and justification for acromioplasty during rotator cuff repairs developed from this hypothesis. Bigliani et al. (1991) further defined subacromial impingement by classifying acromial morphology into three primary types: flat (type I), curved (type II), and hooked (type III) (**Fig. 5.8**). The hooked acromion (type III) is most often associated with impingement and rotator cuff tears. Several recent studies support the relationship between subacromial impingement and development of rotator cuff tears (Flatow et al. 1995; Gill et al. 2002). In a cadaveric study, Flatow et al. (1995) showed a marked increase in contact between the rotator cuff and a type III acromion. On the basis of a review of their patients treated for impingement syndrome, Wang et al. (2000) suggested that acromial morphology has a predictive value in determining the success of conservative measures and the need for surgery.

In general, another source of impingement is enthesophytes located at the coracoacromial ligament insertion on the acromion. In a cadaveric study, Natsis et al. (2007) showed that enthesophytes were significantly more common in type III acromions. Other types of acromions recently described include a type IV (convex) acromion (Vanarthos and Monu 1995) and an acromion with a keel (Tucker and Snyder 2004). There are no data to strongly support an association between type IV acromions and rotator cuff pathology. In an MRI study of rotator cuff disease, Baechler and Kim (2006) reported that the percentage of the humeral head not covered superiorly by the anterolateral acromion may be a factor in the pathogenesis of full-thickness rotator cuff tears. Greater "uncoverage" may allow hinging of the humeral head on the anterolateral edge of the acromion during early shoulder abduction, causing impingement of the supraspinatus tendon between these two structures.

Conversely, on the basis of a radiographic study of patients with rotator cuff disease, Nyffeler et al. (2006) reported a statistically significant association between a large lateral extension of the acromion and full-thickness degenerative rotator cuff tears. In another radiographic study, Torrens et al. (2007) demonstrated that patients with rotator cuff tears have significantly more coverage of the humeral head by the acromion, compared with the control group without tears. Even though research studies support the association between type III acromions and rotator cuff tears, there is an equivalent amount of evidence disputing it (Chang et al. 2006). Several recent clinical studies also suggest that avoiding acromioplasty at the time of rotator cuff repair does not change the clinical or anatomical outcome (De Franco and Cole 2009). Given these studies, the association between acromial morphology and rotator cuff tears may not be as strong as described in the literature. Nevertheless, acromioplasty continues to be used by most shoulder surgeons, except in cases where the coracoacromial arch provides superior stability to prevent escape of the humeral head, as in massive rotator cuff tears. Overall, although a causal interrelationship of impingement syndrome, rotator cuff pathology, and acromial morphology is strongly suggested by published scientific data, the exact sequence of cause and effect between these entities is not well defined (De Franco and Cole 2009).

Coracoacromial ligament

The coracoacromial ligament originates along the distal two-thirds of the lateral aspect of the coracoid process as a broad ligament. It passes posteriorly to insert on to the anteromedial and anteroinferior

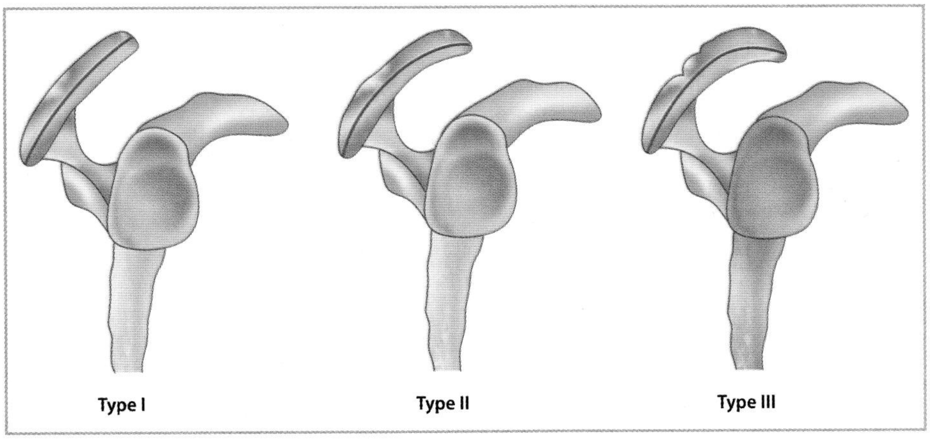

Figure 5.8 Bigliani classification of acromial morphology (left shoulder). Type III was more commonly associated with rotator cuff tears.

surfaces of the acromion. A recent cadaveric study showed variation in the morphology of the coracoacromial ligament. Most commonly, it consists of two distinct bands: anterolateral and posteromedial (Fealy et al. 2005). Spur formation occurs preferentially in the anterolateral band, which is commonly involved in impingement syndrome. If the posteromedial bundle is mistaken for the entire ligament, the surgeon may fail to visualize the anterolateral corner of the acromion and perform an incomplete subacromial decompression (De Franco and Cole 2009).

Despite the conclusions by Fealy et al. (2005) about the role of the coracoacromial ligament in impingement syndrome, Pieper et al. (1997) found no significant relationship between the morphology of the coracoacromial ligament and the incidence of rotator cuff degenerative changes or spur formation. Similarly, Kesmezacar et al. (2008) reported on five anatomical variations of the coracoacromial ligament. On the basis of this study, the Y-shaped ligament is the most common type, and there was no statistically significant association between rotator cuff disease and the type of geometric measurement of the ligament. Fremerey et al. (2000), in a cadaveric study, defined the anatomical and biomechanical properties of the coracoacromial ligament in shoulders with either intact rotator cuff or rotator cuff disease. Specimens from cadavers with rotator cuff disease had a shorter medial and lateral band of the coracoacromial ligament than specimens taken from shoulders with intact rotator cuffs. The cross-sectional area of the lateral band was enlarged in older specimens with rotator cuff degeneration. The authors suggested that substantial alterations in morphological and biomechanical properties occur in the coracoacromial ligament during aging (Fremerey et al. 2000). However, more studies are needed to determine whether variation in the coracoacromial ligament morphology causes or is a consequence of impingement.

Coracoid process

Many anatomical studies define the morphology of the coracoid process. In a relatively recent study Bhatia et al. (2007) used quantitative and statistical analysis of linear and angular dimensions to define the individual pillars of the coracoid process. The pillar anatomy of the coracoid and its effect on subcoracoid space are essential to understand the concept of coracoid impingement. According to Bhatia et al. (2007), impingement of the rotator cuff occurs between the posterolateral coracoid and humeral head. Clinically, this condition manifests itself as anterior shoulder pain with forward flexion, internal rotation, and horizontal adduction of the humerus. Subcoracoid pain is the result of impingement of the subscapularis tendon between the lesser tuberosity and the coracoid process. Changes associated with this impingement include supraspinatus tendon injury, subscapularis tendon injury, changes to the rotator interval, and thickening of the coracoacromial ligament.

Theoretically, an increase in axial angulation of either pillar, a decrease in interpillar angulation, or a decrease in the length of either pillar may predispose an individual to coracoid impingement and place supraspinatus or subscapularis at risk for tearing. In a cadaveric study, Ferreira et al. (2006) showed that women have a smaller distance between the apex of the coracoid process and the lesser tuberosity of the humerus with the arm in internal rotation. This finding suggests that impingement may be more likely between these two bony structures in female patients. Previous studies have also suggested that mechanical bony irritation, caused in part by pathological coracoid morphology, is an important etiological factor in the development of coracoid impingement.

Schulz et al. (2005) correlated coracoid tip position with rotator cuff tears. In a radiographic study they concluded that type I coracoids (in which the tip of the coracoid process projects on to the inferior half of the glenoid surface) are associated with supraspinatus tears. Type II coracoids (in which the tip of the coracoid process projects on to the superior half of the glenoid surface) are associated with subscapularis tears.

Richards et al. (2005) used a retrospective cohort to show a significant relationship between a narrowed coracohumeral distance and subscapularis pathology. In a prospective study by Kragh et al. (2004), coracoplasty resulted in statistically significant relief of pain and improved function in patients with primary coracoid impingement in whom non-surgical management failed. Subcoracoid impingement can also be a problem during the postoperative period.

Suenaya et al. (2000) studied postoperative subcoracoid impingement syndrome in 11 of 216 patients who underwent an acromioplasty and rotator cuff repair. In these 11 patients, the authors identified subcoracoid impingement as the cause of ongoing pain and unsatisfactory clinical outcome. Even though these studies suggest a relationship between subcoracoid stenosis and the development of rotator cuff tendon tears, recent studies are not in agreement with this hypothesis. In a cadaveric study, Radas and Pieper (2004) evaluated coracoid impingement of subscapularis. The distance between the lesser tuberosity and the coracoid was measured at different degrees of humeral rotation. On the basis of this study, coracoid impingement does not seem to be caused by anatomical variations of the coracoid, but rather by a functional problem, such as anterior instability of the shoulder joint, which leads to a functional narrowing of the coracohumeral distance.

Bursae

There are three bursae relevant to shoulder pain and rotator cuff disease: subacromial, subdeltoid, and subcoracoid. The subacromial bursa occupies a space above the rotator cuff and under the acromion. It is a synovium-lined cavity that acts as a gliding surface in two locations: (1) between the rotator cuff tendons and the coracoacromial arch and (2) between the deltoid muscle and the cuff tendon. There may be a connection between the subcoracoid and subacromial bursae. Voloshin et al. (2005) reported that high levels of inflammatory cytokines and enzymes produce a catabolic environment in the bursae of patients with rotator cuff tears. This emphasizes the importance of bursectomy to reduce pain and inflammation associated with rotator cuff disease. Duranthon and Gagey (2001) performed a cadaveric study to define the anatomy and function of the subdeltoid bursa. An increase in thickness of the subdeltoid bursa can contribute to subacromial impingement. The study also found anatomical continuity between the coracoacromial ligament and the subdeltoid bursa, which can mask the outer edge of the coracoacromial ligament.

Recognition of these anatomical findings is helpful in performing a thorough subacromial decompression. Subacromial disease encompasses a spectrum of disease ranging from bursitis to adhesion formation. Rotator cuff tears are often associated with subacromial bursitis, and this bursitis leads to the formation of adhesions, which contribute to impingement. Machida et al. (2004) found that adhesions of the subacromial bursa increase impingement between the acromion and the insertion of the rotator cuff. Funk et al. (2006) studied patients who were diagnosed with a subacromial plica during arthroscopic subacromial decompression. Overall, the prevalence of subacromial plica is 6% in shoulders presenting with subacromial impingement. The impingement changes caused by the plica are not degenerative, but mechanical abrasions due to rubbing between the rotator cuff and the undersurface of the acromion and the coracoacromial ligament.

In younger patients the diagnosis of plica as a reason for impingement should be considered only after secondary impingement due to instability has been ruled out. Overall, the bursae are essential to normal rotator cuff function. Bursectomy and plica removal as part of a thorough subacromial decompression are required to alleviate pain and make an accurate assessment of other structures, such as the acromion, coracoacromial ligament, and rotator cuff. This opinion is not, however, without controversy. There are investigators who recommend bursal preservation at the time of rotator cuff repair because of the theoretical contribution of blood supply to the healing of the tendo-osseous junction (De Franco and Cole 2009).

Long head of biceps

The long head of biceps passes through a tunnel formed by the coracohumeral ligament to reach the supraglenoid tubercle, and has connections through its sheath to the rotator interval capsule as well as to the glenoid labrum. It is considered by some to be part of the rotator cuff mechanism. The long head of biceps, when active, may augment the stability of the glenohumeral joint at the lower degrees of abduction, by centering the humeral head on the glenoid fossa. This is predominantly with abduction and external rotation of the arm in the scapular plane. Its role as a secondary stabilizer of the glenohumeral joint has been put forward after observation of hypertrophy of the long head in the presence of rotator cuff tear.

The biceps pulley is a stabilizer of the long head of biceps in the biceps groove. Rupture of this pulley with a rotator cuff tear leads to medial subluxation of the long head of biceps, and dysfunction. Lesions of the biceps tendon occur frequently with tears of the rotator cuff, and have been identified as a source of persistent pain that can resolve with spontaneous rupture. After spontaneous rupture, loss of elbow flexion strength is up to 16%. Arthroscopic biceps tenotomy in the management of rotator cuff tears in selected patients yields good objective improvement and a high degree of patient satisfaction. Despite these improvements, arthroscopic tenotomy or tenodesis can increase superior translation of the humeral head during active abduction of the shoulder in the scapular plane (Warner and McMahon 1995), and does not appear to alter the progressive radiographic changes that occur with long-standing rotator cuff tears (Boileau et al. 2007; Szabó et al. 2008).

Rotator interval

The rotator interval plays an important role in affecting the proper function of the glenohumeral joint. The rotator interval is an anatomical region in the anterosuperior aspect of the glenohumeral joint that represents a complex interaction of the fibers of the coracohumeral ligament, superior glenohumeral ligament, glenohumeral joint capsule, and supraspinatus and subscapularis tendons. Anatomically, the most superior part of the subscapularis tendon was attached to the upper margin of the lesser tuberosity and extended as a thin tendinous slip to the fovea capitis of the humerus. The superior glenohumeral ligament ran spirally along the biceps tendon. Histologically, the superior glenohumeral ligament was attached to the tendinous slip (Hunt et al. 2007). There was no clear boundary between the superior glenohumeral and coracohumeral ligament. Lesions of the rotator interval may result in glenohumeral joint contractures, shoulder instability, or lesions to the long head of biceps tendon. To keep the biceps tendon in place and stabilized, tension in the superior glenohumeral ligament and buttress support of the most superior insertion point of subscapularis from behind the ligament may be necessary (Arai et al. 2010).

ROTATOR CUFF PATHOANATOMY

Cuff ultrastructure

The fusing of the rotator cuff tendons suggests that they act more as a combined and integrated structure than as single entities. The microstructure of the rotator cuff tendons near the insertions of supraspinatus and infraspinatus has been further described as a five-layer structure:

- **Layer one** is composed of the superficial fibers of the coracohumeral ligament.
- **Layer two**, which is the main portion of the cuff tendons, is seen as closely packed parallel tendon fibers grouped in large bundles extending directly from the muscle bellies to the insertion on the humerus.
- **Layer three** is also a thick tendinous structure but with smaller bundles than in layer two, and a less uniform orientation.
- **Layer four** is composed of loose connective tissues with thick bands of collagen fibers running perpendicular to the primary fiber orientation of the cuff tendons. This layer contains the deep extension of the coracohumeral ligament and has been variously described as a transverse band, a pericapsular band, and a rotator cable. This layer may have a role in the distribution of forces between tendinous insertions and may explain why some rotator cuff tears are clinically asymptomatic.
- **Layer five** is the true capsular layer, and forms a continuous cylinder from glenoid to humerus. The fibers in this layer are, for the most part, randomly oriented.

The fiber orientation also differs along the length of the rotator cuff tendon. Near the musculotendinous junctions, the tendons are composed mainly of parallel homogeneous collagen fibers, but become flat ribbon-like bundles of fibers that cross at an angle of about 45° as they reach insertion into the humerus.

As a result of the orientations of the various fiber and distinct layers within the superior capsular complex, significant shear forces likely exist and may have a role in cuff tears. These intratendinous variations in the cuff structure may explain why intrasubstance tears occur. Shear forces are probably directed to layer four, which is the site of development of intratendinous cuff tears (De Franco and Cole 2009).

Collagen

The midsubstance of the supraspinatus tendon is primarily composed of type I collagen, with relatively small amounts of type III collagen, decorin, and biglycan. The fibrocartilage portion of the insertion has a collagen and proteoglycan content similar to that of tissues that have been subjected to compressive loads. This is partly due to the wrapping of the tendon around the humerus. Therefore, it mainly contains type II collagen and larger proteoglycans such as aggrecan. The histological organization does not, however, resemble mature fibrocartilage. In rotator cuff tendinopathy, an increase in collagen type III, a protein that plays a role in healing and repair, and glycosaminoglycan and proteoglycan content has been observed. These compositional changes may be adaptive, pathological, or both, and are found to be altered in the older population. Furthermore, recent studies have shown increased levels of smooth muscle actin (SMA) in torn rotator cuffs. SMA-positive cells have been shown to contract a collagen–glycosaminoglycan analog in vitro. SMA-containing cells in rotator cuff tears may react with the high levels of glycosaminoglycan and proteoglycan, resulting in retraction of the ruptured rotator cuff and inhibition of potential healing (De Franco and Cole 2009).

Vascularity

The major arterial supply to the rotator cuff is derived from the ascending branch of the anterior humeral circumflex artery, the acromial branch of the thoracoacromial artery, as well as the suprascapular and posterior humeral circumflex arteries.

The pathogenesis of rotator cuff tears was considered to be influenced by the microvascular supply of the rotator cuff tendons. Most cadaver studies have demonstrated a hypovascular area within the critical zone of the supraspinatus tendon, and it has been suggested that this area of hypovascularity plays a clinically relevant role in the attritional lesions of the aging tendon. More recent studies of the microvascular supply to the supraspinatus tendon in symptomatic patients with impingement syndrome suggest that, in the area of greatest impingement, i.e., the critical zone (8 mm proximal to the insertion of the supraspinatus tendon), there is actually hypervascularity. In contrast to the cadaver investigations, these studies seem to imply that hypervascularity or neovascularization is associated with symptomatic rotator cuff disease secondary to mechanical impingement. In vivo analysis using orthogonal polarization spectral imaging has demonstrated that there is good vascularity of supraspinatus, even in the critical zone in intact rotator cuffs (De Franco and Cole 2009).

Mechanical properties of the supraspinatus tendon

The articular side of supraspinatus has a higher modulus of elasticity but a lower yield strain than the bursal side, which is information that contributes to our understanding of regions of tear initiation and progression. The longitudinal tendon bundles composing the bursal side of the tendon are more capable of dispersing tensile loads than the interlaced, thinner fibers found in the articular side of the tendon. Therefore, the fibers on the articular side of the tendon are more likely to experience greater tensile loads than those experienced by the fibers on the bursal side. This effect is further magnified with abduction, because the articular side of the rotator cuff is closer to its yield strain than the bursal side.

Mathematical models further support the experimental findings and imply that the stress concentration moves from the articular surface closer to the insertion site with increasing abduction angle. However, the presence of an articular-sided tear is thought to weaken the remaining intact portion of the insertion site and thus increase the risk of tear progression. Bey et al. (2002) have investigated the use of MRI with image-processing techniques to obtain intratendinous strain information non-invasively. Assuming that an increase in tendon strain indicates an increase in the risk of tear progression, the studies investigated the intratendinous strains in relation to different types of tears in different locations of the tendon. Specifically, they conducted studies examining the effect of joint position on strains in the tendon, in both the presence and the absence of an articular-sided, partial-thickness tear.

The presence of a tear caused an increase in strain at 30°, 45°, and 60° abduction but had no effect at 15°. They also found that the strains of the superior, middle, and inferior portions of the tendon were affected differently by the presence of a tear or the increase in the abduction angle, further supporting the notion that the location of the tear should be considered when prescribing treatment. However, the remaining (intact) rotator cuff tendons had decreased mechanical properties in the presence of rotator cuff tears. The remaining (intact) subscapularis and infraspinatus tendon cross-sectional areas increased, whereas tendon modulus decreased after tears of both one and two tendons. The remaining (intact) tendon cross-sectional areas continued to increase with time after injury. These alterations could potentially lead to further tendon damage and tear progression (Perry et al. 2009).

Articular-sided, partial-thickness rotator cuff tears develop at the attachment of the tendon just lateral to the articular margin. Ellman (1990) described a classification system for partial-thickness tears based on the thickness of the rotator cuff tendon. Degenerative rotator cuff tears most commonly involve a posterior location, near the junction of supraspinatus and infraspinatus. The patterns of tear location across multiple tear sizes suggest that degenerative cuff tears may initiate in a region 13–17 mm posterior to the biceps tendon (Kim et al. 2010). On the basis of data in the literature, the thickness of the rotator cuff varies from 10 mm to 14 mm (De Franco and Cole 2009). A normal margin (1.5 mm) of exposed bone exists between the articular cartilage and supraspinatus insertion. Indeed, Sano et al. (1998) negatively correlated the width of the articular margin with the ultimate tensile strength of supraspinatus. The width of this sulcus is, therefore, a useful clinical indication of the integrity and tensile strength of the supraspinatus tendon. The addition of a medial row-to-rotator cuff repair may help to strengthen fixation and distribute force by increasing surface area and allowing the tendon to heal under less stress.

ETIOLOGY OF CUFF TEARS

There is a high correlation between the onset of rotator cuff tears and increasing age (Yamaguchi et al. 2006) and cigarette smoking (Baumgarten et al. 2010). There are two main theories for the cause of rotator cuff tears (**Fig. 5.9**):

1. **Extrinsic**: from compression and impingement of the rotator cuff from without, such as on the subacromial bursal side from acromial spurs and the coracoacromial ligament (subacromial impingement); and on the articular side from trapping of the tendon between the glenoid and humerus in extreme abduction and external rotation (internal impingement).

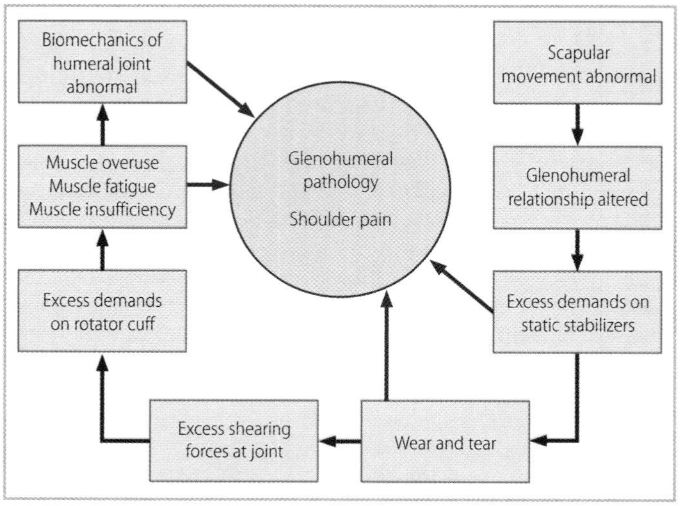

Figure 5.9 Biomechanical reasons for the development of cuff tears.

2. **Intrinsic**: development of tears due to changing properties of the rotator cuff itself.

Subacromial extrinsic impingement

Neer (1972) originally believed that rotator cuff tears arose from a mechanical process secondary to progressive wear. He found the anterior aspect of the acromion to be either involved with or not involved with osteophytes from the acromioclavicular joint. The morphology of the anterior acromion has been found to correlate with cuff tears. A cadaveric study of 140 shoulders showed that 73% of rotator cuff tears found were in type 3 hooked acromions (Bigliani et al. 1991). This has also been demonstrated by recent clinical studies where acromial morphology was found to be a predictor for cuff tears (Gill et al. 2002).

Internal impingement

This syndrome should be clearly differentiated from the classic (external) impingement that is thought to be caused by compression of the subacromial bursa, long head of biceps tendon, and rotator cuff by the coracoacromial arch. Internal impingement syndrome is typified by a painful shoulder from impingement of the soft tissue, including the rotator cuff, joint capsule, and posterosuperior part of the glenoid. The etiology of this syndrome is unclear, but hypotheses include anterior shoulder instability or micro-instability, contracture of the posterior capsule, reduced humeral retroversion, and scapular dyskinesis. The internal impingement occurs when the cuff is pinched between the humeral head and the posterosuperior labrum during extreme abduction and external rotation. This scuffs and abrades the articular surface of the cuff, progressively leading to cuff tears (Walch et al. 1991) (**Fig. 5.10**). Non-surgical therapy represents the first line of treatment for this syndrome and includes the management of pain, stretching of the posterior capsule, and a muscle-strengthening program. Surgical treatment should be considered only when conservative management fails. A number of different surgical procedures have been proposed, but the results are variable. The success rate is generally improved when the subtle instability, associated with internal impingement, is also addressed (Castagna et al. 2010).

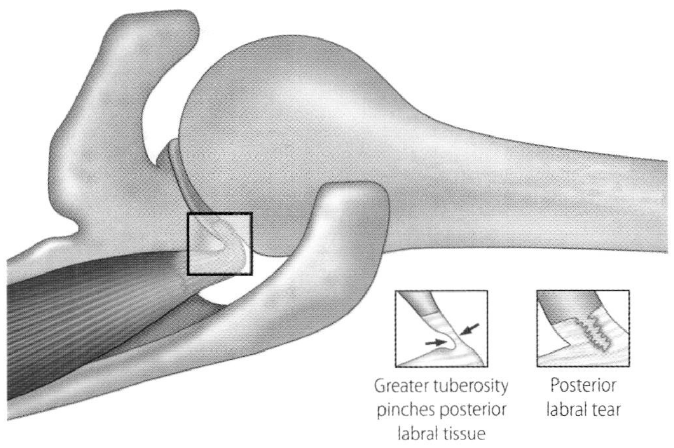

Figure 5.10 The internal impingement (right shoulder). The humeral head moves in a posterosuperior direction with abduction and external rotation during throwing. This results in the articular side of the rotator cuff abutting the posterosuperior glenoid rim and labrum. This has been associated with superior labral anteroposterior (SLAP) lesions, rotator cuff tears, and Bennett's lesions. (Redrawn based on Walch G, Boileau P, Noel E, Donell ST. Internal impingement. J Shoulder Elbow Surg 1992;1:243.)

CONCLUSION

The etiological and pathomechanical factors in the development of rotator cuff tears appear to have multifactorial roots. Understanding the current research is essential to developing surgical principles to treat rotator cuff disease. Application of this knowledge to clinical practice and to future research will result in appropriate care for patients with rotator cuff tears.

REFERENCES

Ahmad CS, Kleweno C, Jacir AM. Biomechanical performance of rotator cuff repairs with humeral rotation: a new rotator cuff repair failure model. Am J Sports Med 2008;36:888–892.

Arai R, Mochizuki T, Yamaguchi K, et al. Functional anatomy of the superior glenohumeral and coracohumeral ligaments and the subscapularis tendon in view of stabilization of the long head of the biceps tendon. J Shoulder Elbow Surg 2010;19:58–66.

Baechler M, Kim D. "Uncoverage" of the humeral head by anterolateral acromion and its relationship to full-thickness rotator cuff tears. Mil Med 2006;171:1035–1038.

Baumgarten KM, Gerlach D, Galatz LM, et al. Cigarette smoking increases the risk for rotator cuff tears. Clin Orthop Relat Res 2010;468:1534–1541.

Bey MJ, Song HK, Wehrli FW, Soslowsky LJ. Intratendinous strain fields of the intact supraspinatus tendon: the effect of glenohumeral joint position and tendon region. J Orthop Res 2002;20:869–874.

Bhatia D, De Beer J, Du Toit D. Coracoid process anatomy: Implications in radiographic imaging and surgery. Clin Anat 2007;20:774–784.

Bigliani L, Ticker J, Flatow E. The relationship of acromial architecture to rotator cuff disease. Clin Sports Med 1991;10:823–838.

Blonna D, Cecchetti S, Tellini A, et al. Contribution of the supraspinatus to the external rotator lag sign: kinematic and electromyographic pattern in an in vivo model. J Shoulder Elbow Surg 2010;19:392–398.

Boehm T, Matzer M, Brazda D, Gholke F. Os acromiale associated with tear of the rotator cuff treated operatively. J Bone Joint Surg Br 2003;85:545–549.

Boehm T, Rolf O, Martetschlaeger F, Kenn W, Gohl F.Rotator cuff tears associated with os acromiale. Acta Orthop 2005;76:241–244.

Boileau P, Baqué F, Valerio L, Ahrens P, Chuinard C, et al. Isolated arthroscopic biceps tenotomy or tenodesis improves symptoms in patients with massive irreparable rotator cuff tears. J Bone Joint Surg Am 2007;89:747–57.

Burkhart SS. Arthroscopic treatment of massive rotator cuff tears. Clin Orthop Relat Res 2001;390:107–118.

Castagna A, Garofalo R, Cesari E, et al. Anterior and posterior internal impingement: an evidence-based review. Br J Sports Med 2010;44:382–388

Chang E, Moses D, Babb J, Schweitzer M. Shoulder impingement: Objective 3D shape analysis of acromial morphologic features. Radiology 2006;239:497–505.

Curtis A, Burbank K, Tierney J, Scheller A, Curran A. The insertional footprint of the rotator cuff: An anatomic study. Arthroscopy 2006;22:603–609.

De Franco MJ, Cole BJ. Current perspectives on rotator cuff anatomy. Arthroscopy 2009;25:305–320.

Duranthon L, Gagey O. Anatomy and function of the subdeltoid bursa. Surg Radiol Anat 2001;23:23–25.

Ellman H. Diagnosis and treatment of incomplete rotator cuff tears. Clin Orthop Relat Res 1990:64–74.

Escamilla RF, Yamashiro K, Paulos L, Andrews JR. Shoulder muscle activity and function in common shoulder rehabilitation exercises. Sports Med 2009;39:663–685.

Fealy S, April E, Khazzam M, Armengol-Barallat J, Bigliani L. The coracoacromial ligament: Morphology and study of acromial enthesopathy. J Shoulder Elbow Surg 2005;14:542–548.
Ferreira Neto A, Almeida A, Maiorino R, Zoppi Filho A, Benegas E. An anatomical study of the subcoracoid space. Clinics 2006;61:467–472.
Flatow E, Coleman W, Kelkar R. The effect of anterior acromioplasty on rotator cuff contact: An experimental computer simulation. J Shoulder Elbow Surg 1995;4:S53–S54.
Fremerey R, Bastian L, Siebert W. The coracoacromial ligament: Anatomical and biomechanical properties with respect to age and rotator cuff disease. Knee Surg Sports Traumatol Arthrosc 2000;8:309–313.
Funk L, Levy O, Even T, Copeland S. Subacromial plica as a cause of impingement in the shoulder. J Shoulder Elbow Surg 2006;15:697–700.
Gates JJ, Gilliland J, McGarry MH, et al. Influence of distinct anatomic subregions of the supraspinatus on humeral rotation. J Orthop Res 2010;28:12–17.
Gill T, McIrvin E, Kocher M, et al. The relative importance of acromial morphology and age with respect to rotator cuff pathology. J Shoulder Elbow Surg 2002;11:327–330.
Hunt SA, Kwon YW, Zuckerman JD. The rotator interval: anatomy, pathology, and strategies for treatment. J Am Acad Orthop Surg 2007;15:218–227.
Ihashi K, Matsushita N, Yagi R. Rotational action of the supraspinatus muscle on the shoulder joint. J Electromyogr Kinesiol 1998;8:337–346.
Kesmezacar H, Akgun I, Ogut T, Gokay S, Uzun I. The coracoacromial ligament: The morphology and relation to rotator cuff pathology. J Shoulder Elbow Surg 2008;17:182–188.
Kim HM, Dahiya N, Teefey SA, et al. Location and initiation of degenerative rotator cuff tears: an analysis of three hundred and sixty shoulders. J Bone Joint Surg Am 2010;92:1088–1096.
Kragh J Jr, Doukas W, Basamania C. Primary coracoid impingement syndrome. Am J Orthop 2004;5:229–232.
Langenderfer JE, Patthanacharoenphon C, Carpenter JE. Variation in external rotation moment arms among subregions of supraspinatus, infraspinatus, and teres minor muscles. J Orthop Res 2006;24:1737–1744.
Liu J, Hughes RE, Smutz WP, Niebur G, Nan-An K. Roles of deltoid and rotator cuff muscles in shoulder elevation. Clin Biomech 1997;12:32–38
Machida A, Sugamoto K, Miyamoto T, et al. Adhesion of the subacromial bursa may cause subacromial impingement in patients with rotator cuff tears: Pressure measurements in 18 patients. Acta Orthop Scand 2004;75:109–113.
Mochizuki T, Sugaya H, Uomizu M. Humeral insertion of the supraspinatus and infraspinatus. New anatomical findings regarding the footprint of the rotator cuff. J Bone Joint Surg Am 2008;90:962–969.
Natsis K, Tsikaras P, Totlis T. Correlation between the four types of acromion and the existence of enthesophytes: A study on 423 dried scapulas and review of the literature. Clin Anat 2007;20:267–272.
Neer CS II. Anterior acromioplasty for the chronic impingement syndrome in the shoulder. J Bone Joint Surg Am 1972;54:41–50.
Nyffeler R, Werner C, Sukthankar A, Schmid M, Gerber C. Association of large lateral extension of the acromion with rotator cuff tears. J Bone Joint Surg Am 2006;88:800–805.
Otis JC, Jiang CC, Wickiewicz TL, et al. Changes in the moment arms of the rotator cuff and deltoid muscles with abduction and rotation. J Bone Joint Surg Am 1994;76:667–676.
Park MC, June BJ, Park CJ. The biomechanical effects of dynamic external rotation on rotator cuff repair compared to testing with the humerus fixed. Am J Sports Med 2007;35:1931–1939.
Park J, Phelps C. Os acromiale associated with rotator cuff impingement: MR imaging of the shoulder. Radiology 1994;193:255–257.
Parsons IM, Apreleva M, Fu FH, Woo SL. The effect of rotator cuff tears on reaction forces at the glenohumeral joint. J Orthop Res 2002;20:439–446.
Perry SM, Getz CL, Soslowsky LJ. After rotator cuff tears, the remaining (intact) tendons are mechanically altered. J Shoulder Elbow Surg 2009;18:52–57.
Pieper H, Radas C, Krahl H, Blank M. Anatomic variation of the coracoacromial ligament: A macroscopic and microscopic cadaveric study. J Shoulder Elbow Surg 1997;6:291–296.
Poppen NK, Walker PS. Forces at the glenohumeral joint in abduction. Clin Orthop Relat Res 1978;135:165–170.
Radas C, Pieper H. The coracoid impingement of the subscapularis tendon: A cadaveric study. J Shoulder Elbow Surg 2004;13:154–159.
Richards D, Burkhart S, Campbell S. Relation between narrowed coracohumeral distance and subscapularis tears. Arthroscopy 2005;21:1223–1228.
Roh MS, Wang VM, April EW. Anterior and posterior musculotendinous anatomy of the supraspinatus. J Shoulder Elbow Surg 2000;9:436–440.
Sano H, Uhthoff H, Backman D. Structural disorders at the insertion of the supraspinatus tendon and relation to tensile strength. J Bone Joint Surg Br 1998;80:720–725.
Schulz C, Anetzberger H, Glaser C. Coracoid tip position on frontal radiographs of the shoulder: A predictor of common shoulder pathologies. Br J Radiol 2005;78:1005–1008.
Su WR, Budoff JE, Luo ZP. The effect of anterosuperior rotator cuff tears on glenohumeral translation. Arthroscopy 2009;25:282–289.
Su WR, Budoff JE, Luo ZP. The effect of posterosuperior rotator cuff tears and biceps loading on glenohumeral translation. Arthroscopy 2010;26:578–586.
Suenaya N, Minami A, Kaneda K. Postoperative subcoracoid impingement syndrome in patients with rotator cuff repair. J Shoulder Elbow Surg 2000;9:275–278.
Szabó I, Boileau P, Walch G. The proximal biceps as a pain generator and results of tenotomy. Sports Med Arthrosc 2008;16:180–186.
Torrens C, Lopez J, Puente I, Caceres E. The influence of the acromial coverage index in rotator cuff tears. J Shoulder Elbow Surg 2007;347–351.
Tucker T, Snyder S. The keeled acromion: An aggressive acromial variant – A series of 20 patients with associated rotator cuff tears. Arthroscopy 2004;20:744–753.
Vahlensieck M, an Haack K, Schmidt HM. Two portions of the supraspinatus muscle: a new finding about the muscles macroscopy by dissection and magnetic resonance imaging. Surg Radiol Anat 1994;16:101–104.
Vanarthos W, Monu J. Type 4 acromion: A new classification. Contemp Orthop 1995;30:227–229
Volk AG, Vangsness CT Jr. An anatomic study of the supraspinatus muscle and tendon. Clin Orthop Relat Res 2001;384:280–285.
Voloshin I, Gelinas J, Maloney M, et al. Proinflammatory cytokines and metalloproteases are expressed in the subacromial bursa in the patients with rotator cuff disease. Arthroscopy 2005;21:1076.e1–1076.e9.
Walch G, Liotard JP, Boileau P, Noël E. Postero-superior glenoid impingement. Another shoulder impingement. Rev Chir Orthop Reparatrice Appar Mot 1991;77:571–4.
Walch G, Boileau P, Noel E, Donell ST. Internal impingement. J Shoulder Elbow Surg 1992;1:243.
Wang J, Horner G, Brown E, Shapiro M. The relationship between acromial morphology and conservative treatment of patients with impingement syndrome. Orthopedics 2000;23:557–559.
Warner JJ, Mc Mahon PJ. The role of the long head of the biceps brachii in superior stability of the glenohumeral joint. J Bone Joint Surg Am 1995;77:366–72.
Weening A, Willems J. Latissimus dorsi transfer for treatment of irreparable rotator cuff tears. Int Orthop 2010;34:1239–1244.
Yamaguchi K, Ditsios K, Middleton WD, et al. The demographic and morphological features of rotator cuff disease. A comparison of asymptomatic and symptomatic shoulders. J Bone Joint Surg Am 2006;88:1699–1704.

Chapter 6 Examination of the shoulder for rotator cuff disease

Edward G. McFarland, Juan Garzon-Muvdi, Jesse Affonso,
Steve A. Petersen

KEY FEATURES

- Unlike in the examination of other joints, the distribution of pain in the shoulder area often does not narrow the diagnosis.
- There are a number of physical findings designed to investigate the status of the rotator cuff muscles, the tendon of the long head of biceps, labrum, and acromioclavicular joint.
- To improve diagnostic accuracy, multiple tests, rather than a single physical finding, should be used during the clinical examination.
- In the authors' opinion, the four most relevant tests to assess rotator cuff disease are elevation of the arm, weakness in abduction, weakness in external rotation, and the external rotation lag sign.

INTRODUCTION

The examination of patients with rotator cuff problems has undergone substantial advancement in the past few years, and there is an increasing appreciation of the importance of integrating the history, physical examination, and imaging findings for determination of the diagnosis. Knowledge about the clinical relevance and limitations of the physical examination of the shoulder is critical for identifying what the examination does and does not reveal.

Examination of the shoulder presents unique challenges: it differs from the examination of other joints in several ways. First, unlike the examination of the knee or ankle, the distribution of pain in the shoulder area often does not narrow the diagnosis. Second, the shoulder is a joint with several moving parts. Shoulder movement includes both glenohumeral and scapulothoracic motion. Both components of total motion must be considered for an accurate examination. Third, the shoulder is covered by large muscles that make palpating specific structures difficult. Fourth, imaging studies can be challenging to interpret. As an example, magnetic resonance imaging (MRI) studies often identify abnormalities that are unrelated to the patient's symptoms.

This chapter reviews the principles of physical examination of the shoulder and explains how the physical findings correlate with specific pathological conditions.

HISTORY AND PRESENTATION

Rotator cuff tendons can be injured by an acute, traumatic event or by a gradual process of unknown cause. The degree of trauma required to produce a rotator cuff injury is quite variable. Common mechanisms of injury include falling on the shoulder or on an outstretched arm, lifting heavy luggage into the overhead bin of an airplane, pulling a lawn mower cord, or simply reaching out and away from the body. The patient will often feel a tear, rip, or pop. Although rotator cuff tears typically do not cause ecchymosis, patients with a bleeding diathesis may have bruising, particularly on the anterior or lateral aspects of the shoulder.

Chronic injuries are typically more insidious in onset. In most cases, the individual cannot recall a specific injury. Rather, there is a gradual increase in shoulder pain and loss of function, a process that we describe to patients as "wearing a hole in the seat of your trousers." This injury pattern increases linearly with age (Uhthoff and Sarkar 1993; Lehman et al. 1995; Yamamoto et al. 2009), and studies have shown that more than half of asymptomatic individuals may have some form of rotator cuff abnormality (Miniaci et al. 1995; Sher et al. 1995).

Various theories have been proposed to explain why the rotator cuff tissue fails. Impingement of the rotator cuff against an acromial spur, attrition secondary to cell senescence, vascular compromise, genetic predisposition, tension overload of the tendons, and differential stress within the layers of the tendons have all been implicated. What is clear is that, as the tendon becomes thinner and weaker, less force is required to tear it. This explains the common clinical presentation of a patient who was completely asymptomatic with an attritional tear, but then experiences a trivial trauma, and develops a much larger and ultimately symptomatic tear.

As the causes can be varied, it is important to obtain an accurate history of not only the specific inciting event, but also any history of previous shoulder problems. Similarly, it is important to determine whether the patient's main complaint is pain, weakness, loss of motion, loss of function, or a combination thereof.

Unfortunately, no one pain pattern is diagnostic of rotator cuff disease. Typically, patients with rotator cuff pathology complain of lateral shoulder pain, but pain in this location is not specific for rotator cuff injury. Other causes of lateral shoulder pain include cervical radiculopathy, visceral pain (**Fig. 6.1**), angina, and, less commonly, acromioclavicular joint pathology (**Fig. 6.2**) (Gerber et al. 1998).

Patients with rotator cuff abnormalities often have pain and/or weakness when using the arm above shoulder level or when lifting objects with the arm extended away from the body. Circular motions with pressure down on the hand, such as wiping a countertop or painting, can cause pain, which typically radiates into the deltoid region.

PHYSICAL EXAMINATION

Basics

The physical examination of the patient with rotator cuff pathology should be part of a more comprehensive upper extremity examination. The examination starts with observation. The patient should change into a gown or other such attire that permits observation of

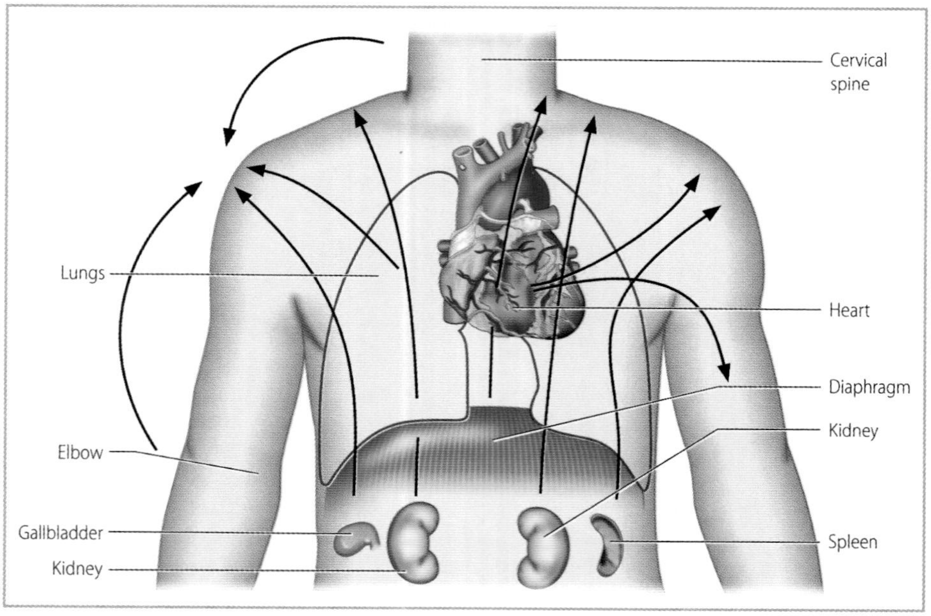

Figure 6.1 Visceral pain can be referred to the shoulder region in a variety of non-specific patterns. (Redrawn, with permission, from Goodman CC, Snyder, TE. Differential Diagnosis in Physical Therapy. Philadelphia: Saunders, 2000: 485).

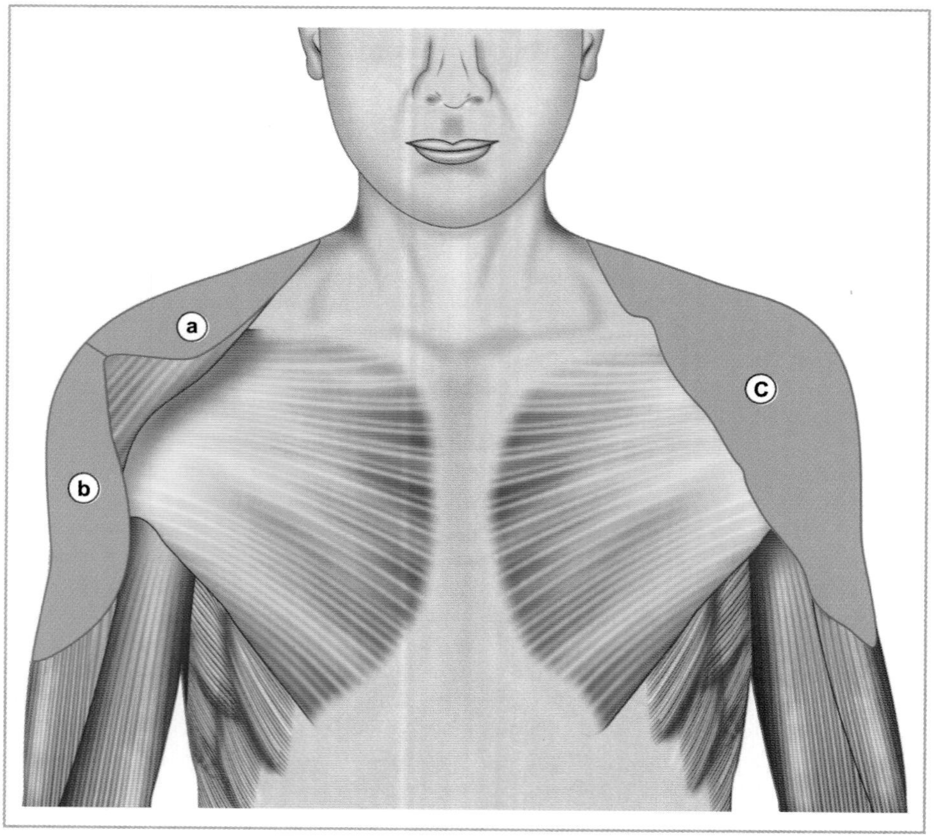

Figure 6.2 AC joint pain is typically located on top of the shoulder (a). Rotator cuff pain is typically located on the outside of the shoulder (b). Pain from a combination of AC joint pathology and rotator cuff disorders can present in both areas (c). (Redrawn, with permission, from McFarland EG. Examination of the Shoulder: The complete guide. New York: Thieme, 2006:3).

the anterior and posterior aspects of the upper extremity. The appropriately attired patient should be examined for atrophy, deformity, or scapular winging (**Fig. 6.3**). These abnormities are more readily detected when one shoulder is compared with the other. Atrophy of the supraspinatus and/or infraspinatus fossa is often indicative of a large, long-standing rotator cuff tear (**Fig. 6.4**). Color changes or excessive swelling suggests vascular conditions such as deep venous thrombosis or arterial comprise.

The next step is to perform a brief vascular and neurological examination. The arm should be inspected for edema, stasis, swelling, and color changes. Capillary refill and pulses should be evaluated. This is particularly important in patients who have complaints of coldness or cramping in their hands. The neurological assessment includes an assessment of light touch sensation and should be performed in all areas corresponding to the distribution of the peripheral nerves and cervical spinal levels (**Table 6.1**). The most reliable method of

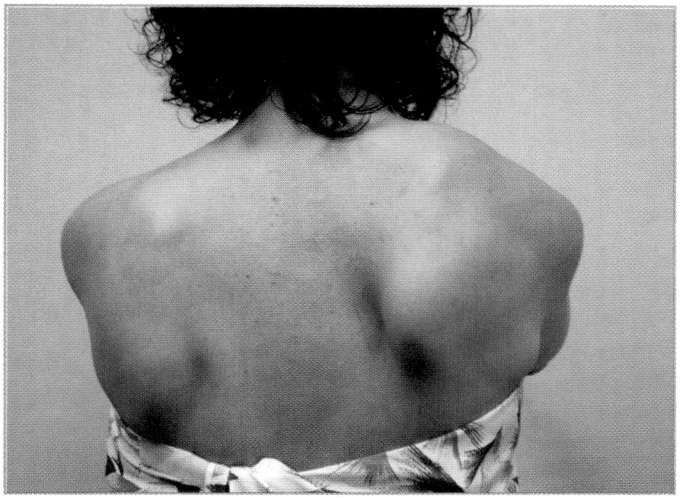

Figure 6.3 Scapular winging can be accentuated by having the patient flex his or her arms in front of the body.

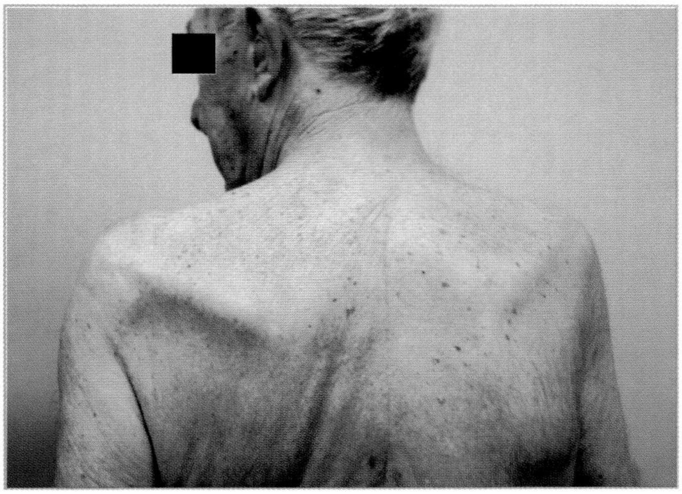

Figure 6.4 In this patient, there is infraspinatus atrophy below and supraspinatus wasting above the scapular spine. (Reprinted, with permission, from McFarland EG. Examination of the Shoulder: The Complete Guide. New York: Thieme, 2006:8).

performing this part of the examination is to touch the same area on each upper extremity simultaneously and ask the patient whether the sensation is the same on each side. A difference indicates that the patient has some nerve involvement, and additional investigation of those symptoms is warranted.

Table 6.1 Basic nerve testing of the upper extremity

Nerve	Root level	Where to test
Axillary	C5–6	The skin covering the inferior region of the deltoid muscle: the "regimental badge" area
Radial	C5, C6, C7, C8, T1	Much of the back of the hand, including the web of skin between the thumb and index finger
Median	C6, C7, C8, T1	Skin of the palm side of the thumb, index, middle finger, and half of the ring finger
Ulnar	C8–T1	Fifth digit and the medial half of the fourth digit

Similarly, it is relatively easy to assess upper extremity strength and motor function. Deltoid, biceps, triceps, wrist flexors, wrist extensors, and interosseus muscle strength should be assessed, graded on a scale of 1–5, and compared with the contralateral side (**Table 6.2**). If the patient is weak, neurological causes should be included in the differential diagnosis.

A thorough upper extremity evaluation should always include an assessment of the joints above and below the area where the patient experiences pain. Shoulder abnormalities frequently coexist with cervical and other upper extremity pathology. Referred pain from neck pathology can be radicular and/or non-radicular in nature. Compressive neuropathies distal to the shoulder can present as a "double-crush" phenomenon and produce pain more proximally.

Range of motion evaluation

An assessment of both active and passive range of motion is an important part of the examination. Subtle changes in range of motion can be helpful in making a diagnosis. Patients with a painful arc of active motion between 90° and 110° of forward elevation often have rotator cuff pathology. Shoulder stiffness (manifested as a loss of passive range of motion) can be indicative of adhesive capsulitis. The patient may present to the clinic with a chief complaint of pain. On further evaluation, however, the loss of motion becomes apparent. For this reason, patients with adhesive capsulitis are not uncommonly diagnosed with rotator cuff tendinopathy. Indeed, in our experience, this is the most common misdiagnosis.

Elevation

Active elevation is always assessed in two positions: in the plane of the body (abduction) (**Fig. 6.5**) and in front of the body (flexion) (**Fig. 6.6**). The clinician should observe the raising motion for bilateral symmetry, to determine whether there is a glitch in the motion on one side compared with that on the other. Particular attention should be directed to

Table 6.2 Basic muscle testing of the upper extremity

Muscle	Nerve	Root level	Test
Deltoid	Axillary	C5–6	Abduction testing (Jobe's)
Biceps	Musculocutaneous	C5–6	Resisted elbow flexion
Triceps	Radial	C7	Resisted elbow extension
Infraspinatus	Suprascapular	C5–6	Strength testing external rotation
Supraspinatus	Suprascapular	C5–6	Jobe's test
Finger abductors/adductors	Ulnar	C7–8	Resisted finger abduction.
Opponens pollicis	Median	C6–7	Test thumb tip to little finger

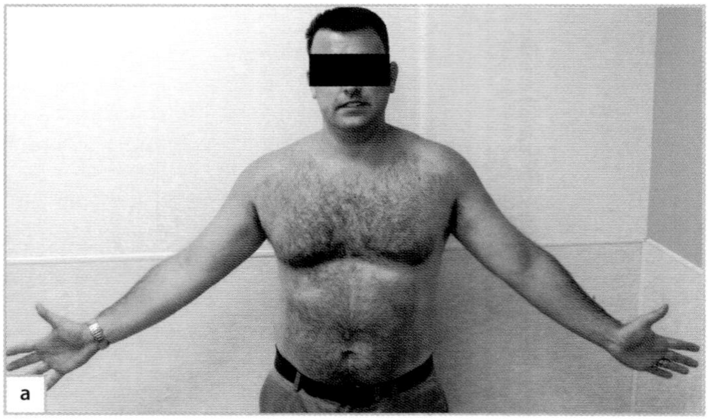

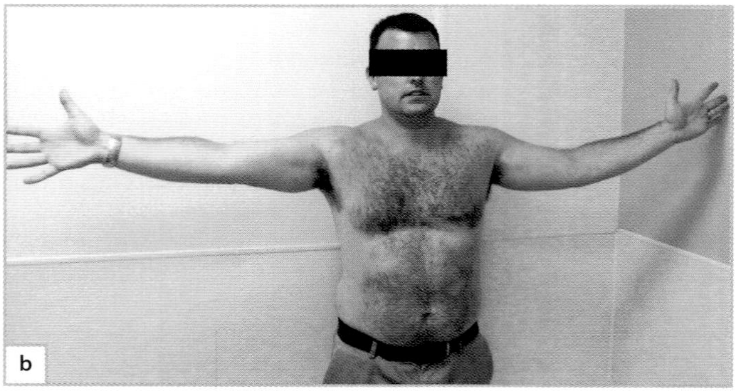

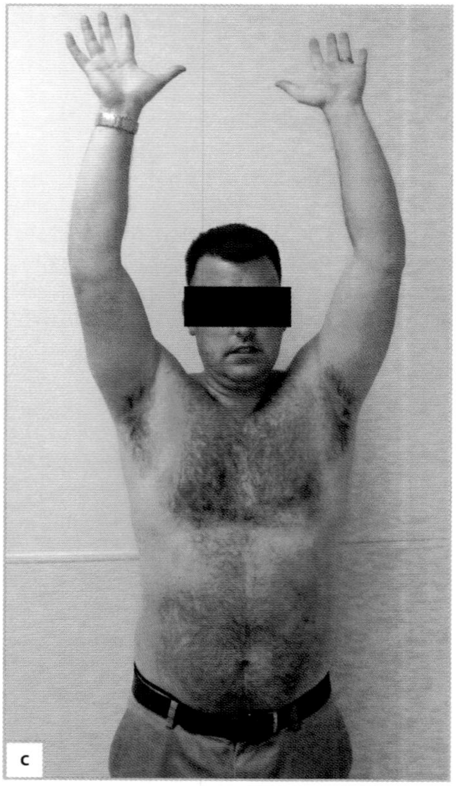

Figure 6.5 Full elevation in the scapular plane is best accomplished with the thumb in an up position so that the humerus is externally rotated as the arm elevates in a continuum of motion from the starting point (a) through the midpoint (b) to the highest point (c) the patient can reach.

shoulder blade motion (Kibler and McMullen 2003). Shoulder blade asymmetry during active forward elevation, best appreciated when viewed from the back, is termed "scapular dyskinesis," and is indicative of muscle weakness. When detected, scapular dyskinesis should prompt a careful evaluation of muscle strength and nerve function.

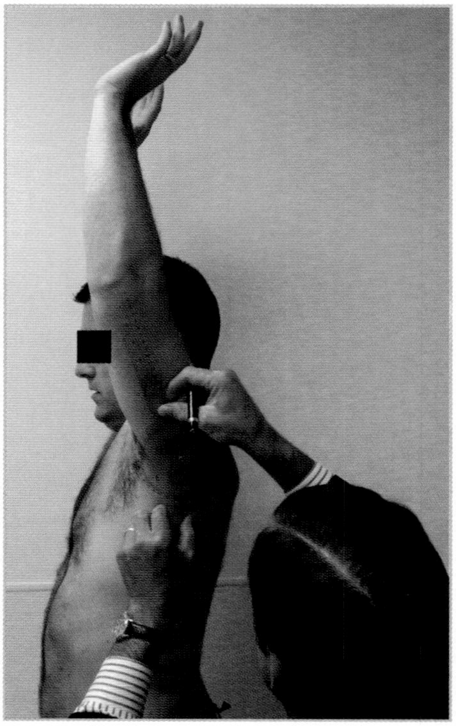

Figure 6.6 Flexion of the arm is measured from the side with the goniometer centered over the glenohumeral joint.

If the patient lacks active elevation, the clinician should attempt to gently elevate the extremity a bit further. If additional elevation is obtained with this passive motion, the previous inability to fully elevate the arm usually indicates a stiff or weak shoulder as opposed to a globally stiff or globally "adherent" shoulder. If passive motion is unsuccessful in elevating the arm beyond the point of active elevation (i.e., there is a firm endpoint beyond which additional motion is not possible), then stiffness is the primary problem.

Painful arc

Some patients experience pain only in certain segments of elevation, most commonly between 70° and 120° (the painful arc) (**Fig. 6.7**) (Kessel and Watson 1977). This pattern is characteristic of rotator cuff conditions, but, alone as an isolated finding, is not diagnostic. Additional demographic and/or examination findings are needed to establish the diagnosis of a rotator cuff disorder (see "Combined tests" below).

Drop-arm sign

This examination maneuver can be accomplished in one of two ways. The patient raises (with or without assistance) the arm above shoulder level to approximately 70° or 80° and is then asked to either hold it against gravity (without assistance) or gradually bring the arm down to the side. It is important that the examiner is careful not to let the arm fall or descend too quickly in an uncontrolled manner because it can be very painful for the patient. If the patient has trouble maintaining elevation, or if the arm falls to the side, the finding is known as a positive drop-arm sign (Codman 1934). This sign may indicate a profound problem secondary to paralysis (neurogenic cause), or massive rotator cuff damage (i.e., large supraspinatus tear or tears of multiple tendons), or both. That said, the inability to maintain elevation may result from pain alone, which must be considered in the differential diagnosis.

Shrug sign

Another non-specific sign of shoulder dysfunction is the shrug sign (McFarland 2006b) (**Fig. 6.8**). This test is performed by asking the

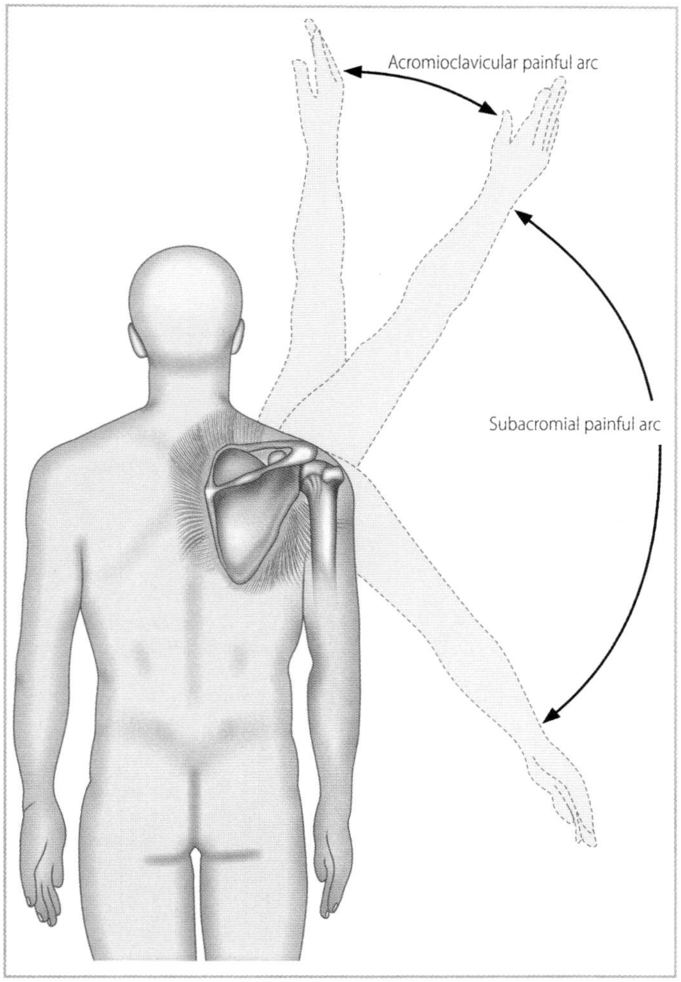

Figure 6.7 The painful arc suggests that pain in different portions of the arc may have different causes. (Reprinted, with permission, from Kessel L, Watson M. The painful arc syndrome: clinical classification as a guide to management. J Bone Joint Surg Br 1977;59:166).

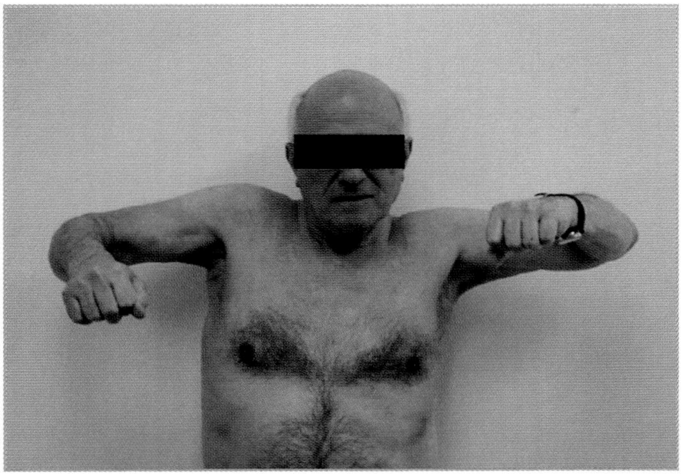

Figure 6.8 The shrug sign is a non-specific sign of shoulder dysfunction that is performed by asking the patient to elevate both arms to 90°. (Reprinted, with permission, from McFarland EG. Examination of the Shoulder: The Complete Guide. New York: Thieme, 2006: 80).

patient to hold the arms parallel to the floor. If this task cannot be done, or if there is asymmetry of the shoulders when performing the test, the patient's shoulder is stiff, weak, or both. This test was originally proposed as an indicator of rotator cuff dysfunction, but, because it can be positive for a wide variety of shoulder conditions, it simply indicates the presence of some abnormality.

Rotation

To test for rotation, the patient is asked to hold the arms at 90° of elevation. The examiner then moves the arm into external (**Fig. 6.9a**) and internal (**Fig. 6.9b**) rotation. Both shoulders are examined, and any

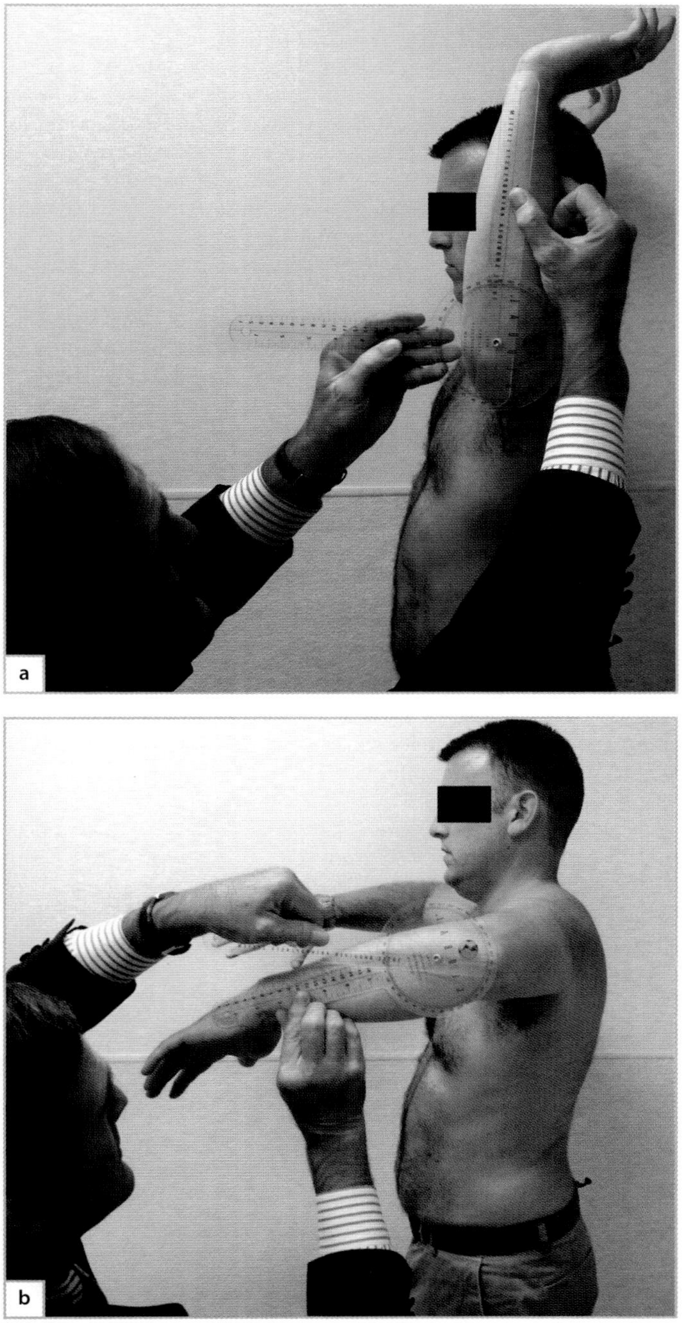

Figure 6.9 External (a) and internal (b) rotation with the arm at 90° of abduction.

differences in rotation are noted. If the patient's shoulder is stiff for any reason, there will be a firm endpoint as the ligaments of the shoulder reach their maximum length. Any movement beyond this point will cause pain or the patient will have to move the scapula or the whole body to accommodate the associated stress. In some athletes, particularly those who have been playing or used to play overhead sports (such as tennis) , there will more external rotation and less internal rotation in the dominant than the non-dominant shoulder (Bigliani et al. 1997; Crockett et al. 2002). This is a normal finding in athletes who play overhead sports, unless it is accompanied by pain. If pain accompanies the loss of motion, the condition is referred to as a glenohumeral internal rotation deficit (Burkhart et al. 2003). Although this phenomenon may be associated with pain in tennis players or swimmers, it is typically not a cause of shoulder pain in patients with rotator cuff disorders.

In another test for external rotation of the shoulder the patient holds the arms at the side with the elbows flexed 90° so that the elbows touch the sides of the body (**Fig. 6.10**). The examiner then compares both sides as the patient rotates the arms externally. Loss of external rotation in this position (i.e., not with the arm elevated as above) is a general sign of a shoulder abnormality. Any asymmetry indicates shoulder stiffness but does not identify the cause of the stiffness.

To further test internal rotation, the patient is asked to place the hand up the back with the thumb up (**Fig. 6.11**). Each arm is done sequentially, and the motions are compared. If one side is different from the other, this asymmetry indicates that the patient's shoulder is stiff or weak, or both, but the cause is not identified by this test.

Strength testing

Probably the most helpful portion of the examination of the shoulder with which to formulate the diagnosis of rotator cuff disease is strength testing. These examinations are quite simple and easy to perform. To perform them correctly, and to prevent the patient from compensating with muscles other than the one being tested, the practitioner needs to understand the functional anatomy of the upper extremity.

In abduction

General comments

One of the myths of rotator cuff disease is that people need the rotator cuff muscles to have full elevation of the shoulder (**Fig. 6.12**).

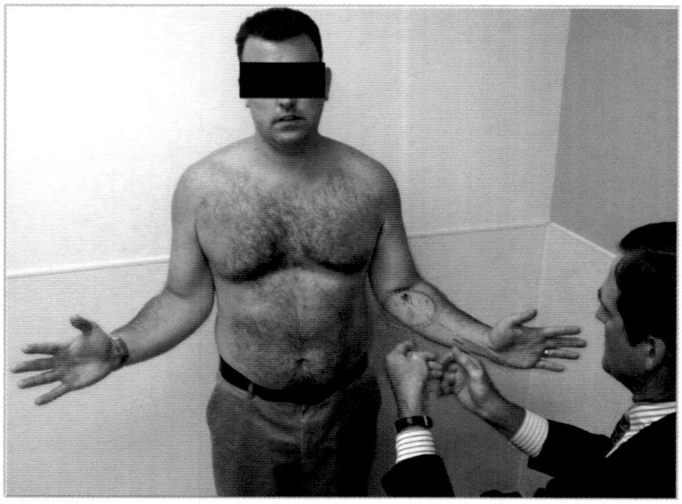

Figure 6.10 External rotation of the arm at the side is performed by having the patient bend the elbows 90°, keeping them close to the body.

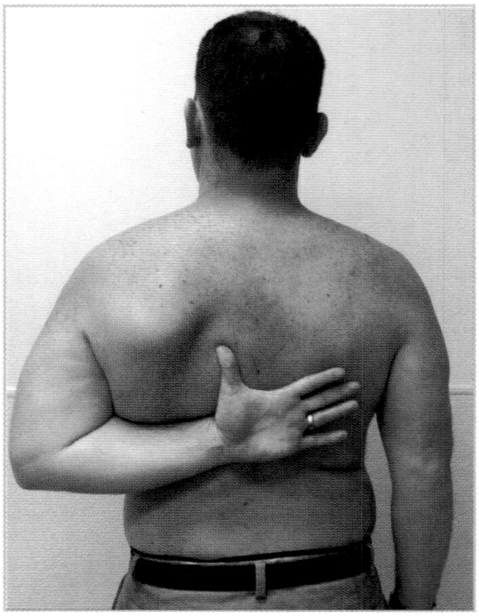

Figure 6.11 For internal rotation of the arm, the patient is asked to place the hand up the back with the thumb up.

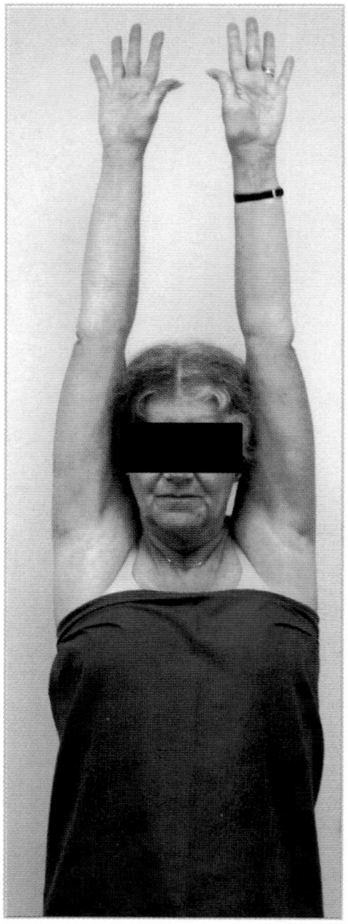

Figure 6.12 Patient with rotator cuff tear and full range of motion.

In reality, the muscles most responsible for arm elevation are deltoid (axillary nerve; C5 nerve root) and supraspinatus (suprascapular nerve; C5–6 nerve roots), and the arm can be fully elevated even if only one of those two muscles is functional. However, if both are injured, the patient will have little or no shoulder abduction (**Fig. 6.13**). In addition, although patients can present excellent range

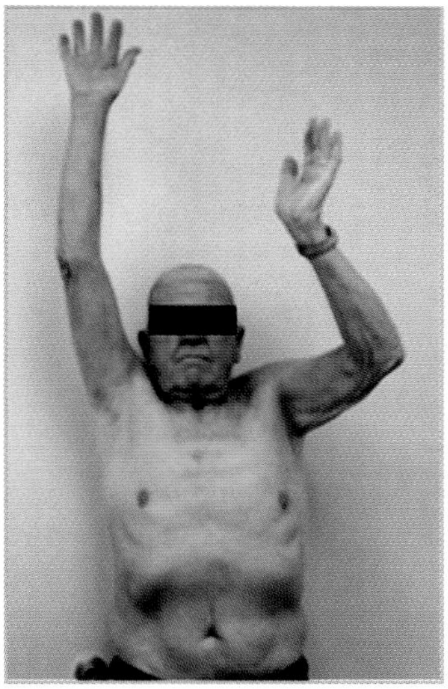

Figure 6.13 Patient with decreased abduction.

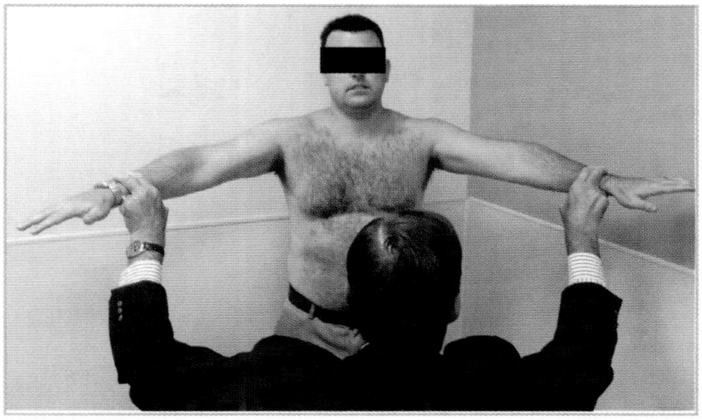

Figure 6.14 The strength of supraspinatus can be tested with the arm abducted in the plane of the scapula with the thumb in a neutral position to the floor.

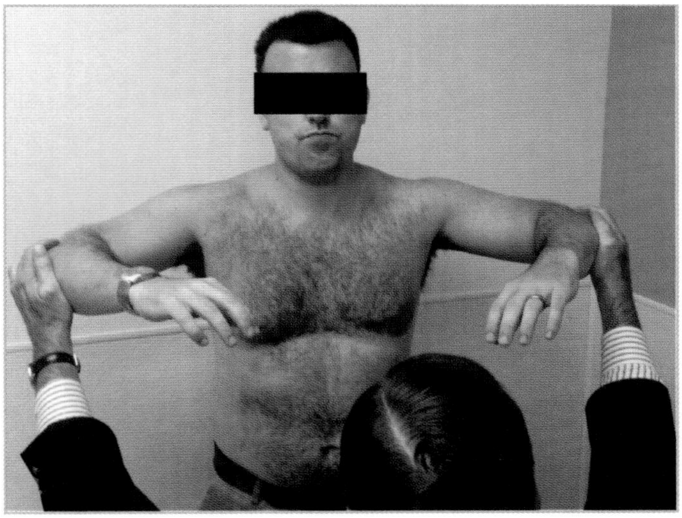

Figure 6.15 The strength of supraspinatus can be tested with the elbows flexed rather than extended to reduce the stress.

of motion and function in the presence of full-thickness tears of the rotator cuff, the shoulder is usually weak on manual muscle testing, with weakness when using the arm above shoulder level or when lifting objects away from the body.

Supraspinatus testing

Although there is no strength test that will completely isolate the supraspinatus muscle and tendon, any weakness with forward elevation suggests injury to this muscle.

For the first test in determining shoulder strength, the patient is asked to fully elevate the arm to ear level. If the patient has a normal deltoid muscle and yet cannot lift the arm against gravity (in other words the patient has a positive "drop-arm sign" as described above), then the weakness is most likely the result of some abnormality in the supraspinatus muscle or tendon.

The second test for supraspinatus is performed by asking the patient to elevate the arms to a position parallel to the ground (**Fig. 6.14**). The arms should be brought forward approximately 30° from the plane of the body (this position is called the "plane of the scapula" because the scapula sits at a 30° angle to the thorax) and, with the patient's elbows flexed, the examiner pushes down on the arms as the patient resists the pressure. Having the patient flex the elbows decreases stress on the shoulder and allows for a more accurate assessment (**Fig. 6.15**). This is especially important in the presence of pain or for patients with rotator cuff abnormality, for whom the extended elbow position can be very painful.

If the arm gives way with this test, the examiner can infer that the weakness is the result of pain alone or injury to supraspinatus itself.

If the patient's shoulder is not weak when this test is performed with the elbows flexed, then the test can be repeated with the elbows extended. This maneuver is commonly referred to as Jobe's test (Moseley et al. 1992). The test can be performed equally effectively with the thumbs down ("empty can" position) (**Fig. 6.16a**) (Jobe et al. 1996), the thumbs up ("full can" position) (**Fig. 6.16b**), or the thumbs in neutral (Kelly et al. 1996) (see **Fig. 6.14**). The examiner pushes down on the arm at the wrist and asks the patient to resist. The test is positive for weakness in abduction when the patient cannot hold the arm in this position against resistance.

Although weakness in abduction is frequently indicative of rotator cuff pathology, it is important to remember that this is not always the case. Other causes of weakness in abduction include nerve injury, biceps tendon injury, and pain from a labral tear (Park et al. 2005). In addition, many patients do not experience shoulder weakness with smaller rotator cuff tears. For this reason, strength testing is not sensitive for partial-thickness rotator cuff tears or for asymptomatic tendinopathy of the rotator cuff (McCabe et al. 2005).

In external rotation

Testing the strength of the shoulder when in external rotation is another important way to assess rotator cuff function. As with strength testing in abduction, shoulder weakness in external rotation is often, but not always, indicative of rotator cuff pathology (McFarland 2006c; McFarland et al. 2006).

Strength testing in external rotation is performed by asking the patient to bend the elbows to 90° while keeping them close to the body (**Fig. 6.17**). It is important that the patient does not lift the arms away from the body because doing so engages the compensatory abductors and other muscles. The examiner then asks the patient to resist an internal rotation force. The test is considered positive if the patient cannot maintain the arm in the starting position. Itoi et al. (2006) have reported that this test is more accurate

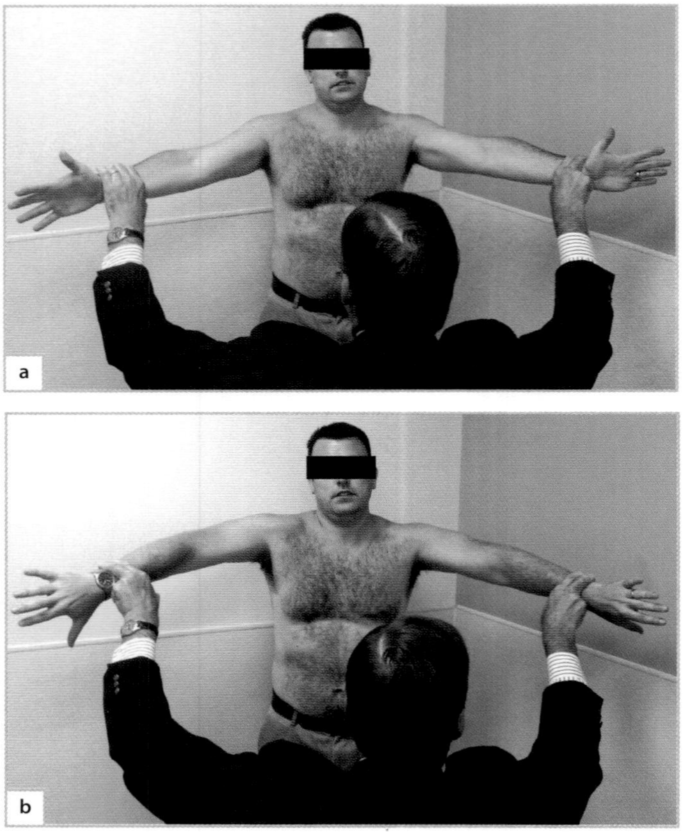

Figure 6.16 The strength of the supraspinatus can be tested with the arm abducted in the plane of the scapula with the thumb down, known as the "empty can" position (a), or the thumb up, known as the "full can" position (b).

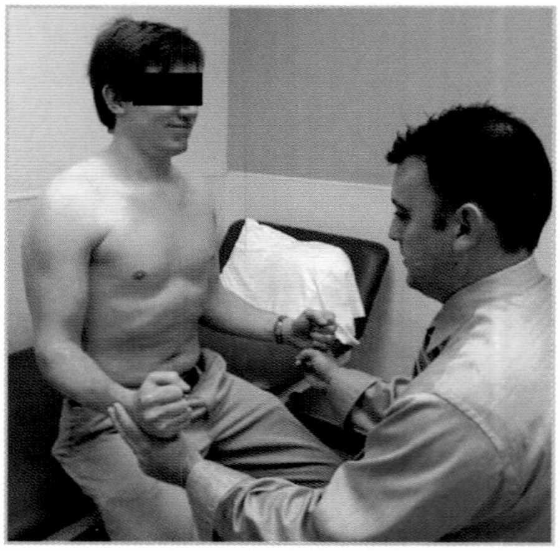

Figure 6.17 Strength testing in external rotation is performed by having the patient bend the elbows 90°, keeping them close to the body.

for determining rotator cuff tears when weakness rather than pain is used as a positive test.

Tests of the subscapularis tendon

Although full-thickness tears of the subscapularis tendon are not as common as tears of the supraspinatus and infraspinatus tendons, they produce fairly consistent findings on physical examination. Partial tears of the subscapularis tendon are relatively common and often do not result in significant physical impairments. In contrast, complete tears of subscapularis can produce profound weakness of internal rotation of the shoulder (Kim et al. 2003). Over the past few decades, clinicians have devised more accurate methods of detecting subscapularis pathology.

Lift-off test

Many believe that the best test for the subscapularis tendon is the lift-off test (Gerber and Krushell 1991). To perform this test, the patient places one hand behind the back in the low lumbar region. The patient is then instructed to lift the hand off the back. The procedure is repeated with the opposite hand. The test is considered positive if the patient cannot lift the hand away from the back. A positive test indicates that the subscapularis tendon is probably completely torn from its insertion site on the proximal humerus (**Fig. 6.18**).

Belly press sign

The belly press sign is another helpful test for subscapularis function (Gerber et al. 1996). When performing the test, the patient places the palm of one hand on the abdomen (**Fig. 6.19**) and then brings the elbow forward, away from the body. The patient is then asked to press the hand into the abdomen. The procedure is repeated with the opposite hand. The test is positive when the wrist flexes as the hand is pushed into the abdomen or when there is marked differences between the two extremities. A positive test usually indicates a full-thickness subscapularis tear.

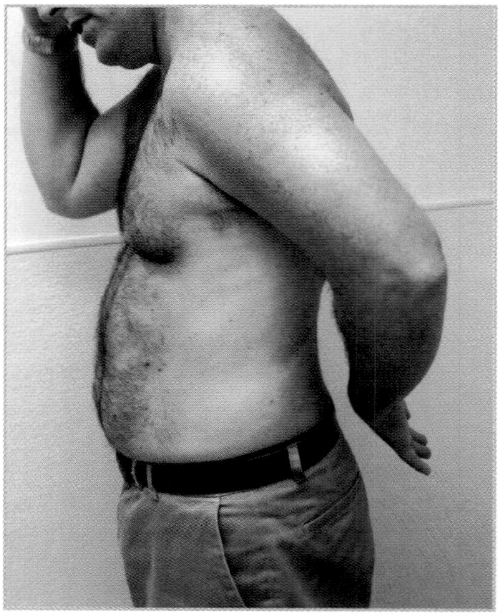

Figure 6.18 In the lift-off test for the subscapularis muscle and tendon integrity, the patient tries to lift the hand off the back.

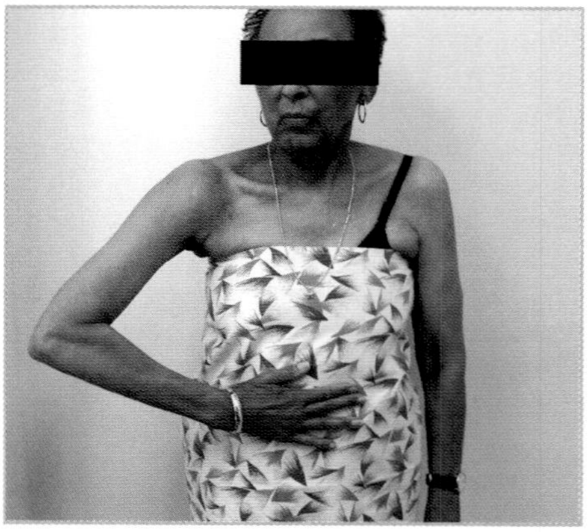

Figure 6.19 The belly press test for the subscapularis muscle and tendon is an alternative test in patients who cannot internally rotate. (Reprinted, with permission, from McFarland EG. Examination of the Shoulder: The Complete Guide. New York: Thieme, 2006: 118).

Superior subluxation of the humeral head

In a patient with extensive rotator cuff tears, shoulder motion can be impaired to the degree that the humeral head may actually subluxate from the glenoid when the patient attempts to elevate the extremity. In such instances, as the patient attempts to elevate the arm, the head of the humerus slides out of the glenoid and produces a prominence in the anterior and superior aspects of the shoulder (**Fig. 6.20**). The shoulders in such patients are often extremely weak in abduction and external rotation. Active motion is extremely limited, but passive range of motion is preserved. This situation is commonly seen in patients for whom surgery for a large rotator cuff tear failed.

Lag signs

Lag signs are shoulder examination tests that are predicated on the observation that the muscles must have a certain amount of strength to hold the arm in one position. When present, these signs typically reflect that either the muscle being tested is extremely weak or the tendon being tested has a very large tear that includes the whole tendon.

External rotation lag sign (supraspinatus tear)

The external rotation lag sign indicates a full-thickness, large supraspinatus rotator cuff tear (Hertel et al. 1996; Blonna et al. 2010). The test is performed by having the patient position the arm at 15–20° abduction and the elbow at 90° flexion (**Fig. 6.21**). The examiner holds the patient's elbow in this position and externally rotates the arm until an endpoint or resistance to external rotation is felt. The examiner then asks the patient to hold the arm in that position. A test is considered positive when the patient cannot hold the arm in this position, i.e., when the arm falls back into internal rotation. If

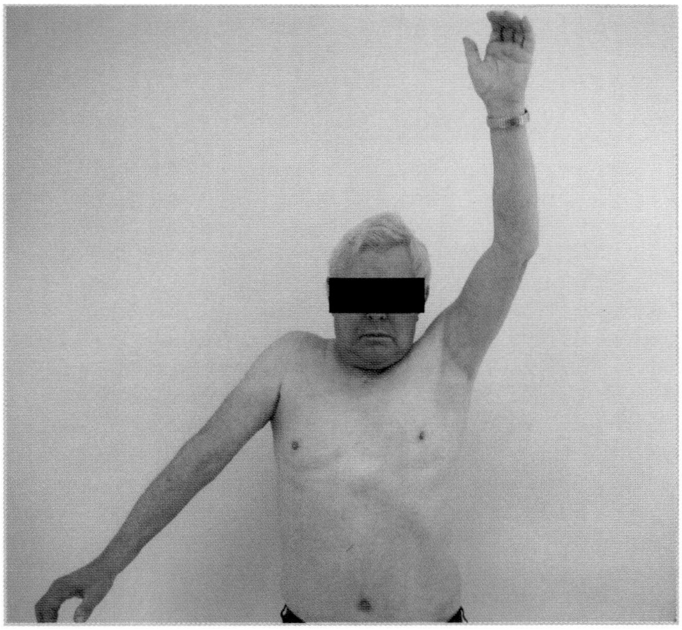

Figure 6.20 Superior and anterior subluxation of the humeral head. In this patient with a massive rotator cuff tear, the humeral head "escapes" in a superior and anterior direction with attempted forward elevation.

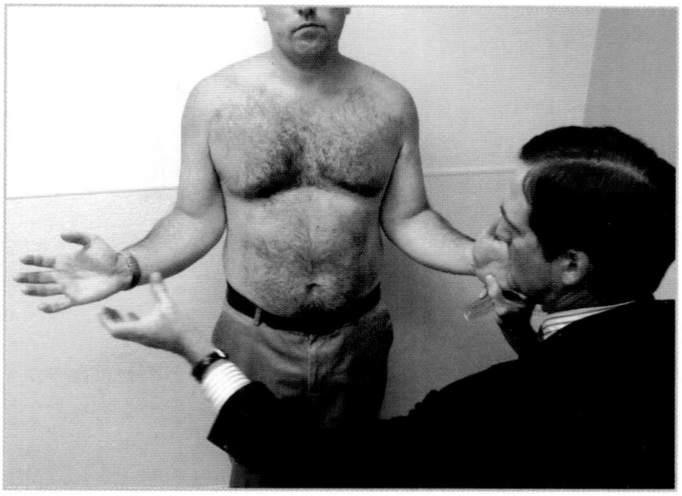

Figure 6.21 The external rotation lag sign is performed by externally rotating the arm at the side and asking the patient to hold that position. The test is positive if the arm falls back into internal rotation.

this happens, it is a sign that the muscles providing external rotation to the shoulder (supraspinatus and infraspinatus) are torn or not functioning properly.

Dropping lag sign (infraspinatus and teres minor tear)

The "dropping sign" (Walch et al. 1998) should be distinguished from the drop-arm sign (Codman 1934). The latter indicates that the patient cannot hold the arm against gravity (see earlier for description of the drop-arm sign). The dropping sign is performed by asking the patient to abduct the arm 90° with the elbow flexed 90°. The examiner supports the elbow in this position, and externally rotates the arm to 90° of external rotation. The examiner then asks the patient to hold the arm in that position. A positive test is noted when the patient cannot hold that position and the arm drops into internal rotation (**Fig. 6.22**). A positive test is indicative of an injury to infraspinatus and/or teres minor (Walch et al. 1998).

Lift-off lag sign (subscapularis tendon)

This test is performed in a manner similar to that of a lift-off test. For this test, a patient is asked to place each hand sequentially in the small of the back as if performing a lift-off test (**Fig. 6.23**). The examiner supports the elbow and pulls the hand off the back by the wrist, and then asks the patient to hold this position with the hand off of the back. If the hand falls to the back or toward the buttocks, the test is positive, indicating that there is a full-thickness tear of the subscapularis tendon (Gerber and Krushell 1991).

Provocative maneuvers

Neer's sign

Neer's sign, described by Charles Neer in 1972 (Neer 1972), is perhaps the most commonly recognized and performed test for rotator cuff pathology. This test is performed with the patient standing and the examiner to the patient's side (**Fig. 6.24**). The examiner stabilizes the scapula with one hand and, with the other, passively flexes the arm until the patient reports pain or full flexion is reached. The test is considered

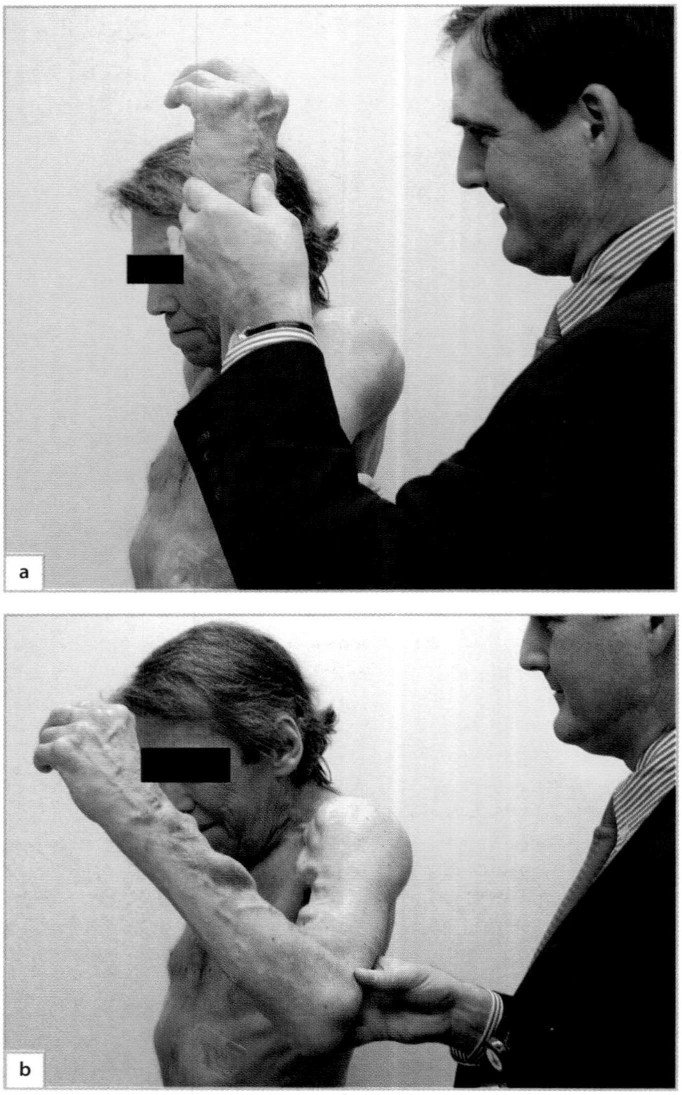

Figure 6.22 The drop sign: This test is performed by placing the arm in abduction and external rotation and asking the patient to hold the arm in that position (a). The test is positive if the arm falls back into internal rotation (b). (Reprinted, with permission, from McFarland EG. Examination of the Shoulder: The Complete Guide. New York: Thieme, 2006: 155).

positive if the patient reports pain into the anterior or lateral aspect of the shoulder.

Unfortunately, Neer's sign is not always indicative of a rotator cuff problem. A positive Neer's sign is often elicited in a wide variety of shoulder conditions, especially stiffness.

Neer himself recognized this point in his original description of the test: "It also causes pain in patients with many other shoulder conditions, including stiffness (partial frozen shoulder), instability (e.g., anterior subluxation), arthritis, calcium deposits, and bone lesions" (Neer 1983).

Studies of this and other physical tests for shoulder pathology have substantiated this observation (Park et al. 2005; McFarland 2006a; Hegedus et al. 2008). Neer's test has a specificity for rotator cuff disease of any type (painful tendinopathy to massive tears) of just 43.4–59.9% (Jia et al. 2009) and a sensitivity of 59.3–75.4% (Hegedus et al. 2008; Jia et al. 2009). Therefore, a positive Neer's sign does not necessarily indicate a rotator cuff tear unless it is considered in conjunction with other tests.

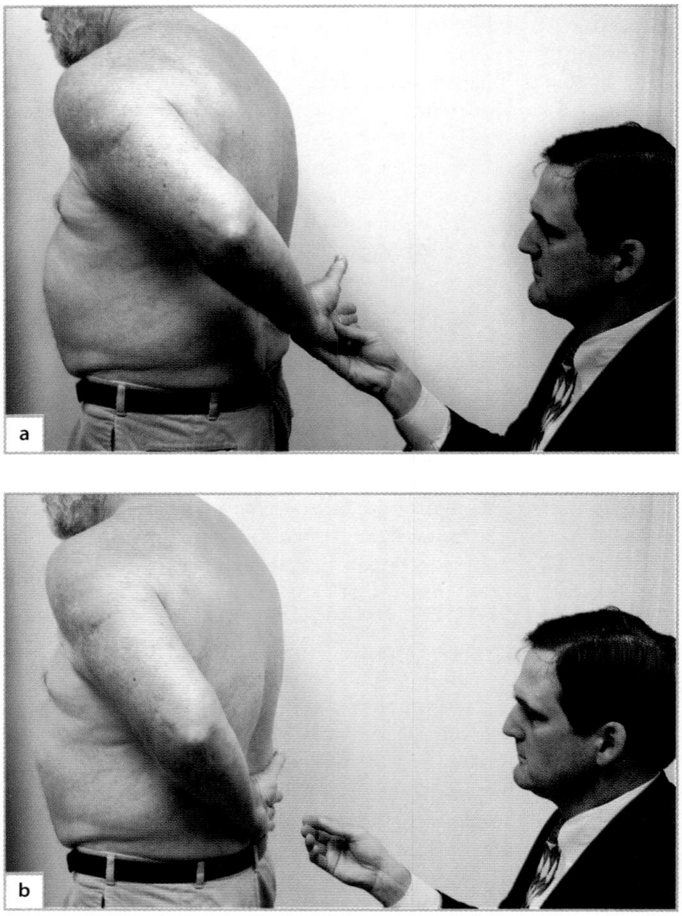

Figure 6.23 The subscapularis lag sign: This sign is elicited by placing the arm in a position similar to that of the lift-off test (a). The patient is asked to hold the arm away from the body. A positive test occurs when the hand falls to the patient's back (b). (Reprinted, with permission, from McFarland EG. Examination of the Shoulder: The Complete Guide. New York: Thieme, 2006: 156).

Kennedy–Hawkins sign

The Kennedy–Hawkins sign for rotator cuff abnormality was described by Richard Hawkins, who ascribed the sign to his colleague John Kennedy (Hawkins and Kennedy 1980). This test is performed with the patient standing and the examiner standing at the patient's side (**Fig. 6.25**). The examiner stabilizes the scapula and then elevates the patient's arm passively with the elbow flexed to 90°. For best results, the arm should be flexed and not abducted (Park et al. 2005). The arm is elevated until resistance is met and then the arm is carefully internally rotated. A test is considered positive if the maneuver elicits pain in the anterior or lateral shoulder region. Pain elicited in other locations, such as the posterior shoulder, is not considered a positive finding.

The limitations of this test are similar to those of Neer's sign. The Kennedy–Hawkins test can be positive for a wide variety of shoulder conditions. Its specificity has been found to be 44.5% for painful tendinopathy, 48.3% for full-thickness supraspinatus tears, and 35.6% for massive rotator cuff tears (Jia et al. 2009); its sensitivity for rotator cuff abnormality of any type is 71.2% (Jia et al. 2009). For this reason, a positive Kennedy–Hawkins test, in the absence of other positive confirmatory tests such as a positive Neer's test, should be interpreted with caution. Indeed, both these tests may be more useful when considered together with other tests (Park et al. 2005; Hegedus et al. 2008).

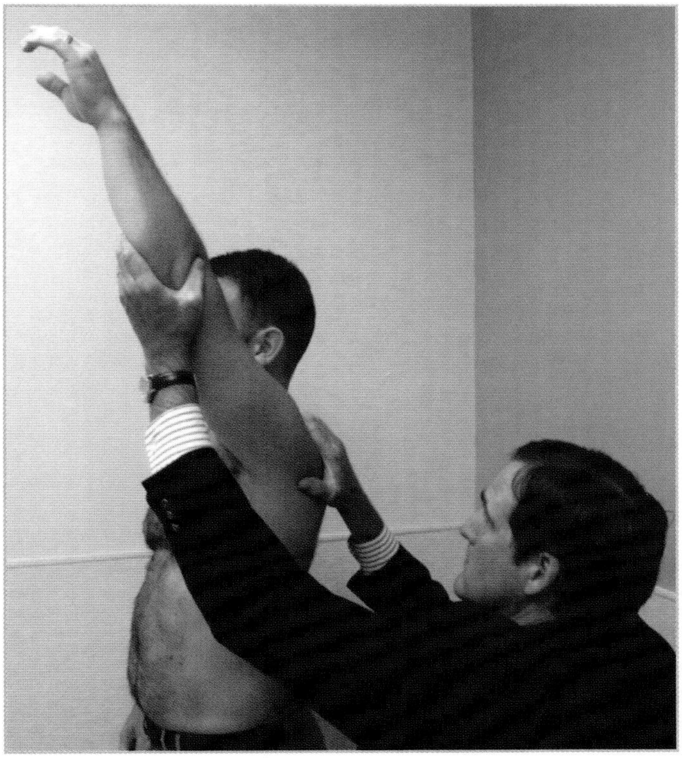

Figure 6.24 Neer's sign is passive forward flexion of the arm, which should produce anterior or lateral shoulder pain.

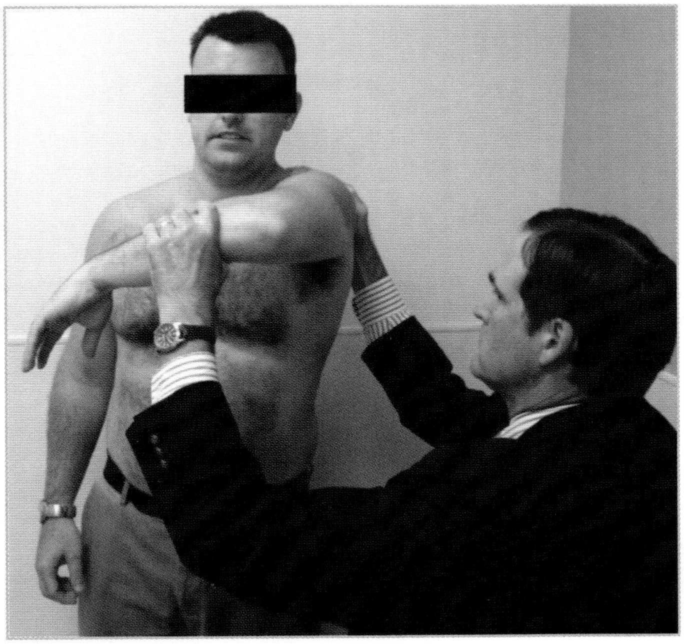

Figure 6.25 The Kennedy–Hawkins sign is performed with the arm in forward flexion and internal rotation.

Combined tests

Two studies have shown that using multiple tests is the best method for determining if a patient has a rotator cuff tear (Murrell and Walton 2001; Park et al. 2005). Murrell and Walton (2001) reported that, if a patient was >60 years old, had weakness in abduction, and had a positive impingement sign (Neer's or Kennedy–Hawkins), then there is a 98% chance that the patient has a torn rotator cuff. Park et al. (2005) similarly found that a patient >60 years old, with a positive painful arc sign, weakness in abduction, and weakness in external rotation has a 90% chance of having a full-thickness rotator cuff tear.

Biceps tendon examination

General comments

Many tests for the biceps function have been described. However, it is still difficult to reliably make the diagnosis of biceps tendon abnormality on physical examination alone because the biceps tendon does not produce a unique pain pattern, is difficult to palpate reliably, and rarely presents as an isolated abnormality, and patients with a biceps tendon abnormality usually have coexisting rotator cuff disease.

Although the biceps tendon is anatomically located in the proximal anterior shoulder, no pain pattern is distinctive for the tendon. In addition, biceps pathology is just one cause of anterior shoulder pain. Indeed, many conditions such as rotator cuff disease, stiffness of the shoulder, and glenohumeral joint arthritis can produce pain in a similar distribution. Therefore, the practitioner should not assume that anterior shoulder pain is the result of an abnormality of the biceps tendon.

Examination of the biceps tendon may be more challenging than one might expect. With the arm in internal rotation, the biceps tendon is at the level of the anterior shoulder joint. To remove biceps from the anterior joint, the arm should be externally rotated approximately 30°. The examiner can then flex and extend the elbow and palpate biceps. In thin patients, the biceps can often be felt moving in the anterior shoulder. Tenderness with this maneuver suggests a problem with the biceps. However, it should be remembered that the tendons of supraspinatus and subscapularis insert in this location of the anterior shoulder. For this reason, anterior shoulder tenderness is not diagnostic for biceps tendon abnormality (Gill et al. 2007).

Full-thickness tears of the biceps tendon can produce the typical "Popeye" deformity of the proximal arm (**Fig. 6.26**). Clinically, when a patient experiences an acute tear of the biceps tendon, there is often a perceptible "pop," sudden deformity in the arm, and tenderness where the lump occurs. Ecchymosis in the upper arm may occur, particularly if the patient is on anticoagulants.

Speed's test

The most widely performed test for the biceps tendon is Speed's test (Crenshaw and Kilgore 1966; Bennett 1998). For this test, the arm is flexed 90° and horizontally extended 10°, and the elbow is extended with the palm of the hand facing upward (**Fig. 6.27**). The examiner

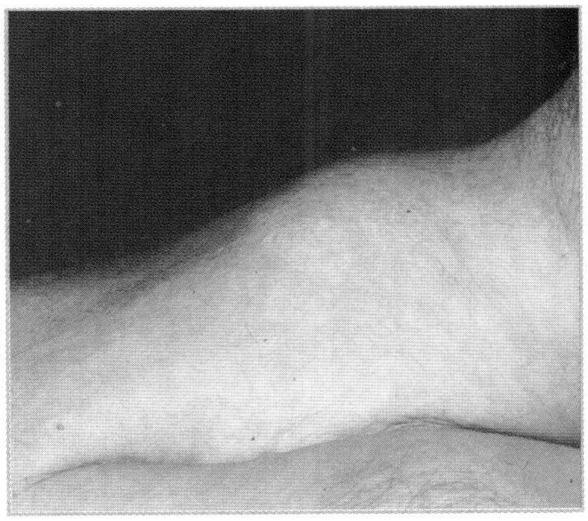

Figure 6.26 Full-thickness tear of the biceps tendon produces a lump in the arm or "Popeye" deformity.

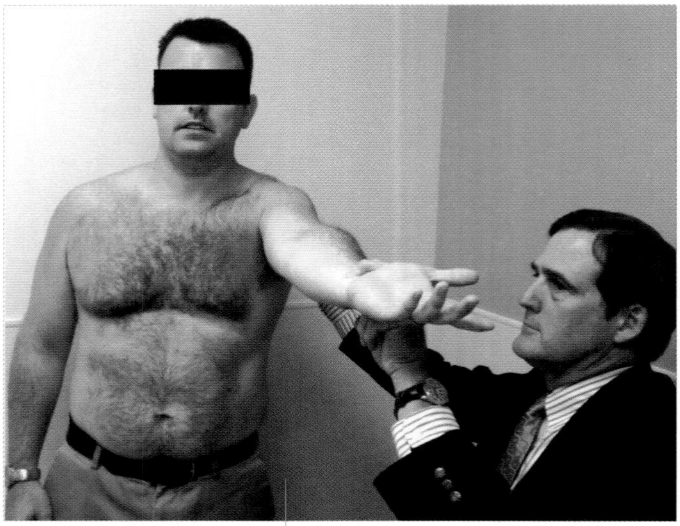

Figure 6.27 Speed's test has been described as a test for biceps abnormality.

then applies pressure down on the arm. The test is considered positive when the patient reports pain into the anterior shoulder; pain elsewhere is not indicative of a positive test. This test has not been found to be clinically useful for determining the presence of partial tears of the biceps tendon (Gill et al. 2007).

Acromioclavicular joint tests

Pathology of the acromioclavicular (AC) joint can result in pain in the anterior, lateral, and sometimes posterior aspects of the shoulder (Gerber et al. 1998). Therefore, the practitioner should always consider the AC joint when evaluating a patient for a shoulder problem.

The most important physical finding on physical examination of a pathological AC joint is tenderness directly on the joint. The AC joint can be found by palpating the clavicle in the distal third, and then progressively moving in a lateral direction until a soft spot is felt between the clavicle and the acromion. Tenderness in this location is usually indicative of an AC joint disorder. The pain is often increased as the arm is positioned across the body while applying an adduction stress. Indeed, the combination of point tenderness directly over the joint with a positive adduction stress maneuver is highly suggestive of pathology in the AC joint.

The four most important tests for rotator cuff evaluation

Although a complete and thorough examination of the rotator cuff is the goal, in clinical practice it is not necessary for the general practitioner to know every test and its accuracy. An examination has some merit as long as the findings are interpreted correctly and the subsequent clinical decision-making is based on the findings.

In our opinion, the four most important tests for a patient with suspected rotator cuff disease are elevation of the arm, weakness in abduction, weakness in external rotation, and the external rotation lag sign.

Elevation of the arm

The patient should have a sufficiently active range of motion so that the arm reaches the ear (see **Fig. 6.6**). If full elevation is not obtained, the shoulder is weak or stiff, or both. The inability to fully elevate warrants additional evaluation first with radiographs and then, depending on the findings, referral or additional study with MRI or ultrasonography.

Weakness in abduction (Jobe's strength testing)

Inability to hold the arm in elevation against gravity (the drop-arm test) or against resistance is a frequent sign of rotator cuff disease (see **Fig. 6.13**). That said, it is important to realize that nerve injury, cervical spine disc disease, myopathy, or neuropathy can cause these tests to be positive.

Weakness in external rotation

Weakness in external rotation (see **Fig. 6.17**) indicates that there is a rotator cuff tear or a neurological problem. This sign indicates a possible abnormality that might need additional investigation if other physical findings do not point to rotator cuff disease.

External rotation lag sign

The external rotation lag sign (see **Fig. 6.21**) indicates severe weakness in external rotation and means that the patient most likely has at least a tear of supraspinatus and probably also of infraspinatus tendons.

REFERENCES

Bennett WF. Specificity of the Speed's test: arthroscopic technique for evaluating the biceps tendon at the level of the bicipital groove. Arthroscopy 1998;14:789–796.

Bigliani LU, Codd TP, Connor PM, et al. Shoulder motion and laxity in the professional baseball player. Am J Sports Med 1997;25:609–613.

Blonna D, Cecchetti S, Tellini A, et al. Contribution of the supraspinatus to the external rotator lag sign: kinematic and electromyographic pattern in an in vivo model. J Shoulder Elbow Surg 2010;19:392–398.

Burkhart SS, Morgan CD, Kibler WB. The disabled throwing shoulder: spectrum of pathology. Part I: pathoanatomy and biomechanics. Arthroscopy 2003;19:404–420.

Codman EA. Calcified deposits in the supraspinatus tendon. In: The Shoulder. Rupture of the supraspinatus tendon and other lesions in or about the subacromial bursa. Boston, MA: Thomas Todd, 1934: 178-215.

Crenshaw AH, Kilgore WE. Surgical treatment of bicipital tenosynovitis. J Bone Joint Surg Am 1966;48:1496–1502.

Crockett HC, Gross LB, Wilk KE, et al. Osseous adaptation and range of motion at the glenohumeral joint in professional baseball pitchers. Am J Sports Med 2002;30:20–26.

Gerber C, Krushell RJ. Isolated rupture of the tendon of the subscapularis muscle. Clinical features in 16 cases. J Bone Joint Surg Br 1991;73:389–394.

Gerber C, Hersche O, Farron A. Isolated rupture of the subscapularis tendon. Results of operative repair. J Bone Joint Surg Am 1996;78:1015–1023.

Gerber C, Galantay RV, Hersche O. The pattern of pain produced by irritation of the acromioclavicular joint and the subacromial space. J Shoulder Elbow Surg 1998;7:352–355.

Gill HS, El Rassi G, Bahk MS, et al. Physical examination for partial tears of the biceps tendon. Am J Sports Med 2007;35:1334–1340.

Hawkins RJ, Kennedy JC. Impingement syndrome in athletes. Am J Sports Med 1980;8:151–157; discussion 157–158.

Hegedus EJ, Goode A, Campbell S, et al. Physical examination tests of the shoulder: a systematic review with meta-analysis of individual tests. Br J Sports Med 2008;42:80–92.

Hertel R, Ballmer FT, Lambert SM, Gerber C. Lag signs in the diagnosis of rotator cuff rupture. J Shoulder Elbow Surg 1996;5:307–313.

Itoi E, Minagawa H, Yamamoto N, et al. Are pain location and physical examinations useful in locating a tear site of the rotator cuff? Am J Sports Med 2006;34:256–264.

Jia X, Petersen SA, Khosravi AH, et al. Examination of the shoulder: the past, the present, and the future. J Bone Joint Surg Am 2009;91:10–18.
Jobe CM, Pink MM, Jobe FW, Shaffer B. Anterior shoulder instability, impingement, and rotator cuff tear. Section A: Theories and concepts. In: Jobe FW (ed.), Operative Techniques in Upper Extremity Sports Injuries. St Louis, MO: Mosby, 1996: 164–176.
Kelly BT, Kadrmas WR, Speer KP. The manual muscle examination for rotator cuff strength. An electromyographic investigation. Am J Sports Med 1996;24:581–588.
Kessel L, Watson M. The painful arc syndrome. Clinical classification as a guide to management. J Bone Joint Surg Br 1977;59:166–172.
Kibler WB, McMullen J. Scapular dyskinesis and its relation to shoulder pain. J Am Acad Orthop Surgeons 2003;11:142–151.
Kim TK, Rauh PB, McFarland EG. Partial tears of the subscapularis tendon found during arthroscopic procedures on the shoulder: a statistical analysis of sixty cases. Am J Sports Med 2003;31:744–750.
Lehman C, Cuomo F, Kummer FJ, Zuckerman JD. The incidence of full thickness rotator cuff tears in a large cadaveric population. Bull Hosp Joint Dis 1995;54:30–31.
McCabe RA, Nicholas SJ, Montgomery KD, et al. The effect of rotator cuff tear size on shoulder strength and range of motion. J Orthop Sports Phys Ther 2005;35:130–135.
McFarland EG. Rotator cuff disease and impingement. In: Kim TK, Park HB, El Rassi G, et al. (eds), Examination of the Shoulder: The Complete Guide. New York: Thieme, 2006a:126–161.
McFarland EG. Shoulder range of motion. In: Kim TK, Park HB, El Rassi G, et al. (eds), Examination of the Shoulder: The Complete Guide. New York: Thieme, 2006b: 15–87.
McFarland EG. Strength testing. In: Kim TK, Park HB, El Rassi G, et al. (eds). Examination of the Shoulder: The Complete Guide. New York: Thieme, 2006c: 88–125..
McFarland EG, Selhi HS, Keyurapan E. Clinical evaluation of impingement: what to do and what works. Instr Course Lect 2006;55:3–16.
Miniaci A, Dowdy PA, Willits KR, Vellet AD. Magnetic resonance imaging evaluation of the rotator cuff tendons in the asymptomatic shoulder. Am J Sports Med 1995;23:142–145.
Moseley JB Jr, Jobe FW, Pink M, et al. EMG analysis of the scapular muscles during a shoulder rehabilitation program. Am J Sports Med 1992;20:128–134.
Murrell GAC, Walton JR. Diagnosis of rotator cuff tears. Lancet 2001;357:769–770.
Neer CS, II. Anterior acromioplasty for the chronic impingement syndrome in the shoulder: a preliminary report. J Bone Joint Surg Am 1972;54:41–50.
Neer CS, II. Impingement lesions. Clin Orthop Relat Res 1983;173:70–77.
Park HB, Yokota A, Gill HS, et al. Diagnostic accuracy of clinical tests for the different degrees of subacromial impingement syndrome. J Bone Joint Surg Am 2005;87:1446–1455.
Sher JS, Uribe JW, Posada A, et al. Abnormal findings on magnetic resonance images of asymptomatic shoulders [see comments]. J Bone Joint Surg Am 1995;77:10–15.
Uhthoff HK, Sarkar K. The effect of aging on the soft tissues of the shoulder. In: Matsen FA, III, Fu FH, Hawkins RJ (eds), The Shoulder: A balance of mobility and stability. Rosemont, IL: American Academy of Orthopaedic Surgeons, 1993: 269–278.
Walch G, Boulahia A, Calderone S, Robinson AHN. The "dropping" and "hornblower's" signs in evaluation of rotator-cuff tears. J Bone Joint Surg Br 1998;80:624–628.
Yamamoto A, Takagishi K, Osawa T, et al. Prevalence and risk factors of a rotator cuff tear in the general population. J Shoulder Elbow Surg 2010;19:116–120.

Chapter 7 Imaging of the rotator cuff

Varand Ghazikhanian, John Furia, Javier Beltran

KEY FEATURES

- Although there are different modalities available for the assessment of rotator cuff integrity, MRI remains the most complete modality, and is the examination of choice for the evaluation of the shoulder and suspected rotator cuff pathology.
- Ultrasonography is accurate, but is user dependent, and does not always allow for assessment of the internal structures as accurately as MRI.
- MR arthrography is the preferred method for the assessment of partial-thickness rotator cuff tears, the labrum, and glenohumeral ligaments.
- CT arthrography is a very useful alternative when MR arthrography is contraindicated. It is very sensitive and specific in identifying complete rotator cuff tears, but not nearly as accurate for identifying partial-thickness rotator cuff tears.

CLINICAL SCENARIO 1

AS is a 53-year-old woman who fell while waterskiing. Her primary complaint was anterior lateral shoulder pain, worse with pushing, pulling, and lifting overhead. She related weakness when performing overhead activities and had pain with sleeping at night. Her symptoms did not respond to relative rest, activity modification, medication, or physical therapy.

Physical examination revealed tenderness over the anterolateral aspect of the acromion. There was pain with active forward elevation. Impingement signs were positive, and there was significant weakness with resisted external rotation.

There are multiple different imaging modalities available for evaluation of the rotator cuff. Although these different modalities are used for specific clinical scenarios, magnetic resonance imaging (MRI) remains the most complete modality and examination of choice for the evaluation of the shoulder and suspected rotator cuff pathology. In this chapter, the advantages and limitations of different imaging modalities are briefly described, with emphasis on the indications and contraindications of MRI, fundamental signal characteristics of MRI, normal rotator cuff anatomy on MRI, and rotator cuff pathology on MRI.

IMAGING MODALITIES

Ultrasonography

High-resolution, real-time ultrasonography is a very useful imaging modality for evaluation of rotator cuff tears. With multiple advances in ultrasound technology and the use of high-frequency (12 MHz) linear array transducers, much more accurate images of the rotator cuff may be obtained. The advantages of ultrasonography are that it is inexpensive and widely available. A meta-analysis by De Jesus et al. (2009) showed that ultrasonography is comparable to MRI in sensitivity and specificity for detection of partial- and full-thickness rotator cuff tears. Also, ultrasonography is a dynamic study and may demonstrate impingement syndromes in real time. Although ultrasonography is not the diagnostic procedure of choice in the USA, it is widely utilized in other parts of the world and, in experienced hands, can be very reliable (Rumack et al. 2005; Bin Bilal et al. 2010).

Plain film radiography and arthrography

Although plain film radiography is not very sensitive or specific for rotator cuff tears, it is usually the first examination performed, especially in the setting of trauma or for evaluation of chronic massive rotator cuff tears (which can be diagnosed confidently by radiography alone). Radiography also helps evaluate the mineralization of bone, calcifications (e.g., hydroxyapatite deposition in calcific tendinosis), and degenerative changes, and can demonstrate the shape of the acromion.

Arthrography can demonstrate complete rotator cuff tears by the presence of contrast material in the subacromial–subdeltoid bursa, but is usually combined with computed tomography (CT) arthrography. Air or iodine may be used as a contrast medium. Usually, 8–12 mL of iodine contrast or 3–4 mL iodine contrast and 10–12 mL of air are injected to distend the capsule, and multiple images are obtained (Bin Bilal et al. 2010).

CT arthrography

CT arthrography is a very useful alternative when MR arthrography is contraindicated. It is very sensitive and specific in identifying complete rotator cuff tears, and is useful for evaluation of the surrounding soft tissues, labrum, glenohumeral ligaments, long head of biceps tendon, and bony structures. However, it is not very sensitive for evaluation of partial-thickness tears or tendinopathy. The contrast injection (air or iodine contrast) technique is similar to plain film arthrography in preparation.

CLINICAL SCENARIO 2

An MRI study of AS's shoulder was obtained. The study revealed an abnormal signal on the STIR and T2-weighted images in the supraspinatus tendon. Discontinuation of the tendon with fluid filling the gap between the fragments was noted. Fluid was also noted in the surrounding subacromial and subdeltoid bursal tissues. The findings were consistent with a full-thickness rotator cuff tear.

Magnetic resonance imaging

MRI is the modality of choice for complete evaluation of the shoulder. Lambert et al. (2009) prospectively showed a 100% positive predictive value of 3.0 T MRI when compared with arthroscopy for the detection of rotator cuff tendon tears requiring surgery. With MRI, the bone marrow, tendons, muscles, ligaments, capsule, bursa, and labrum can be evaluated in multiple planes. MRI can identify tendinopathy, partial tears, intratendon tears, and tears of the bursal aspect of the tendon. MRI is effective for the detection of factors contributing to rotator cuff disease, such as structural causes of impingement syndromes. It can also demonstrate muscle atrophy, extent of muscle retraction, and bursitis, and is very sensitive to any bone marrow abnormalities that may be associated with rotator cuff disease (such as bone marrow edema and contusion).

MR arthrography is the most sensitive and specific imaging study for detection of complete or partial rotator cuff tears and best characterizes the type and morphology of rotator cuff tears. It is the study of choice for evaluation of the labrum and glenohumeral ligaments (Waldt et al. 2007; Bin Bilal et al. 2010). In the next section, the contraindications, sequences, and a guide for interpretation of MR scans, are reviewed.

MRI of the shoulder

Fundamentals of shoulder MRI

Before being able to identify pathology in the shoulder with MRI, one must have a fundamental understanding of the multi-planar shoulder anatomy and characteristics of MR signals on different pulse sequences, both of which are beyond the scope of this chapter. A short fundamental review of MRI signal characteristics is provided here.

On T1-wieghted pulse sequences, methemoglobin (subacute hematoma), melanin, fat, and gadolinium appear as high signal whereas fluid (edema) appears as low signal. On "fluid-sensitive" images such as STIR (short T1 inversion recovery) or T2-weighted images (including T2*), fluid appears as high signal. Therefore, most pathology such as edema, inflammation (tendinopathy and tendon tears), and most tumors usually appear as high signal on T2-weighted images and low signal on T1-weighted images. Fatty infiltration of muscles, which results from chronic atrophy, appears as high signal on T1-weighted images.

Cortical bone and calcifications appear as low signal on all pulse sequences. Bone marrow consists of red and yellow marrow: yellow marrow has the same signal characteristics as subcutaneous fat on T1- (high signal) and T2-weighted (intermediate signal) images and is completely suppressed on STIR or fat-saturated, T2-weighted pulse sequences. Red marrow appears as an intermediate signal on T1- and T2-weighted images. Red marrow can be differentiated from yellow marrow by the decrease in signal on T1-weighted images, and lack of suppression on fat-saturated, T2-weighted or STIR images. As red marrow also contains fat cells, it should always be higher in signal intensity than normal muscle or intervertebral disks on T1-weighted images. STIR and fat-suppressed, T2-weighted images are useful sequences for evaluating bone marrow pathology and T1-weighted sequences may be used for evaluation of tumors.

Normal articular cartilage is gray on proton density and dark gray on STIR and fat-saturated, T2-weighted images. These sequences can be particularly helpful for evaluation of the articular surface.

Fibrocartilage is also dark on all pulse sequences. The best sequences to evaluate the labrum are T1-weighted images after intra-articular gadolinium injection and gradient echo (T2*) images (Helms et al. 2001).

Tendons and ligaments usually appear as low signal on all pulse sequences. There are a few situations in which a normal tendon may display high signal. One cause is the magic angle phenomenon, which may occur in the supraspinatus tendon, approximately 1 cm proximal to the insertion of the tendon into the greater tuberosity, in the region that was previously described as the "critical zone." The magic angle phenomenon manifests as intermediate signal on short TE (echo time) sequences (such as T1-weighted, T2*, proton density) when collagen fibers are oriented at 55° to the constant magnetic induction field. If such a signal is present, one may check different sequences with longer echo times (such as T2-weighted images) and, if there is no abnormal signal, then a magic angle artifact can be confirmed. Tendons are best evaluated with T2*, T1-weighted and STIR or fat-saturated, T2-weighted images (Timins et al. 1995; Helms et al. 2001).

Finally, muscle gives intermediate signal on all sequences. T1-weighted images may be used for evaluation of muscle architecture and fatty infiltration of muscle, such as in chronic atrophy. STIR images may be used to detect edema and other intramuscular pathology.

Sequences

Most institutions use a slight variation of the widely accepted standard imaging sequences of the shoulder. Different sequences are used for imaging with and without contrast. In either procedure, a surface coil is required because the coil significantly enhances detail and resolution for any kind of imaging to obtain adequate detail and resolution. Small field of view (12–14 cm) and 3- to 4-mm thick slices are obtained in the coronal, oblique, axial, and sagittal oblique planes. In standard non-contrast MRI, the patient is placed supine with the arm on the side in neutral position or slight external rotation. With MR arthrography, especially for further evaluation of the labrum, glenohumeral ligaments, and impingement syndrome, the arm is also placed in abduction and external rotation (ABER).

Standard pulse sequences for non-contrast MRI include coronal oblique proton density (PD) or T1-weighted or gradient echo (T2*) and fat-saturated, T2-weighted or STIR images, axial fat-saturated PD or gradient echo images, and T1-weighted images, and sagittal fat-saturated PD or gradient echo images, STIR, and T2-weighted images.

Contrast-enhanced MRI may be obtained by the indirect method in which gadolinium is injected intravenously and delayed images are obtained, or by the direct method, in which gadolinium is injected into the joint capsule with fluoroscopic guidance. The advantage of direct injection is the ability to distend the joint. Usually, 0.1 mL gadolinium is mixed with 10 mL 0.9% saline and 3 mL iodine contrast, and approximately 10–12 mL of this solution injected intra-articularly.

Standard pulse sequences for contrast-enhanced MRI include coronal oblique, fat-saturated, T1- and T2-weighted or STIR images (for evaluation of fluid in the subacromial–subdeltoid bursa or other extra-articular fluid collections), sagittal oblique, fat-saturated, T1-weighted and non-fat-saturated, T1-weighted images (to evaluate muscle atrophy), and T1-weighted axial images with or without fat suppression to evaluate the labrum. An ABER view with fat-saturated, T1-weighted images greatly enhances detection of labrum and glenohumeral ligament pathology as well as the diagnosis of impingement syndrome (Kwak et al. 1998; Helms et al. 2001).

Contraindications for MRI

With the refinement of biological materials, more and more MRI-friendly surgical implants are being developed, reducing the need to obtain alternative imaging. However, many patients still have surgical implants that may prevent them from undergoing MRI.

Contraindications to MRI include electronically, magnetically, and mechanically stimulated implants, ferromagnetic hemostatic materials in the central nervous system, ferromagnetic materials such as automatic implantable cardioverter defibrillators, cardiac pacemakers, and ocular metallic foreign objects. Other contraindications for MRI include cochlear implants, other pacemakers such as carotid sinus pacemakers, insulin pumps, and nerve stimulators, lead wires, certain drug delivery patches, prosthetic heart valves (especially with suspicion of dehiscence), hemostatic materials in the body, and non-ferromagnetic stapedial implants. Many of the above contraindications are considered relative by the American College of Radiology, so each situation should be reviewed on a case-by-case basis with a radiologist and/or MRI safety officer to document when and exactly what type of hardware is present, to better assess whether a particular MRI examination may or may not be performed.

The presence of other implants including non-ferromagnetic implants and the date of implantation also need to be communicated to the MRI operator. Some patients are claustrophobic and may either receive mild sedation before examination or, as an alternative, obtain their imaging study with an open MRI.

Finally, in patients with chronic renal insufficiency, especially with a glomerular filtration rate of <30 mL/min per 1.73 m^2, there is a risk of developing nephrogenic systemic fibrosis with the use of intravenous gadolinium. Contrast must be used with caution when treating these patients (Flyer and Ghazikhanian 2008).

ROTATOR CUFF IMAGES

Normal anatomy

The rotator cuff is made up of the tendons of supraspinatus, infraspinatus, teres minor, and subscapularis (**Figs 7.1** and **7.2**). The tendinous fibers of supraspinatus, infraspinatus, and teres minor blend together from their lateral margins before they insert on to the greater tuberosity. The supraspinatus tendon fibers insert on to the superior aspect of the greater tuberosity and infraspinatus and teres minor insert posteriorly, whereas the subscapularis tendon inserts on to the lesser tuberosity anteriorly. The rotator cuff interval, i.e., the gap between the subscapularis and supraspinatus tendons, contains the coracohumeral ligament and superior glenohumeral ligament. It also allows the long head of biceps tendon to pass from the bicipital groove through the glenohumeral joint, before inserting on to the superior glenoid. The coracohumeral ligament traverses from the coracoid process to insert on to the lesser and greater tuberosities and the transverse ligament. The rotator cuff tendons are not surrounded by either a synovial sheath or a paratenon.

The supraspinatus tendon travels between the undersurface of the acromion and above the humeral head, and it inserts on to fibrocartilage superiorly on the greater tuberosity. The entire length of supraspinatus is well visualized on coronal oblique images. The supraspinatus muscle and tendon travel at about 45° relative to the coronal plane and are visualized on the images that also best demonstrate the acromioclavicular joint. The musculotendinous junction is located just lateral to the acromioclavicular joint. More posteriorly, infraspinatus is also best visualized longitudinally on coronal oblique

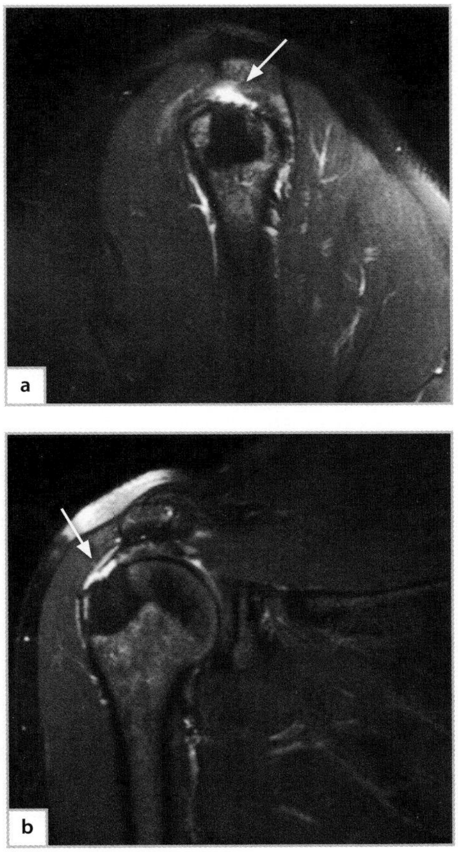

Figure 7.1 MRI of the ahoulder of AS: full thickness supraspinatus tendon tear. Sagittal (a) and coronal (b) fat saturated T2 weighted images of the shoulder demonstrate a high signal (fluid) gap in the posterior insertional fibers of the supraspinatus (and anterior infraspinatus) tendon at its insertion (arrows), with uncovering of the articular surface, compatible with a full thickness tear. There is no tendinous retraction or muscle atrophy.

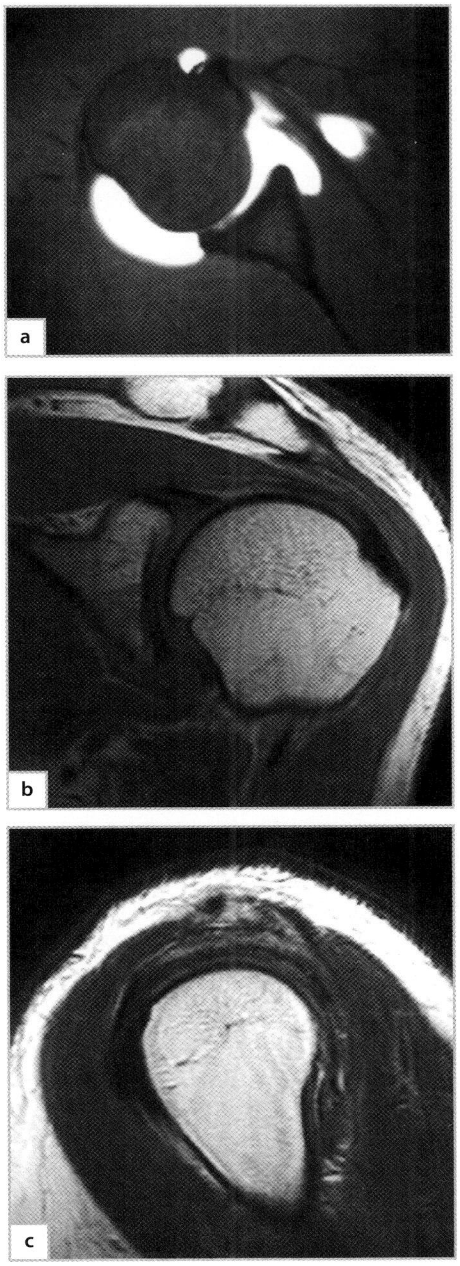

Figure 7.2 Normal rotator cuff. (a) Axial, fat-saturated, T1-weighted arthrogram, (b) coronal oblique, T1-weighted , and (c) sagittal oblique, T1-weighted images demonstrating the normal rotator cuff.

images. The infraspinatus tendon travels obliquely in a craniocaudal direction, also at about a 45° angle, and attaches to the posterior aspect of the greater tuberosity. On sagittal oblique images, tendons of all four rotator cuff muscles are visualized in cross-section and are surrounded by their respective muscles. The proximal portion of the long head of biceps tendon is also visualized in cross-section on this view, which is used to confirm pathology suspected in other planes where the muscles and tendons are seen longitudinally (Helms et al. 2001; Tuite and Sanford 2010).

The subscapularis muscle and tendon, which travel anterior to the shoulder, are demonstrated longitudinally on axial images. The subscabularis tendon attaches to the lesser tuberosity and blends with the transverse humeral ligament. Again, the sagittal oblique views can be used to confirm pathology in cross-section, when suspected in other planes.

The origin of the long head of biceps tendon, at its attachment on the superior labrum, and the portion of the tendon inferior to the bicipital groove are visualized longitudinally on coronal oblique images. The portion of the long head of biceps tendon located in the bicipital groove is visualized transversely on axial images, appears as a round or oval structure, and may have a small amount of fluid on the dependent side of the tendon sheath, which is a normal finding. If a joint effusion is present, fluid will be seen around the entire tendon, because the tendon sheath is in direct communication with the glenohumeral joint.

The portion of the deltoid tendon that attaches to the superior and inferior margins of the acromion is visualized on coronal oblique images. Finally, the rotator interval is best visualized on sagittal oblique views.

The coracoacromial arch is formed by the humeral head posteriorly, the acromion superiorly, and the coracoid process and coracoacromial ligament anteriorly. The subacromial–subdeltoid bursa, the supraspinatus tendon and muscle, and the long head of biceps tendon are located in the coracoacromial arch. Symptoms of impingement can be seen with narrowing of the coracoacromial arch. The coracoacromial ligament is visualized on sagittal oblique images and can be seen in coronal oblique images. The acromion is evaluated on coronal and sagittal oblique planes. The anterior and posterior aspects of the inferior cortical line of the acromion on sagittal oblique views should be horizontal or curved, paralleling the humeral head, whereas on coronal oblique images the anterior aspect of the acromion should be horizontal and at the level of the clavicle. Also, the undersurface of the acromioclavicular joint and acromion should be smooth and horizontal. The subacromial–subdeltoid bursa may have a small amount of fluid within it but should not be distended with fluid (Farley et al. 1994; Vangsness et al. 1994).

Rotator cuff and related structure pathology

The goal of MRI is to identify the location, size, and extension (or retraction) of rotator cuff tears.

Supraspinatus

Supraspinatus tendon degeneration and partial tears usually coexist and are sometimes difficult to distinguish on MRI. On T1-weighted images, they both appear as intermediate signal focally or diffusely in the tendon. On T2-weighted images, degeneration usually has the same signal intensity as muscle and a partial-thickness tear has the signal intensity of fluid. Again, differentiation may be very difficult on MRI. Partial-thickness tears occur on the bursal or articular surface, or are intrasubstance. These are graded as low (<50%), medium (50%), and high (>50%) (**Fig. 7.3**). Partial-thickness tears on the articular surface of the tendon usually fill with injected gadolinium and demonstrate high T1 signal on MR arthrography. Partial-thickness tears on the bursal surface (or intrasubstance tears) are not visualized with MR arthrography because the intra-articular gadolinium cannot reach this area; they are therefore evaluated with regular MRI sequences. Partial-thickness tears mostly start on the articular surface of the distal anterior supraspinatus tendon (given the relative lack of vascularity in these fibers and the fact that superficial fibers are more resistant to tensile forces) and travel posteriorly. At this stage, the articular layers may retract whereas the bursal layers remain intact.

Full-thickness tears of the supraspinatus tendon are diagnosed with direct and secondary findings on MRI (**Fig. 7.4**). Direct findings include discontinuation of the tendon with fluid filling the gap between the fragments on T2-weighted images. It may be difficult to visualize tendon disruption on MRI because of the presence of granulation tissue, debris, far anterior location, or small size of a tear. Secondary signs may be used to aid the diagnosis in these situations, and include medial retraction of the musculotendinous junction and focal thinning or irregularity of the tendon. Subacromial–subdeltoid bursal fluid and atrophy of supraspinatus may also be present, but these are more non-specific findings. Preoperative fatty degeneration index values can also be used to predict the success rate of arthroscopic repair of large to massive rotator cuff tears.

MR arthrography has the highest sensitivity and specificity for detection of supraspinatus tendon partial or complete tears. On MR arthrography, high signal on T1-weighted images is seen in the subacromial–subdeltoid bursa due to discontinuity of the tendon, and high signal is also seen between the disrupted tendon fragments. MR arthrography

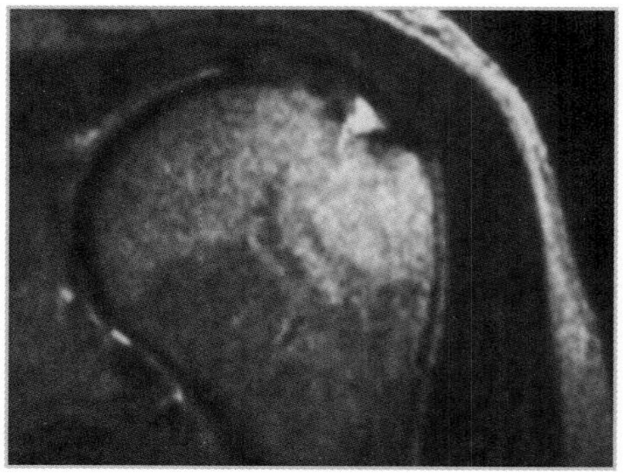

Figure 7.3 Partial supraspinatus tendon tear. Coronal oblique T2-weighted image of the shoulder demonstrating a partial articular surface tear of the supraspinatus tendon (arrow), with focal high signal (edema) at the site of the tear.

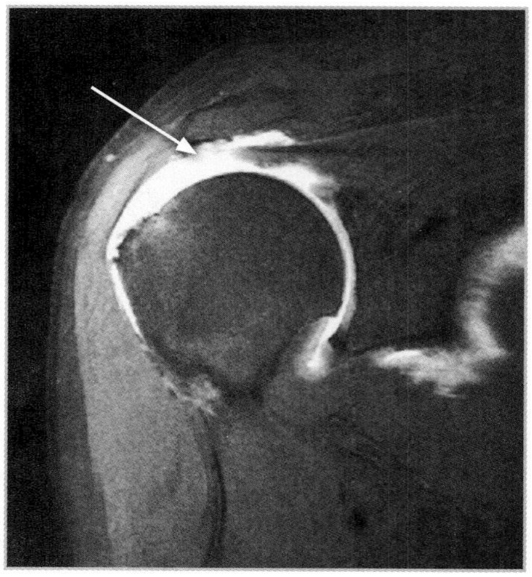

Figure 7.4 Full-thickness supraspinatus tendon tear. Coronal oblique, fat-saturated, T1-weighted arthrogram demonstrating a full thickness tear of the supraspinatus tendon (arrow), with contrast extending into the subacromial-subdeltoid bursa.

can also accurately identify morphological classification of the torn tendon (Carrino et al. 1997; Shahin-Akyar et al. 1998; Helms et al. 2001; Goutallier et all 2003; Ardic et al. 2006; Dinter et al. 2008; Yoo et al. 2009).

Many causes of supraspinatus tendon impingement can be identified on MRI. The shape of the acromion may contribute to impingement of supraspinatus. A type I acromion has a flat undersurface, a type II has a concave undersurface, a type III has an inferiorly projecting anterior hook that narrows the space between the acromion and humerus (and is most associated with impingement), and finally a type IV acromion has a convex undersurface. The shape of the acromion is determined on the sagittal oblique plane just lateral to the acromioclavicular joint. The slope of the acromion is evaluated on coronal oblique and sagittal oblique images and its lateral aspect is usually horizontal on sagittal oblique images.

An anterior and downsloping acromion occurs when the inferior cortex of the anterior acromion is located more caudally than the inferior cortex of the posterior aspect of the acromion. Inferolateral tilt of the acromion is detected on coronal oblique images, and occurs when the lateral aspect of the acromion is tilted inferiorly relative to the clavicle. The normal inferior cortex of the acromion is at the same level as the inferior cortex of the clavicle on coronal oblique images. In a low-lying acromion the inferior cortex is below the inferior cortex of the clavicle. An os acromiale is an accessory ossification center of the acromion that does not fuse by age 25; it occurs in 15% of the population, and is best seen on axial images.

Degenerative changes of the acromioclavicular joint, including osteophytosis and capsule overgrowth, may project inferiorly and cause impingement. Although this can be identified on plain radiographs, MRI demonstrates the extent of the impingement. Focal thickening of the coracoacromial ligament also causes impingement and may be caused by chronic anterior instability. It is best seen on sagittal oblique views. Another cause of impingement is post-traumatic deformity of the bony structures close to the coracoacromial arch. Even with normal anatomy, hypertrophy of supraspinatus from overuse may cause impingement. Finally, shoulder instability can contribute to impingement and commonly coexists with it. Impingement of the supraspinatus tendon may cause partial or complete tendon tears. However, many of the same tendon abnormalities exist without evidence of impingement, and most partial-thickness tears of the supraspinatus tendon occur on the articular surface, where most of the above-mentioned abnormalities are present (Helms et al. 2001; Tuite et al. 2010).

Infraspinatus

Infraspinatus tendon tears are seen after trauma, in association with supraspinatus tendon tears, and with posterosuperior impingement of infraspinatus and supraspinatus tendons between the humeral head and the posterior glenoid rim during overhead movements, such as in overhead throwing sports. When arising from a posterosuperior impingement syndrome, MRI findings include partial or complete infraspinatus tear (with or without supraspinatus tendon tear), degenerative cysts on the posterior aspect of the humeral head near the insertion of the infraspinatus tendon, and fraying or tears of the posterior glenoid labrum.

Subscapularis

Subscapular tendon tears may be caused by acute trauma when the arm is adducted in external rotation, anterior dislocation of the shoulder, or subcoracoid impingement from narrowing of the space between the tip of the coracoid process and humerus, and may be associated with massive rotator cuff tears (**Fig. 7.5**). MRI best demonstrates tears in the axial plane, confirmed on sagittal views, which are also best seen with T2-weighted images or T1-weighted MR arthrography images. Again, tears may be seen as discontinuation of the tendon with gadolinium

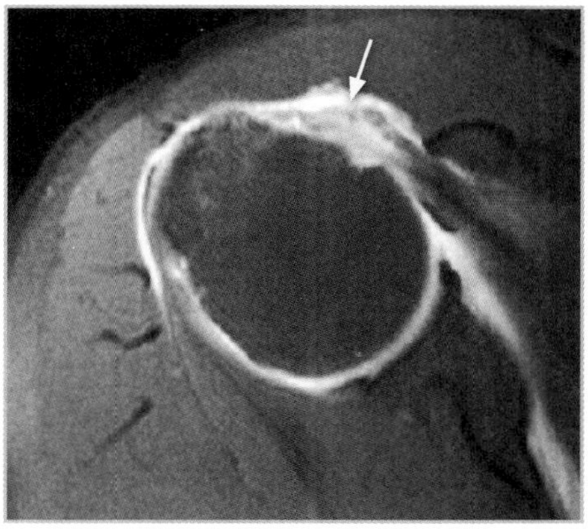

Figure 7.5 Subscapularis tendon tear. Axial, fat-saturated, T1-weighted arthrogram demonstrating a subscapularis tendon tear (arrow), with contrast extending into and around the disrupted tendon.

entering the tendon substance, intrasubstance abnormal tendon signal, abnormal tendon caliber, and abnormal position of the tendon. Gadolinium may also be seen under the insertion of the tendon on to the lesser tuberosity along with muscle atrophy. Finally, subluxation and dislocation of the long head of biceps tendon are usually associated with subscapularis tendon tears (Patte 1990; Patten 1994; Helms et al. 2001).

Long head of biceps tendon

The long head of biceps tendon is abnormal in up to 33% of patients with supraspinatus tendon tears, given its proximity to the supraspinatus tendon, which is affected by impingement (**Fig. 7.6**). These tendon tears usually occur proximal to the bicipital groove in older patients, with the muscle and tendon retracting distally, and leaving an empty bicipital groove on axial images on MRI. Acute tears occur in younger patients and also occur more distally, near the musculotendinous junction. The tendon of the long head of biceps may also be subluxed or dislocated after acute trauma which produces disruption of the transverse humeral ligament. A subscapularis tendon tear is also usually present. When it dislocates, the tendon may be displaced anteromedially, which could be associated with a subscapularis tendon tear. A medial dislocation is always associated with a tear of the subscapularis tendon at its attachment to the lesser tuberosity. This is best demonstrated on axial images that show an empty bicipital groove and the presence of the tendon medial to the groove, deep or superficial to the subscapularis tendon (Cervilla et al. 1991, Chan et al. 1991, Tuckman 1994).

Massive rotator cuff tear

Finally, massive rotator cuff tears are usually present in older patients with diabetes, inflammatory arthritis, marked tendon degeneration, or steroid therapy (**Fig. 7.7**). MRI usually reveals complete tears of multiple rotator cuff tendons with musculotendinous retraction

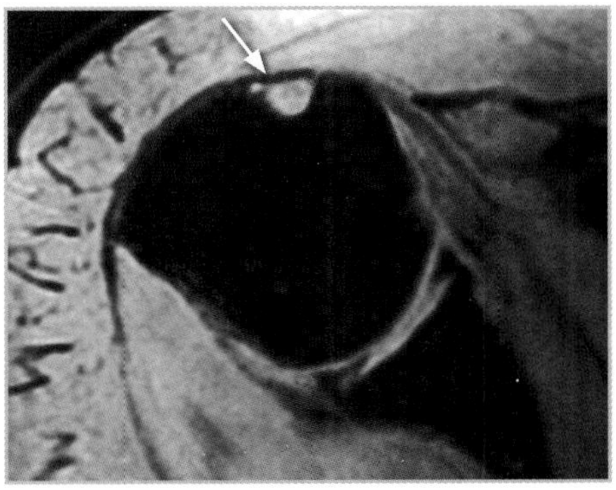

Figure 7.6 Long head of the biceps tendon tear. Axial, gradient-echo image demonstrating a long head of the biceps tendon tear. The normally low-signal tendon that is usually seen in cross-section on axial images is not present in the bicipital groove (arrow).

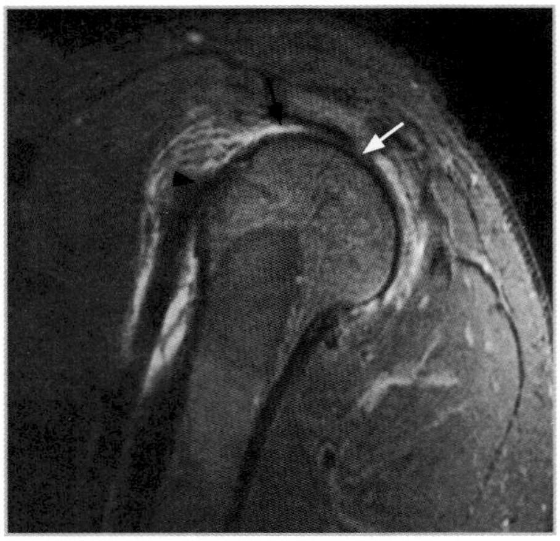

Figure 7.7 Massive rotator cuff tear. Sagittal oblique STIR image demonstrating a massive rotator cuff tear with retraction of the supraspinatus tendon (black arrow) and infraspinatus tendon (white arrow). The long head of the biceps tendon is also torn (arrowhead).

and muscle atrophy. There is a large communication between the joint and subacromial–subdeltoid bursa. Sometimes a synovial cyst is seen extending through the acromioclavicular joint and forming a soft-tissue mass on the superior aspect of the shoulder. There is usually proximal migration of the humeral head with marked associated degenerative changes, usually seen on plain radiographs.

CONCLUSION

Multiple modalities can be used to evaluate the rotator cuff and rotator cuff pathology. Ultrasonography is very accurate in the detection of rotator cuff tears, but cannot evaluate many of the internal structures as accurately as MRI. MRI is the most complete study for evaluation of the shoulder, and MR arthrography is the most accurate modality to detect rotator cuff tears and evaluate the labrum and glenohumeral ligaments. CT arthrography may be used for rotator cuff pathology if MRI is contraindicated, but is also limited in the evaluation of partial tears.

CLINICAL SCENARIO 3

AS elected to undergo arthroscopic repair of her rotator cuff tear. A 1 × 2 cm full-thickness tear of the distal anterior aspect of the supraspinatus tendon was identified (see **Fig. 7.8**). After acromioplasty and subacromial decompression, the tear was repaired directly to bone using a single-row, suture-anchor technique.

Postoperatively, the extremity was immobilized in a sling for a period of 3 weeks. Physical therapy was initiated, and gradually the patient was introduced to passive motion first, and active mobilization afterwards. By 8 weeks after the operation, AS had regained full active range of motion. By 16 weeks post-surgery, AS had regained full strength and returned to unrestricted activity.

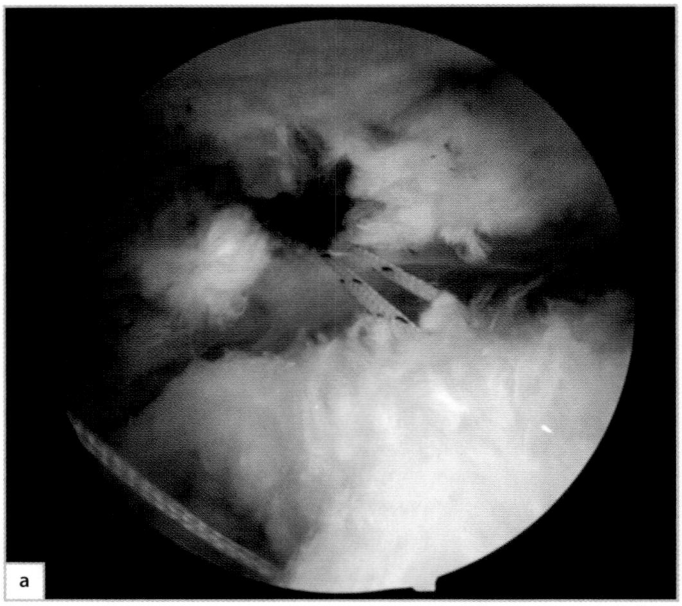

a

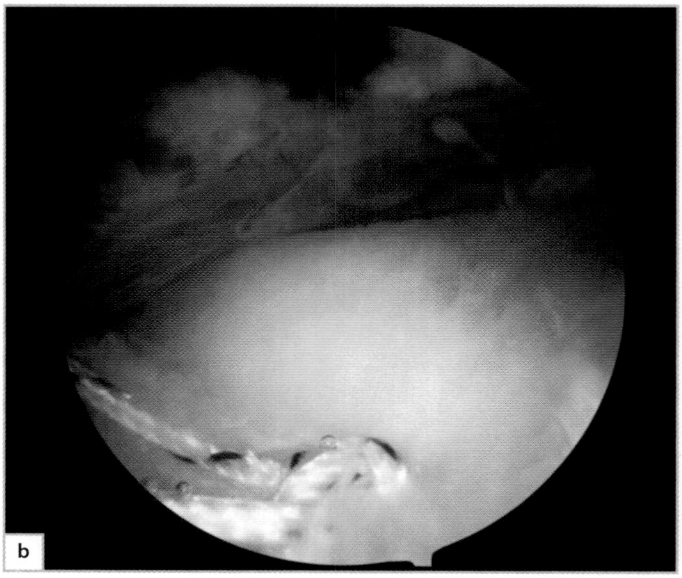

b

Figure 7.8. Full thickness supraspinatus tendon tear. Intraoperative arthroscopic image demonstrating a full-thickness, non-retracted tear of the supraspinatus tendon. (a) Note the sutures positioned at the leading edge of the tear and through the rotator cuff tissue. (b) Final repair.

REFERENCES

Ardic F, Kahraman Y, Kacar M, et al. Shoulder impingement syndrome: relationships between clinical, functional, and radiologic findings. Am J Phys Med Rehabil 2006;85:53–60.

Bin Bilal RH, Duffy PJ, Shafi BBB, Hafi BB. Rotator Cuff Pathology. Emedicine, 2010. Available at: http://emedicine.medscape.com/article/1262849-overview (accessed October 2010).

Chan TW, Dalinka MK, Kneeland JB, et al. Biceps tendon dislocation: evaluation with MR imaging. Radiology 1991;179:649–652.

Carrino JA, McCauley TR, Katz LD, Smith RC, Lange RC. Rotator cuff: evaluation with fast spin-echo versus conventional spin-echo MR imaging. Radiology 1997;202:533–539.

Cervilla V, Schweitzer ME, Ho C, et al. Medial dislocation of the biceps brachii tendon: appearance at MR imaging. Radiology 1991;180:523–526.

De Jesus JO, Parker L, Frangos AJ, Nazarian LN. Accuracy of MRI, MR arthrography, and ultrasound in the diagnosis of rotator cuff tears: a meta-analysis. AJR Am J Roentgenol 2009;192:1701–1707.

Dinter DJ, Martetschläger F, Büsing KA, et al. Shoulder injuries in overhead athletes: utility of MR arthrography. Sportverletz Sportschaden. 2008;22:146–152.

Farley TE, Neumann CH, Steinbach LS, et al. The coraco-acromial arch: MR evaluation and correlation with rotator cuff pathology. Skeletal Radiol 1994;23:641–645.

Flyer M, Ghazikhanian V. Enhanced MRI and the nephrogenic systemic fibrosis debate: Practical perspectives. Medscape 2008. Available at: http://cme.medscape.com/viewarticle/708576 (accessed October 2010).

Goutallier D, Postel JM, Gleyze P, Leguillox P, Van Driessche S. Influence of cuff muscle fatty degeneration on anatomic and functional outcomes after simple suture of full thickness tears. J Shoulder Elbow Surg 2003;12:550–554.

Helms CA, Major NM, Anderson MW, Kaplan P, Dussault R. Musculoskeletal MRI. Philadelphia, PA: Saunders, 2001:169–223.

Kanal E, Barkovich AJ, Bell C, et al. ACR guidance document for safe MR practices: 2007. AJR Am J Roentgenol. 2007;188:1447–1474.

Kwak SM, Brown RR, Trudell D, et al. Glenohumeral joint: comparison of shoulder positions at MR arthrography. Radiology 1998;208:375–380.

Lambert A, Loffroy R, Guiu B, et al. Rotator cuff tears: value of 3.0T MRI. J Radiol 2009;90(5 Pt 1):583–588.

Patte D. The subcoracoid impingement. Clin Orthop 1990;254:55–59.

Patten RM. Tears of the anterior portion of the rotator cuff (the subscapularis tendon): MR imaging findings. AJR Am J Roentgenol 1994;162:351–354.

Rumack CM, Wilson SR, Charboneou JW, Levine D. Diagnostic Ultrasound, Vol. 1, 3rd edn. St Louis, MO: Mosby, 2005: 889–908.

Sahin-Akyar G, Miller TT, Staron RB, McCarthy DM, Feldman F. Gradient-echo versus fat-suppressed fast spin-echo MR imaging of rotator cuff tears. AJR Am J Roentgenol 1998;171:223–227.

Timins ME, Erickson SJ, Estkowski LD, et al. Increased signal in the normal supraspinatus tendon on MR imaging: diagnostic pitfall caused by the magic angle effect. AJR Am J Roentgenol 1995;165:109–114.

Tuckman GA. Abnormalities of the long head of the biceps tendon of the shoulder: MR imaging findings. AJR Am J Roentgenol 1994;163:1183–1188.

Tuite M, Sanford MF. Shoulder, rotator cuff injury (MRI). Emedicine, 2010. Available at: http://emedicine.medscape.com/article/401714-overview (accessed October 2010).

Vangsness CT Jr, Jorgenson SS, Watson T, et al. The origin of the long head of the biceps from the scapula and glenoid labrum: an anatomical study of 100 shoulders. J Bone Joint Surg Br 1994;76:951–954.

Waldt S, Bruegel M, Mueller D, et al. Rotator cuff tears: assessment with MR arthrography in 275 patients with arthroscopic correlation. Eur Radiol 2007;17:491–581.

Yoo JC, Ahn JH, Yang JH, et al. Correlation of arthroscopic repairability of large to massive rotator cuff tears with preoperative magnetic resonance imaging scans. Arthroscopy 2009;25:573–582.

Chapter 8 Partial rotator cuff tears

Rocco Papalia, Francesco Franceschi, Sebastiano Vasta, Biagio Zampogna, Nicola Maffulli, John Furia, Vincenzo Denaro

KEY FEATURES

- Partial-thickness rotator cuff tears are defined as a partial disruption of the fibers of the tendon, but with no communication between the subacromial bursa and the glenohumeral joint.
- Partial-thickness tears of the rotator cuff are classified as bursal, interstitial, and intra-articular.
- Tear depth is the key factor when determining definitive treatment.
- Rotator cuff repair is indicated for patients in whom more than 50% of the tendon thickness is involved; debridement is preferred for tears involving less than 50% of the tendon.
- With regard to repair of partial-thickness tears, transtendon repair and subacromial repair after conversion to full-thickness tear provide comparable outcomes.

INTRODUCTION

Definition and classification

Partial-thickness rotator cuff tears are a frequent cause of a painful shoulder. They are defined as a partial disruption of the fibers of the tendon with no communication between the subacromial bursa and the glenohumeral joint (Fukuda 2003). The main feature in considering a partial-thickness tear is the depth of the lesion more than the width of the involved area (Ellman 1990; Snyder et al. 1991). There are three major subtypes: (1) "bursal-sided tear" when the bursal surface of the tendon is involved; (2) "intratendinous tear" if the disruption of the fibers occurs within the tendon; and (3) "joint-sided tear" when the lesion involves the surface of the tendon adjacent to the joint (Codman 1934).

Among the tendons, supraspinatus is the most frequently involved, sometimes together with the tendon of infraspinatus although rarely with subscapularis. Isolated lesions of infraspinatus, teres minor, or subscapularis tendons are not uncommon (Fukuda 2003). Neer (1972) classified rotator cuff pathology into three stages: stage I considers the presence of pain, inflammation, edema, and hemorrhage, stage II when tendon fibrosis is present, and stage III initial disruption of the fibers. The Neer staging system has been revised by different authors (Fukuda et al. 1983, 1987a, 1987b; Olsewski and Depew 1994). The modified stage I is characterized by pain, inflammation, edema, hemorrhage, and chronic fibrosis; modified stage II includes partial-thickness tears and modified stage III full-thickness tears. In still another classification scheme, Ellman (1990) used location and size as factors for assessing the degree of the tear. Considering 8–12 mm the mean thickness of the supraspinatus tendon, Ellman classified grade I tears as having a depth of <3 mm or 25% of the tendon thickness, grade II tears of 3–6 mm or 50%, and grade III tears >6 mm or >50%. The grade is determined intraoperatively using an arthroscopic probe.

Snyder et al. (1991; Snyder 1994) introduced a separate entity for the partial articular supraspinatus tendon avulsion or "PASTA lesion." Also, they proposed a new classification for cuff lesions in which partial articular-sided lesions are indicated as "A," partial bursal-sided lesions as "B," and full-thickness are addressed as "C." The letter is associated with a number (from 0 to 4) indicating the size and the severity of the lesions (**Table 8.1**).

Incidence and prevalence

The exact incidence of partial-thickness rotator cuff tears (PTRCTs) remains unknown. Many lesions, especially the intratendinous ones, are identified only intraoperatively, and many asymptomatic partial tears remain unknown until MRI demonstrates their presence (Sher

Table 8.1 Classification of partial-thickness rotator cuff tears patterns

Authors	Type	Fields	Year
Neer (1972)	Pathological progression of the anatomical findings	Stage I: inflammation, hemorrhage, edema, and pain Stage II: tendon fibrosis Stage III: progressive tearing	1972
Ellman (1990)	Grade of lesion defined in terms of the depth with an arthroscopic measurement	Grade I: depth tears <3 mm or 25% of thickness Grade II: for 3–6 mm or 50% Grade III: >6 mm or >50%.	1990
Snyder et al. (1991); Snyder (1994)	Modification of the classification system for partial-thickness lesion with location and tear severity. The "PASTA lesion" is listed separately	Location of tear: A articular B bursal C full thickness Grade: 0: normal cuff 1: inflamed synovium and superficial fraying <1 cm 2: moderate tear with actual fiber disruption 1–2 cm 3: disruption and fragmentation of tissues 2–3 cm 4: complex PTRCT (flap formation and retraction) >3 cm	1991

PASTA, partial articular-sided tendon avulsion; PTRCT, partial-thickness rotator cuff tear.

et al. 1995). What is clear is that the incidence of PTRCTs increases with age. In a cadaveric study of 1934, Codman reported an incidence rate of complete ruptures of 10–20%, which must be doubled if partial-thickness tears were included. These data have been confirmed by successive cadaveric studies. Lohr and Uhthoff (1987) showed a rate of 32% for partial-thickness tears and of 19% for full-thickness tears occurring in the supraspinatus tendon of 306 cadaveric shoulders. Yamanaka and Fukuda (1987) studied 249 cadavers, reporting an incidence rate of 13% for partial-thickness tears, whereas complete tears accounted for 7%. Of the PTRCTs 55% were intratendinous, 27% were articular sided, and 18% were bursal sided.

Others have had different results. Several studies show (Itoi and Tabata 1992; Ryu 1992; Olsewski and Depew 1994; Gartsman and Milne 1995; Weber 1997; McConville and Ianotti 1999) a rate of articular-sided tears that was two to three times more than bursal-sided tears, whereas intratendinous-sided tears were less frequent. PTRCTs are probably underdiagnosed, hence the small prevalence in several series (Fukuda 2003). A systematic review addressing incidence rate of rotator cuff tears as determined by cadaveric exam, ultrasonography, and magnetic resonance imaging (MRI) reports that, in a cadaveric population of 4629 shoulders with a mean age of 70 years, the prevalence of partial-thickness tears was 18.49% compared with 11.75% for full-thickness tears. US-based studies found a prevalence of PTRCTs of 17.2% for asymptomatic patients and 6.7% for symptomatic patients, whereas an MRI-based study reported a prevalence of 15.9% and 8.9% for asymptomatic and symptomatic patients, respectively. The authors concluded that about 5–10% of patients presenting with shoulder pain have symptomatic PTRCTs and that full-thickness rotator cuff tears (FTRCTs) are more symptomatic than PTRCTs (Reilly et al. 2006).

Rotator cuff lesions are particularly common in throwing (or overhead) athletes. Connor et at (2003) found a prevalence of PTRCTs of 40% (8/20) in 20 asymptomatic overhead athletes. Payne et al. (1997) reported that, in their case series of young athletes, 92% (39/42) of the lesions were articular-sided tears.

PATHOGENESIS/PATHOLOGY (TABLE 8.2)

The pathogenesis of rotator cuff lesions is complex and multifactorial. Traditionally, it has been related to intrinsic and extrinsic factors or to a traumatic mechanism.

Extrinsic factors

Extrinsic compression of the rotator cuff by the acromion is commonly referred to as the impingement syndrome. Bigliani et al. (1991) classified the acromion shape into three types: type I flat (17% of cuff tears), type II curved (43% of cuff tears), and type III hooked (39% of cuff tears). Each type of acromion, under the correct circumstances, can contribute to extrinsic impingement. Anterior instability is also associated with rotator cuff tearing. Anterior instability can result from many different conditions such as thinning of the anterior band of the inferior glenohumeral ligament, or a posterior capsular contracture (Kvitne et al. 1995; Burkhart et al. 2003). Repetitive microtrauma can result in excessive humeral motion and eventual attrition of the rotator cuff tendons. Instability is probably the cause of many of the rotator cuff injuries identified in the overhead athlete (Walch et al. 1992; Neer 1972; Davidson et al. 1995; Jobe 1996; Sonnery-Cottet et al. 2002; Meister et al. 2003).

Intrinsic factors

Pathological factors occurring within the cuff itself are globally called intrinsic factors. The *degeneration–microtrauma theory* (Yadav et al. 2009) considers the association of age-related degenerative changes and microtraumatism. In a cadaveric study Hashimoto et al. (2003) identified seven features: thinning and disorientation of the collagen fibers (one of the main features is the loss of the wavy shape of the fibers that become linear), myxoid degeneration, hyaline degeneration, vascular proliferation, fatty infiltration, chondroid metaplasia, and calcification. Kannus and Jozsa (1991) describe how vascular proliferation and fatty infiltration are more frequent at the bursal side of the tendons and probably represent the signs of a healing process. Soslowsky et al. (2000), in a histological and biomechanical study of an animal model, demonstrated that repetitive microtrauma leads to an increased expression of inflammatory molecules (cyclooxygenase 2 or COX-2, prostaglandin E_2 or PGE_2), metalloproteases (MMP1–3 and -13) and an increased oxidative stress. Cuff vascularity may also have a role in rotator cuff tearing.

Traditionally, a critical hypovascular zone of the footprint of supraspinatus was described. Many authors (Lohr and Uhthoff 1987; Fukuda 2003; Uhthoff and Sano 1997; Ide et al. 2005) have suggested that the hypovascular zone may contribute to the pathogenesis of rotator cuff pathology. This hypothesis is still controversial. Moseley and Goldie (1963) demonstrated in a cadaveric rotator cuff study that no zone of hypovascularity was present in injured specimens. In a subsequent histological study by Brooks et al. (1992) injured specimens were noted to have a diminished number and diameter of vessels and no significant hypovascularity. Indeed, intraoperatively Doppler flowmetry studies performed by Fukuda et al. (1990) and Swiontkowski et al. (1990) demonstrated areas of hypervascularity in correspondence to the critical zone. Uhthoff et al. (1992) suggested that the hypervascularity should be related to the synovitis occurring because of the repetitive microtrauma.

Traumatic factors

Rotator cuff tears related to traumatic mechanisms are less common than degenerative tears. Traumatic tears are more common in younger

Table 8.2 Overview on risk factors for rotator cuff tears.

Intrinsic factors	Extrinsic factors	Traumatic factors
Age-related degenerative changes: decreased cellularity, fascicular thinning and disruption, and dystrophic calcification Metabolic changes: accumulation of granulation tissue Vascular changes: relative frequency of articular-sided versus bursal-sided partial-thickness tears may potentially be related to this difference in vascularity	Classic subacromial impingement Shoulder instability (typically anterior) Internal impingement Anterior instability Posterior capsular contracture Decreased humeral retroversion Tension overload Poor throwing mechanics Scapular muscle imbalance	Single traumatic injury Repetitive microtrauma Excessive tensile load of the cuff

people and can occur secondary to direct trauma (i.e., a fall) or non-direct trauma from a sudden contraction of the shoulder muscles after a fall (Blevins et al. 1996).

CLINICAL PRESENTATION

One of the main clinical features of the PTRCTs is pain, especially nocturnal pain. However, not all PTRCTs are symptomatic. Indeed in a series of 58 patients followed longitudinally with a PTRCT, Yamaguchi (1998) reported that 51% became symptomatic over a period of 2.8 years. Reilly et al. (2006) suggested that the lesions detectable only by radiological assessment may represent a presymptomatic stage. Gschwend et al. (1988) and Fukuda (2003) suggested that this should be kept in mind because PTRCTs may be more painful than full-thickness tears. The relationship between hand dominance and painful rotator cuff lesions is still controversial, some studies showing significant correlation (Jay 2010) and others reporting the contrary (Milgrom et al. 1995).

Fukuda et al. (1996) divided symptoms associated with rotator cuff disease into two groups: category A symptoms related to inflammation of the subacromial bursa and tendinopathy and category B symptoms resulting from a torn tendon. Group A (pain, signs of fluid, a painful arc, an impingement sign, a positive procaine test, and contracture) may be reversible after conservative measures; group B (drop-arm sign, crepitus, muscle weakness, and atrophy of the spinati) are irreversible after conservative measures alone. The same authors noticed that, of the subtypes of PTRCTs, the most symptomatic was the bursal-sided one, suggesting an early surgical management to decrease symptoms and recovery function.

Physical examination

Clinical examination starts with a careful history taking to determine when symptoms arose, if they were related to a traumatic events, and the presence of pain and its features (nocturnal, location, referral, relationship to shoulder motion). A visual analogue scale (VAS) is generally used to assess degree of pain. A functional score may be helpful to evaluate the shoulder's response to intervention. The physical exam includes inspection and palpation (of the acromial arc and the region corresponding to the long head of biceps) to determine pain and muscle atrophy, assessment of motion and strength, and provocative tests. Range of movement (ROM) testing, both passive and active, are performed and compared with the contralateral side. Assessment of cervical spine function should be performed to exclude a compressive neuropathy that may be responsible for radicular involvement in the shoulder region.

Inspection and palpation of the cervical region, active and passive cervical range of motion, and provocative tests, such as Sperling's maneuver, are important aspects of the physical exam. Once the intrinsic shoulder origin has been ascertained, specific tests for rotator cuff function are performed. Rotator cuff testing includes Jobe's test for the supraspinatus tendon, Patte's test and the drop sign of infraspinatus, and the lift-off or Napoleon's test for subscapularis function. Neer's sign and test, Yocum's test, and Hawkins' test are the commonly performed impingement tests. Each can be performed with or without subacromial local anesthetic injection.

It is difficult to differentiate partial- and full-thickness rotator cuff tears by clinical tests alone. Hertel et al. (1996) described the lag sign which may be useful in differentiating a full-thickness from a partial-thickness tear; the external rotation lag sign (ERLS) for supraspinatus and infraspinatus tendons is generally negative in the presence of partial-thickness tears although it is positive in full-thickness lesions. Muscle strength is generally decreased when a full-thickness tear occurs, whereas absence of pain and preserved muscle strength performing a supraspinatus test suggest a modified stage I or II rotator (especially articular-sided or intratendinous PTRCTs) cuff disease (Matava et al. 2005). Shoulder instability should be also investigated, especially in younger patients and/or athletes because of the possible coexistence of these two disorders. Many clinical tests are available, and they are divided into laxity tests (anterior drawer test, Jahnke's test, sulcus sign, Gagey's test) and apprehension tests (Rockwood's test, fulcrum test, relocation test). Finally, the long head of biceps is evaluated (O'Brien's test, Yergason's test, Speed's test) to assess its role in producing shoulder pain.

DIAGNOSIS (TABLE 8.3)

Clinical assessment is often insufficient to diagnose partial-thickness rotator cuff tears. The use of imaging diagnostic tools is necessary. Ultrasonography and MRI are most helpful, with both being very accurate for detecting full-thickness rotator cuff tears, but less accurate for detecting partial-thickness tears.

Shoulder radiographs, arthrography, and bursography

Shoulder radiographs are generally not essential for the diagnosis of partial-thickness rotator cuff tears. However, radiographs can furnish indirect signs of conditions related to the development of rotator cuff pathology (such us a type I, II, or III acromion of Bigliani) or indirect signs of rotator cuff lesions (a subchondral cyst in the greater tuberosity

Table 8.3 Features of different diagnostic tools available for rotator cuff tears diagnosis

Technique	Accuracy	Costs	Invasiveness	Time
Shoulder treatment	From 15% (Gartsman and Milne 1995) to 83%. (Lohr and Uhthoff 1990)	Normal	–	Fast
Bursography	67% (Fukuda et al. 1987b), although Itoi and Tabata (1992) reported a success rate of only 25%	Normal	–	Fast
Ultrasonography	Higher accuracy to diagnose full-thickness tears than tears (Wiener and Seitz 1993)	Low	–	Fast
MRI	Traughber and Goodwin (1992) gave a sensitivity of 56–72% and a specificity of 83–85% for arthroscopically proven, partial-thickness lesions	High	–	Slow
MRA (contrast RM arthrography)	The use of MRA, fat-suppression techniques, and positional variation have been introduced to improve diagnostic accuracy (Quinn et al. 1995; Reinus et al. 1995)	Very High	+	Very slow
Diagnostic arthroscopy	Arthroscopy is an excellent support in the diagnosis and treatment of partial-thickness rotator cuff tears	Very high	++	Very slow

MRA, magnetic resonance arthroscopy; MRI, magnetic resonance imaging.

or, in throwing athletes, a greater tuberosity notch has been correlated with the presence PTRCTs). Arthrography of the shoulder evaluates the integrity of the undersurface of the rotator cuff (Nakagawa et al. 2001). In the past, arthrography was considered the standard diagnostic test to distinguish between a full or partial tear in the rotator cuff. Studies of double-contrast arthrography reported sensitivity and specificity ranging from 0.71 to 1.0, and the use of conventional single- or double-contrast arthrography is still considered to be highly accurate in detecting PTRCTs (Farin et al. 1996). Its use has, however, been widely replaced by ultrasonography and MRI. The role of bursography is limited to the diagnosis of a bursal-sided, partial-thickness tear. The range of accuracy is wide, ranging from 25% (Itoi et al. 1992) to 67% (Fukuda et al. 1987b). Similar to radiographs and arthrography, the clinical use of bursography is strongly reduced in diagnosing PTRCTs.

Ultrasonography

More than 25 years ago, Matsen and Kilcoine (1984) introduced the use of ultrasonography for the diagnosis of rotator cuff lesions. Its sensitivity and specificity are high in diagnosing full-thickness tears whereas their values decrease in detecting partial-thickness rotator cuff lesions. In a systematic review (Dinnes et al. 2003) of 38 studies evaluating the diagnostic features of ultrasonography, the overall sensitivity and specificity for full-thickness rotator cuff tears were 0.87 (95% confidence interval [CI] 0.84–0.89) and 0.96 (95% CI 0.94–0.97). For partial-thickness tears, the sensitivity of ultrasonography is 0.67 (95% CI 0.61–0.73). The difficulty of differentiating an articular-sided, partial-thickness tear from a tendinopathy may be a source of error, both appearing as a hypoechoic area, and the greater the size of a bursal-sided tear the greater the possibility to mistake it for a full-thickness tears (Teefey et al. 2005). Currently, ultrasonography is a powerful diagnostic tool, but outcomes are strongly dependent on the operator's competence and experience because of the long learning curve needed to acquire the technique.

MRI (Fig. 8.1)

Advances in technologies (shoulder coils, imaging software, data-capturing techniques) have made MRI the diagnostic tool of choice for the assessment of rotator cuff lesions. For a thorough description of MRI technology, see Chapter 7. In simple terms, the T1-weighted images produced by MRI allow assessment of overall rotator cuff morphology. T2-weighted images allow the detection of edema and tissue fluids arising when an inflammatory process is present. More recent sequences (fast-spin echo, fat suppression) have improved the accuracy of MRI. A systematic review (Dinnes et al. 2003) of 20 studies evaluating MRI for the diagnosis of rotator cuff tears reported, as the overall pooled sensitivity, 0.83 (95% CI 0.79–0.86) and specificity as 0.86 (95% CI 0.83–0.88) for any cuff lesions (full- or partial-thickness rotator cuff), but both were statistically heterogeneous, with sensitivity ranging from 0.41 to 1.00, and specificity from 0.48 to 1.00.

Considering only full-thickness lesions, overall pooled sensitivity and specificity become higher, whereas they decrease as only partial-thickness tears are investigated (the pooled sensitivity is 0.44 [95% CI 0.36–0.51], specificity 0.90 [95% CI 0.87–0.92]). The sensitivity of diagnosing PTRCTs may be improved in throwing athletes by the use of the throwing or the abducted and externally rotated position (ABER). As mentioned earlier, rotator cuff lesions are not always symptomatic. Sher et al. (1995) reported on a series of 96 asymptomatic patients. Of these 96, 34% (33/96) had a rotator cuff lesion. The frequency of full- and partial-thickness tears increased significantly with age. Rotator cuff lesions were present in 54% (25/46) of patients aged >60 years, in 28% (7/25) of patients aged between 40 and 60, and in 4% (1/25) of patients aged between 19 and 39 years. Although MRI was less sensitive compared with ultrasonography in diagnosing PTRCTs, it has the advantages of being non-operator dependent and MRI can address coexisting pathologies (Olsewski et al. 1994).

Contrast MRA

Contrast MR arthrography (MRA) been developed to increase diagnostic accuracy (Reinus et al. 1995). A systematic review (Dinnes et al. 2003) of six studies ascertaining the accuracy of MRA reported that it may be very accurate for the detection of full-thickness rotator cuff tears (overall pooled sensitivity 0.95 [95% CI 0.82–0.98] and specificity 0.93 [95% CI 0.84–0.97]), whereas, with regard to partial-thickness tears (only three of the six studies consider PTRCTs), sensitivity is 0.62 (95% CI 0.40–0.80) and specificity 0.92 (95% CI 0.83–0.97). Lee and Lee (2002) demonstrated that MRA sensitivity increases up to 100% when changing from a coronal oblique view (sensitivity 21%) to an ABER position. Two studies comparing MRI and MRA show that higher outcomes are reached with the latter. Hodler et al. (1992) found a higher accuracy for MRA in detecting partial-thickness tears whereas MRI and MRA showed no difference in detecting full-thickness tears. Yagci et al. (2001) found better performance of MRA than MRI regardless of the thickness of the rotator cuff lesion. In conclusion MRA is a reliable and highly sensitive diagnostic tool, although its weakness points are invasiveness and elevated costs.

Diagnostic arthroscopy

The development of arthroscopic surgery furnishes a better diagnosis and management of rotator cuff pathology. When a clinically and radiologically based diagnosis is inconclusive, arthroscopy allows excellent examination of both the articular and the bursal sides of the rotator cuff. Many techniques have been developed to improve the diagnostic accuracy of arthroscopy. The first step is thorough inspection and palpation of the cuff's footprint, which is often diagnostic. With regard to articular surface tears, the Fukuda color test using methylene blue (Fukuda et al. 1987a) and the Snyder suture marking technique (Snyder et al. 1991) are available. Both can confirm or rule out a full-thickness lesion. The Lo and Burkhart (2002) "bubble sign" is also useful. This test is performed by injecting 0.5 mL of saline solution through a 18 gauge spinal needle, from the bursal surface directly into the tendon area suspected of being involved by the lesion. The presence of an intratendinous tear is suggested if the solution results in dilation of that tendon's area.

MANAGEMENT

The management of partial-thickness rotator cuff is still controversial. The lack of clinical trials based on large populations and the dearth of clinical trials analyzing the outcomes of the different treatment options make it difficult to establish a widely shared management algorithm. Conservative management is usually the first approach to partial tears of the rotator cuff. Physical therapy, activity modification, and synergistic muscle strength may all help improve the clinical situation.

However, hypovascularity of the critical zone of the injured tendon, together with the mechanical stresses to which tendons are subjected, may contribute to poor spontaneous healing (Ellman and Kay 1991) and poor success rate with non-surgical management. The low rate of tendon healing (less than 50% according to Breazeale and Craig [1997]) associated with conservative management has made some professionals adopt a more aggressive approach.

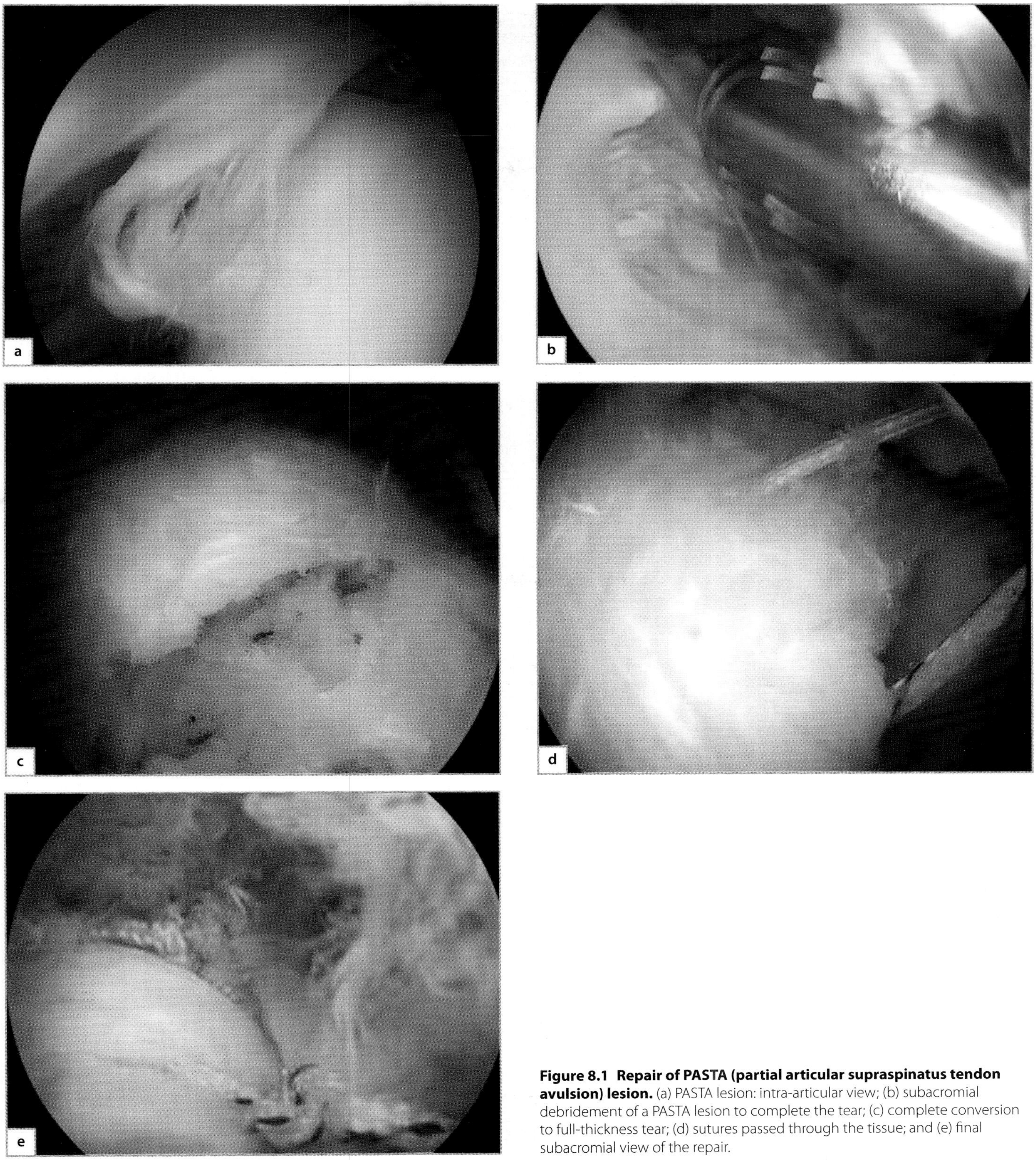

Figure 8.1 Repair of PASTA (partial articular supraspinatus tendon avulsion) lesion. (a) PASTA lesion: intra-articular view; (b) subacromial debridement of a PASTA lesion to complete the tear; (c) complete conversion to full-thickness tear; (d) sutures passed through the tissue; and (e) final subacromial view of the repair.

Table 8.4 Description, indication, outcomes, and complications for each surgical technique

Surgical procedure	Technique	Surgical steps	Results	Complications
Debridement with or without subacromial decompression	1. Examine the subacromial space 2. Assess the integrity of the bursal side of the cuff 3. Evaluated for subacromial impingement 4. Facilitate visualization and working space, when performing an arthroscopic cuff repair	1. The bursa can be distended with 10 mL of 0.25% bupivacaine with epinephrine 2. A blunt obturator is used to "pop" into the space from the posterior glenohumeral scope portal 3. To facilitate assessment of the cuff on the corresponding bursal side, a spinal needle is used to percutaneously pass a monofilament marking suture (PDS) into the cuff defect before withdrawing the scope from the glenohumeral joint	Budoff et al. (1998): 79 shoulders treated with arthroscopic debridement at 25 to 93 months of follow-up 77% had associated labral pathology, 89% showed good to excellent results in with less than 5 years of follow-up based on the UCLA rating scale. With longer follow-up, 5-year good and excellent results decreased to 81%	In an incorrect entrance, the prominent posterior subacromial bursal can mistakenly show that there is bursal hypertrophy and subacromial impingement. and lead to unnecessary bursectomy or subacromial decompression Inadvertently cutting the marking suture
Conversion to full-thickness tears	Bursal-sided, partial-thickness tears are usually completed to full-thickness tears with or without a subacromial decompression	Repair using suture anchors	Park et al. (2004): 22 patients with arthroscopic repair and decompression compared with 20 patients with full-thickness rotator cuff tears in 34 months of average follow-up Both groups had similar improvements in pain, motion, and function by ASES scores, and 93% of all patients had good-to-excellent results with a 95% rate of satisfactory outcome with regard to pain reduction and functional outcome	
Transtendon repair	Debridement and repair	The articular tear, including a intratendinous extension, is debrided back to healthy tissue, and a monofilament-marking suture is placed percutaneously into the center of the defect	Waibl and Buess (2005)) reported 91% (22 consecutive non-athlete patients) overall good and excellent results Ide et al. (2005) reported, in 17 patients, at an average of 39 months follow-up, finding 14 good, 1 fair, and no poor results. Of 6 overhead athletes, 2 returned to their previous level, 3 to a lower level, and 1 did not return Duralde and Kimmerly (2005) reported good or excellent results in 20 of 24 patients at 14 months Conway (2001) reported his experience repairing deep intratendinous partial-thickness tears using a transtendinous technique in a group of 14 baseball players (13 pitchers and 1 outfielder) Of the 9 players followed more than 1 year after surgery (7 professionals and 2 college students), 8 (89%) returned to play at the same or higher level	
Intratendinous repair	Intratendinous suture imbrication repair	A spinal needle is introduced off the acromial edge and directed across the cuff's intratendinous split. Monofilament suture (#1 PDS) is shuttled through the needle, retrieved, and withdrawn from the anterior interval portal	Brockmeier et al. (2008) presented a technique of arthroscopic intratendinous repair for delaminated partial-thickness tears in high-level overhead athletes. In this study at early follow-up of 5 months, the investigators noted encouraging results and reported that longer-term follow-up is necessary	

Contd...

Contd...

Surgical procedure	Technique	Surgical steps	Results	Complications
Mini-open technique	Surgeon can obtain greater exposure by detaching anterior deltoid for 2.0 cm	Combined arthroscopic and open surgical approach that allows a reduction in the morbidity to anterior deltoid This technique is performed using the short deltoid-splitting approach	Weber (1997) reviewed the outcomes after arthroscopic debridement and acromioplasty (14 good and no excellent results) versus acromioplasty and mini-open repair (28 good and 3 excellent results) at 2- to 7-year follow-up Mazouè and Andrews (2006): results of mini-open rotator cuff repair in 16 professional baseball players (12 pitchers) at an average 67-month follow-up This cohort included patients with full-thickness tears; they found that only two players (one pitcher and one position player) with repairs of their dominant shoulder were able to return to a high competitive level of baseball Only 1 of the 12 pitchers was able to return to competitive professional baseball	Avulsion of deltoid from the anterior acromion by overzealous retraction

Non-surgical management

There is general agreement that conservative management should be undertaken as the initial treatment in those patients in whom the partial tear involves less than 50% of the tendon thickness (Liem et al. 2008). The duration of non-surgical treatment should be adapted to the patient's features, such as clinical and radiological findings, degree of impaired function, and physical needs. Conventional non-surgical measures include relative rest, application of cold or heat, massage, oral non-steroidal anti-inflammatory drugs (NSAIDs), modification of activities, and gentle exercises for maintaining and increasing the range of movement (Fukuda 2003). The initial approach is pain control. Oral NSAIDs and two or three intra-articular injections of corticosteroids (no more because of the steroid's possible detrimental effects on soft tissues) can be helpful to control the pain (Matava et al. 2005). As pain is reduced, physical therapy is mandatory to regain muscle strength and avoid shoulder stiffness. Stretching of contracted capsular structures is paramount to improvement.

The anterior capsular tightness is treated with external rotation stretching while the shoulder is an adducted position. This method avoids positioning the arm in an impingement position (60–120° abduction). Internal rotation with adducted shoulder and horizontal adduction or cross-body adduction exercises are recommended to release the posterior capsule (Matava et al. 2005). As pain decreases and range of movement increases, it is necessary to introduce strengthening exercises for the rotator cuff and periscapular musculature to restore the normal kinematics of the shoulder girdle and normal scapulothoracic mechanics (Fukuda 2003; Matava et al. 2005). Although these measures may lead to improvement for articular-sided or intratendinous partial-thickness lesions, less benefit is obtained when treating bursal-sided tears. This is probably due to the major relationship between bursal-sided tears and subacromial impingement. For this reason, when bursal-sided pathology is established by clinical and radiological proof, Fukuda et al. (1987a) recommend surgical intervention.

Surgical management (Table 8.4)

Many surgical treatment options are available for the management of PTRCTs, including:

- Debridement
- Subacromial decompression (with or without debridement)
- Tendon repair.

The decision for debridement versus repair is patient and pathology specific. Selective surgical repair for bursal-sided tears and articular tears involving more than 50% of tendon thickness are generally recommended (Ellman grade III), whereas debridement is usually recommended when the tear involves less than 50% of thickness (Ellman grades I and II).

Arthroscopic debridement with or without subacromial decompression (Fig. 8.2)

The objective of surgical debridement is to remove unstable and degenerative tissue that could be responsible for creating pain. Standard anterior and posterior portals are used to address articular- and bursal-sided tears as well as intratendinous ones. Lesions are identified and debrided with soft-tissue resectors. We advocate the use of the Snyder suture marking technique (Snyder et al. 1991) to assess the effective thickness of the lesion. This technique consists of passing a monofilament suture through a spinal needle into the tendon, before introducing the arthroscope into the subacromial space. If an intratendinous lesion is identified, debridement is recommended. Bursectomy is often necessary to better visualize the lesion or when the bursa is thickened and edematous.

Coexisting pathologies (labral disruptions, long head of biceps tendinopathy, or chondral lesions) should also be visualized. When a subacromial pathology is identified, a subacromial decompression is usually performed. An electrosurgical knife is used to remove the acromial insertion of the coracoacromial ligament. Bursectomy is performed. As the acromion is exposed, an acromioplasty is performed using a resector or powered burr to remove the deleterious bone spurs and osteophytes.

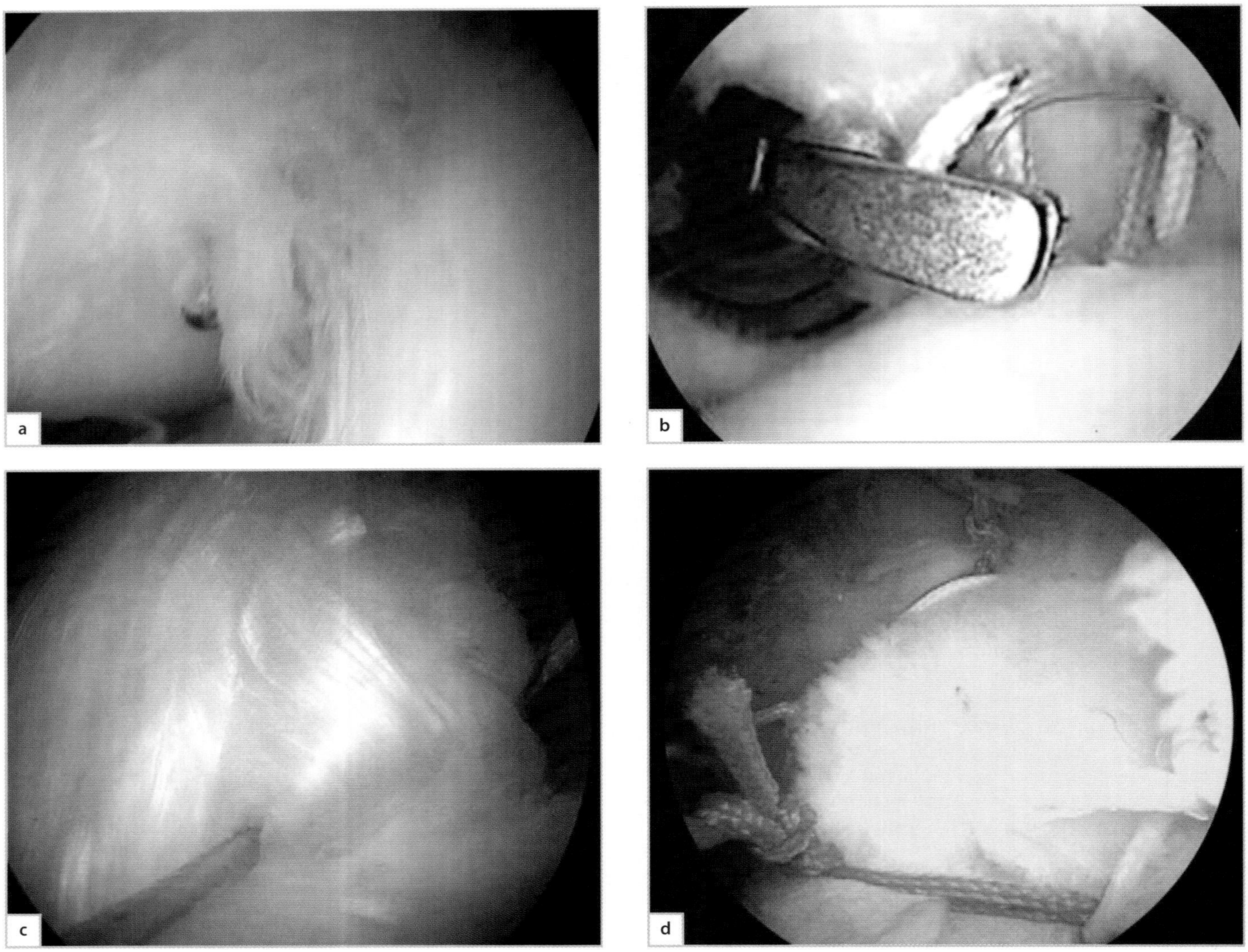

Figure 8.2 Repair of lesion. (a) Intra-articular PASTA (partial articular supraspinatus tendon avulsion) lesion; (b) intra-articular repair: the sutures are passed through the healthy tissue as indicated by the line; (c) intra-articular repair: subacromial view of the sutures passed through the tissue; and (d) intra-articular rotator cuff repair: final subacromial view.

Arthroscopic repair of partial-thickness tears

There is an increasing trend for repair of partial-thickness rotator cuff tears. Tear depth is a key factor, but precise depth measurement is difficult. Surgeons have to use indirect measurement techniques, such as comparing a known reference (e.g., a shaver blade with established length) with the uncovered area of the footprint fibers, bearing in mind that the mean cuff thickness is 12 mm in depth (Ellman 1990). Bursal-sided partial tears can be repaired after a conversion to a full-thickness tear. Articular-sided tears can also be completed and repaired as a full-thickness lesion or directly repaired via the "transtendon" technique. Intratendinous tears may be repaired by débriding and then reapproximating the diseased area using a suture placation technique.

Conversion to full-thickness tears (see Fig. 8.1)

After converting the partial-thickness tear to a full-thickness one, the lesion is repaired directly to bone using a suture anchor technique. Two pairs of non-absorbable sutures are passed through the tendon and tightened using a sliding knot. The procedure can be performed via a mini-open or arthroscopic technique.

Transtendon repair (see Fig. 8.2)

Conversion to a full-thickness tear and direct repair have been widely used over time and have led to good results. However, excising normal tissue and excessive tendon advancement with the resultant excessive repair strain are potential disadvantages of this technique.

Lo and Burkhart (2004) proposed a new technique named "the transtendon" repair, in which the lateral aspect of the tendon footprint is preserved while the medial one is restored by placing transtendon anchors. The transtendon repair starts with acromioplasty and a complete bursectomy to obtain adequate visualization necessary for placing the anchors. As the subacromial decompression is completed, the arthroscope is reintroduced into the glenohumeral space. The transtendon anchors are placed adjacent to the lateral aspect of the acromion with a 45° angle into the bone at the medial margin of the tendon footprint. Two anchors are used if the anteroposterior width of the lesion is

>1.5 cm. The sutures are passed through the residual tendon fibers into the subacromial space, where the sutures are tightened using a sliding knot. The procedure is finished with a general evaluation of both the subacromial and the intra-articular space (Lo and Burkhart 2004).

Intratendinous repair

Intratendinous repair is generally used to repair intratendinous, partial-thickness tears of overhead athletes. Goals of the techniques are to restore the articular surface of the torn tendon, to repair the disrupted fibers, and to eliminate shoulder over-constriction. Standard anterior and posterior portals are utilized, although an additional lateral portal may also be useful to adequately work in the subacromial space. The first step of the procedure is a thorough exam of the entire glenohumeral joint. Particular attention should be paid to the anterosuperior labrum and the capsuloligamentous structures. Once the diagnostic overview of the glenohumeral joint is completed, the intratendinous defect is addressed. A tissue grasper is introduced through the footprint without excessive tension. The injured tendon footprint area can then by debrided by a motorized shaver stimulating a healing process. Next the arthroscope is placed in the subacromial space, where the bursal surface is examined and a bursectomy is performed. Two spinal needles, percutaneously introduced throughout the entire thickness of the tendon, are used to pass two or more sutures. The sutures are retrieved and then tied to each other to obtain a mattress suture that attaches the articular-sided injured area to the healthy surrounding tissue (Brockmeier et al. 2008).

DISCUSSION

Non-surgical management

There is a paucity of data regarding the outcome of non-surgically treated, partial-thickness rotator cuff tears. In a histological cadaver study on 35 surgical specimens Fukuda (2003) found no evidence of active repair in any of the specimens examined. Rather, there were many instances of impending full-thickness tears on histological sections, which showed only narrow tissue connections.

Yamanaka and Matsumoto (1994) followed for 2 years, through arthrographic exam, 40 articular-sided partial tears managed non-surgically: 80% of the lesions progressed to a full-thickness lesion.

Surgical management

Debridement with or without decompression

Snyder et al. (1991) treated 31 patients with combined debridement of partial-thickness tears and concomitant subacromial decompression (only 18/31 patients). They reported 84% good-to-excellent results. Budoff and colleagues (1998) treated with debridement 79 shoulders affected by partial-thickness tears. Follow-up was for 25–93 months. The UCLA (University of California at Los Angeles) shoulder score was used to assess outcomes. Results were 89% good to excellent. However, after the fifth year of follow-up the good-to-excellent results decreased to 81%. Esch et al. (1988) reported on 71 patients with either a full- or partial-thickness rotator cuff tear. Patients were available for follow-up for at least 1 year, and were treated by arthroscopic subacromial decompression. Results showed that 76% of patients had satisfactory UCLA scores (pain, function, active forward flexion, and strength were improved), and 82% of the patients were satisfied. There was no difference in outcome between the partial- and the full-thickness lesions.

Cordasco et al. (2002) analyzed the outcomes from 162 patients who had either normal rotator cuffs, grade 1 (frayed tendon) partial-thickness tears, or grade 2 (<50% of the tendon) partial-thickness tears treated with arthroscopic acromioplasty and debridement. Although no differences were observed between patients with normal cuffs and those with partial-thickness tears of the rotator cuff comprising <50% of the tendon (grade 1 and 2), the subgroup of patients with grade 2B partial tears (bursal-sided tears affecting <50% of tendon thickness) had a significantly higher failure rate. The authors suggested that PTRCTs of >50% of tendon thickness are best treated surgically.

Payne et al. (1997) treated 43 athletes aged <40 years who had partial-thickness tears with arthroscopic debridement and subacromial decompression. Patients were divided into two groups according to the tear pathogenesis, traumatic and atraumatic. In the traumatic group, 12/14 (86%) had satisfactory outcomes, and 9/14 (64%) returned to pre-injury sports. Among atraumatic patients a 66% satisfactory rate (19/29 patients) and a 45% return to pre-injury sports (13/29 patients) were observed.

Surgical repair

Itoi and Tabata (1992) repaired, using open surgery with and without anterior acromioplasty, 38 shoulders with partial-thickness rotator cuff tears: 82% (31/38) good-to-excellent results were obtained. With regard to performing optional acromioplasty or coracoacromial ligament resection, no statistical difference between the groups was noted.

Conversion to full-thickness tears

Park et al. (2004) treated, with arthroscopic repair and decompression, 22 patients with partial-thickness tears (bursal or articular sided) and 20 patients with full-thickness rotator cuff tears, comparing their outcomes after surgery at an average follow-up of 34 months. The ASES rating system was used to assess the results. Pain, motion, and shoulder function were improved in both groups with no statistical differences, and good or excellent results were found in 39/42 (93%) of all patients. Overall satisfactory outcome with regard to pain reduction and functional outcome were reported in 40/42 (95%) patients. Deutsch (2007) treated 41 patients affected by a partial lesion of the rotator cuff of >50% of thickness using arthroscopic conversion of the PTRCT to a full-thickness tear and single-row suture anchor repair. After a mean follow-up of 38 months, significant improvements were demonstrated. The mean ASES score improved from 42 points (range 8–65 points) preoperatively to 93 points (range 62–100 points) postoperatively. Of the 41 patients, 40 (98%) were satisfied with their outcome.

Transtendon repair

Lo and Burkhart (2004) reported their experience with the transtendon repair in a cohort of 25 patients. At a minimum of 1-year follow-up, the mean UCLA shoulder rating scale score increased from 15 preoperatively to 32 postoperatively. Waibl and Buess (2005) reported the early results of their first 22 patients treated by transtendon repair: 91% overall good and excellent results were achieved. Ide et al. (2005) reported their experience with 17 patients treated by transtendon repair. The results, at an average of 39 months of follow-up, showed 14 good, 1 fair, and no poor results. Duralde and Kimmerly (2005) treated 24 patients with a similar technique. After an average follow-up of 14 months, good or excellent results were obtained in 20 of 24 patients. Conway (2001) used the transtendon repair technique to repair the partial-thickness lesions of 14 baseball players. Only nine patients were available at more than

1 year of follow-up and, among these, eight (89%) returned to play at the same or a higher level.

Intratendinous repair

Brockmeier et al. (2008), in a technical note, reported encouraging results after a mean follow-up of 5 months (range 1.5–8.5 months) in eight patients (five baseball players and three tennis players).

Mini-open technique

Weber (1997) reported on a population of 65 patients affected by partial-thickness rotator cuff tears. He compared the postoperative outcomes of 32 patients treated with debridement and acromioplasty with 33 patients with mini-open repair. Using the UCLA shoulder score as the outcome criterion, 14 good and no excellent results were achieved after arthroscopic debridement and acromioplasty. In contrast, 28 good and 3 excellent results were achieved after acromioplasty and mini-open repair. Follow-up was at 2–7 years. The author concluded that, although the arthroscopic approach leads to less early surgical morbidity, the mini-open repair technique favored better long-term results and decreased reoperation rates.

CONCLUSIONS

Conservative measures have been demonstrated to be an effective treatment for less than 50% of PTRCTs. The reason for this unsuccessful trend might be related to poor vascularity, especially on the articular surface of the cuff. This hypovascularity probably contributes to degenerative changes over time. It is a finding that is more common in older athletes. That said, this hypothesis remains controversial.

Arthroscopic debridement with or without subacromial decompression seems to be effective in managing patients whose partial tears approach 50% of the tendon's thickness. Different surgical techniques are available to repair PTRCTs, including transtendon repair, intratendinous repair, and conversion to full-thickness tears. The paucity of randomized, prospective studies specifically addressing the optimal management of partial-thickness rotator cuff tears does not allow an accurate determination of optimal technique.

Further studies are necessary to optimize the management of PTRCTs. In the meantime, we advocate that treatment should be strictly chosen according to the specific features of each patient.

REFERENCES

Bigliani LU, Ticker JB, Flatow EL, Soslowsky IJ, Mow VC. The relationship of acromial architecture to rotator cuff disease. Clin Sports Med 1991;10:823–838.

Blevins FT, Hayes WM, Warren RF: Rotator cuff injury in contact athletes. Am J Sports Med 1996;24:263–267.

Breazeale NM, Craig EV. Partial-thickness rotator cuff tears. Pathogenesis and treatment. Orthop Clin North Am 1997;28:145–155.

Brockmeier SF, Dodson CC, Gamradt SC, et al. Arthroscopic intratendinous repair of the delaminated partial-thickness rotator cuff tear in overhead athletes. Arthroscopy 2008;24:961–965.

Brooks CH, Revell WJ, Heatley FW. A quantitative histological study of the vascularity of the rotator cuff tendon. J Bone Joint Surg Br 1992;74:151–153.

Budoff JE, Nirschl RP, Guidi EJ. Debridement of partial-thickness tears of the rotator cuff without acromioplasty. Long-term follow-up and review of the literature. J Bone Joint Surg Am 1998;80:733–748.

Burkhart SS, Morgan CD, Kibler WB. The disabled throwing shoulder: spectrum of pathology. Part I: pathoanatomy and biomechanics. Arthroscopy 2003;19:404–420.

Codman EA. Rupture of the supraspinatus tendon. In: The shoulder rupture of the supraspinatus tendon and other lesions in and about the subacromial bursa. Boston, MA: Thomas Todd Publishing Co., 1934: 123–177.

Connor PM, Banks DM, Tyson AB, et al. Magnetic resonance imaging of the asymptomatic shoulder of overhead athletes: a 5-year follow-up study. Am J Sports Med 2003;31:724–727.

Conway JE. Arthroscopic repair of partial-thickness rotator cuff tears and SLAP lesions in professional baseball players. Orthop Clin North Am 2001;32:443–456.

Cordasco FA, Backer M, Craig EV, et al. The partial-thickness rotator cuff tear: is acromioplasty without repair sufficient? Am J Sports Med 2002;30:257–260.

Davidson PA, Elattrache NS, Jobe CM, et al. Rotator cuff and posterior-superior glenoid labrum injury associated with increased glenohumeral motion: a new site of impingement. J Shoulder Elbow Surg 1995;4:384–390.

Dinnes J, Loveman E, McIntyre L, et al. The effectiveness of diagnostic tests for the assessment of shoulder pain due to soft tissue disorders: a systematic review. Health Technol Assess 2003;7:1–166.

Deutsch A. Arthroscopic repair of partial-thickness tears of the rotator cuff. J Shoulder Elbow Surg 2007;16:193–201.

Duralde XA, Kimmerly S. The technique of arthroscopic repair of partial thickness rotator cuff tears. Techn Shoulder Elbow Surg 2005;6:116–123.

Ellman H. Diagnosis and treatment of incomplete rotator cuff tears. Clin Orthop Relat Res 1990;254:64–74.

Ellman H, Kay SP. Arthroscopic subacromial decompression for chronic impingement. Two- to five-year results. J Bone Joint Surg Br 1991;73:395–398.

Esch JC, Ozerkis LR, Helgager JA, et al. Arthroscopic subacromial decompression: results according to the degree of rotator cuff tear. Arthroscopy 1988;4:241–249.

Farin PU, Kaukanen E, Jaroma H, et al. Site and size of rotator-cuff tear. Findings at ultrasound, double-contrast arthrography, and computed tomography arthrography with surgical correlation. Invest Radiol 1996;317:387–394.

Fukuda H. The management of partial-thickness tears of the rotator cuff. J Bone Joint Surg Br 2003;85:3–11.

Fukuda H, Mikasa M, Ogawa K, Yamanaka K, Hamada K. The partial thickness tear of the rotator cuff. Orthop Trans 1983;7:137.

Fukuda H, Craig EV, Yamanaka K. Surgical treatment of incomplete thickness tears of rotator cuff: long-term follow-up. Orthop Trans 1987a;11:237–238.

Fukuda H, Mikasa M, Yamanaka K. Incomplete thickness rotator cuff tears diagnosed by subacromial bursography. Clin Orthop 1987b;223:51–58.

Fukuda H II, Hamada K, Yamanaka K. Pathology and pathogenesis of bursal-side rotator cuff tears viewed from en bloc histologic sections. Clin Orthop Relat Res 1990;254:75–80.

Fukuda H, Hamada K, Nakajima T, et al. Partial-thickness tears of the rotator cuff: a clinicopathological review based on 66 surgically verified cases. Int Orthop 1996;20:257–265.

Gartsman GM, Milne JC. Articular surface partial-thickness rotator cuff tears. J Shoulder Elbow Surg 1995;4:409–415.

Gschwend N, Ivosevic-Radovanovic D, Patte D. Rotator cuff tear: relationship between clinical and anatomopathological findings. Arch Orthop Trauma Surg 1988;107:7–15.

Hashimoto T, Nobuhara K, Hamada T. Pathologic evidence of degeneration as a primary cause of rotator cuff tear. Clin Orthop Relat Res 2003;415:111–120

Hertel R, Ballmer FT, Lombert SM, Gerber C. Lag signs in the diagnosis of rotator cuff rupture. J Shoulder Elbow Surg 1996;5:307–313.

Hodler J, Kursunoglu-Brahme S, Snyder SJ, et al. Rotator cuff disease: assessment with MR arthrography versus standard MR imaging in 36 patients with arthroscopic confirmation. Radiology 1992;182:431–436.

Ide J, Maeda S, Takagi K. Arthroscopic transtendon repair of partial-thickness articular-side tears of the rotator cuff: anatomical and clinical study. Am J Sports Med 2005;33:1672–1679.

Itoi E, Tabata S. Incomplete rotator cuff tears: results of operative treatment. Clin Orthop 1992;284:128–135.

Jay D. Keener Asymptomatic rotator cuff tears: Patient demographics and baseline shoulder function J Shoulder Elbow Surg 2010;19:1191–1198.

Jobe CM. Superior glenoid impingement: current concepts. Clin Orthop Relat Res 1996;330:98–107.

Kannus P, Jozsa L. Histopathological changes preceding spontaneous rupture of a tendon. A controlled study of 891 patients. J Bone Joint Surg Am 1991;73:1507–1525.

Kvitne RS, Jobe FW, Jobe CM. Shoulder instability in the overhand or throwing athlete. Clin Sports Med 1995;14:917–935.

Lee SY, Lee JK. Horizontal component of partial-thickness tears of rotator cuff: imaging characteristics and comparison of ABER view with oblique. Radiology 2002;224:470–476.

Liem D, Alci S, Dedy N, Steinbeck J, Marquardt B, Mollenhoff G. Clinical and structural results of partial supraspinatus tears treated by subacromial decompression without repair. Knee Surg Sports Traumatol Arthrosc 2008;16:967–972.

Lo IKY, Burkhart SS. Transtendon arthroscopic repair of partial-thickness, articular surface tears of the rotator cuff. Arthroscopy 2004;20:214–220.

Lo IK, Gonzalez DM, Burkhart SS. The bubble sign: an arthroscopic indicator of an intratendinous rotator cuff tear. Arthroscopy 2002;18:1029–1033.

Lohr JF, Uhthoff HK. The pathogenesis of degenerative rotator cuff tears. Orthop Trans 1987;11:237.

Lohr JF, Uhthoff HK. The microvascular pattern of the supraspinatus tendon. Clin Orthop Relat Res 1990;254:35–38.

McConville OR, Ianotti JP. Partial-thickness tears of the rotator cuff: evaluation and management. J Am Acad Orthop Surg 1999;7:32–43.

MacDonald PB, Clark P, Sutherland K. An analysis of the diagnostic accuracy of the Hawkins and Neer subacromial impingement signs. J Shoulder Elbow Surg 2000;9:299–301.

Matava MJ, Purcell DB, Rudzki JR. Partial-thickness rotator cuff tears. Am J Sports Med 2005;33:1405–1417.

Matsen FA, Kilcoine RF. Sonographic evaluation of the rotator cuff. Orthop Trans 1984;8:42.

Mazouè CG, Andrews JR. Repair of full-thickness rotator cuff tears in professional baseball players. Am J Sports Med 2006;34:182–189.

Meister K, Seroyer S. Arthroscopic management of the thrower's shoulder: internal impingement. Orthop Clin North Am 2003;34:539–547.

Milgrom C, Schaffler M, Gilbert S, van Holsbeeck M. Rotator-cuff changes in asymptomatic adults. The effect of age, hand dominance and gender. J Bone Joint Surg Br 1995;77:296–298.

Moseley HF, Goldie I. The arterial pattern of the rotator cuff of the shoulder. J Bone Joint Surg Br 1963;45:780–789.

Nakagawa S, Yoneda M, Hayashida K, et al. Greater tuberosity notch: an important indicator of articular-side partial rotator cuff tears in the shoulders of throwing athletes. Am J Sports Med 2001;29:762–770.

Neer CS. Anterior acromioplasty for the chronic impingement syndrome in the shoulder: a preliminary report. J Bone Joint Surg Am 1972;67:41–50.

Olsewski JM, Depew AD. Arthrscopic subacromial decompression and rotator cuff debridement for stage II and stage III impingement. Arthroscopy 1994;10:61–68.

Park JY, Chung KT, Yoo MJ. A serial comparison of arthroscopic repairs for partial- and full-thickness rotator cuff tears. Arthroscopy 2004;20:705–711.

Payne LZ, Altchek DW, Craig EV, Warren RF. Arthroscopic treatment of partial rotator cuff tears in young athletes. A preliminary report. Am J Sports Med 1997;25:299–305.

Quinn SF, Sheley RC, Demlow TA, Szumowski J. Rotator cuff tendon tears: evaluation with fat-suppressed MR imaging with arthroscopic correlation in 100 patients. Radiology 1995;195:497–500.

Reilly P, Macleod I, Macfarlane R, et al. Dead men and radiologists don't lie: a review of cadaveric and radiological studies of rotator cuff tear prevalence. Ann R Coll Surg Engl 2006;88:116–121.

Reinus WR, Shady KL, Mirowitz SA, Totty WG. MR diagnosis of rotator cuff tears of the shoulder: value of using T2-weighted fat-saturated images. AJR Am J Roentgenol 1995;164:1451–1455.

Ryu RKN. Arthroscopic subacromial decompression: a clinical review. Arthroscopy 1992;8:141–147.

Sher JS, Uribe JW, Posada A, et al. Abnormal findings on magnetic resonance images of asymptomatic shoulders. J Bone Joint Surg Am 1995;77:10–15.

Snyder SJ, Pachelli AF, Del Pizzo W, et al. Partial thickness rotator cuff tears: results of arthroscopic treatment. Arthroscopy 1991;7:1–7.

Snyder SJ, II. Arthroscopic evaluation and treatment of the rotator cuff. In: Pennington J, McCurdy P (eds), Shoulder Arthroscopy. New York: McGraw-Hill, 1994:148–149.

Sonnery-Cottet B, Edwards TB, Noel E, et al. Results of arthroscopic treatment of posterosuperior glenoid impingement in tennis players. Am J Sports Med 2002;30:227–232.

Soslowsky LJ, Thomopoulos S, Tun S, et al. Neer Award 1999. Overuse activity injures the supraspinatus tendon in an animal model: a histologic and biomechanical study. J Shoulder Elbow Surg 2000;9:79– 84.

Swiontkowski MF, Iannotti JP, Boulas HJ, Esterhai JL. Intraoperative assessment of rotator cuff vascularity using laser Doppler flowmetry. In: Post M, Morrey BF, Hawkins RJ (eds), Surgery of the Shoulder. St Louis, MO: Mosby, 1990: 208–212.

Teefey SA, Middleton WD, Payne WT, Yamaguchi K. Detection and measurement of rotator cuff tears with sonography: analysis of diagnostic errors. AJR Am J Roentgenol 2005;184:1768–1773.

Traughber PD, Goodwin TE. Shoulder MRI: arthroscopic correlation with emphasis on partial tears. J Comput Assist Tomogr 1992;16:129–133.

Uhthoff HK, Sano H. Pathology of failure of the rotator cuff tendon. Orthop Clin North Am 1997;28:31–41.

Uhthoff HK, Sarkar K. Periarticular soft tissue conditions causing pain in the shoulder. Curr Opin Rheumatol 1992;4:241–246.

Waibl B, Buess E. Technical note: partial-thickness articular surface supraspinatus tears: a new transtendon suture technique. Arthroscopy 2005;21:376–381.

Walch G, Boileau P, Noel E, Donell ST. Impingement of the deep surface of the supraspinatus tendon on the posterosuperior glenoid rim: an arthroscopic study. J Shoulder Elbow Surg 1992;1:238–245.

Weber SC. Arthroscopic debridement and acromioplasty versus mini-open repair in the management of significant partial-thickness tears of the rotator cuff. Orthop Clin North Am 1997;28:79–82.

Wiener SN, Seitz WH Jr. Sonography of the shoulder in patients with tears of the rotator cuff: accuracy and value for selecting surgical options. Am J Roentgenol 1993;160:103–107.

Wright SA, Cofield RH. Management of partial-thickness rotator cuff tears. J Shoulder Elbow Surg 1996;5:458–466.

Yadav H, Nho S, Romeo A, MacGillivray JD. Rotator cuff tears: pathology and repair. Knee Surg Sports Traumatol Arthrosc 2009;17:409–421.

Yagci B, Manisali M, Yilmaz E, et al. Indirect MR arthrography of the shoulder in detection of rotator cuff ruptures. Eur Radiol 2001;11:258–262.

Yamaguchi K. Natural history of rotator cuff tears. In: Tetro A, Blam O, Teefey SA, Middleton WD (eds), A Longitudinal Analysis of Asymptomatic Tears Detected Sonographically. Proceedings of the 7th ICSS, Sydney, 1998.

Yamanaka K, Matsumoto T. The joint side tear of the rotator cuff. A followup study by arthrography. Clin Orthop Relat Res 1994;304:68–73.

Yamanaka K, Fukuda H. Pathologic studies of the supraspinatus tendon with reference to incomplete partial thickness tear. In: Takagishi N (ed.), The Shoulder. Tokyo: Professional Postgraduate Services, 1987: 220–224.

Chapter 9 The overhead athlete

Michael Thomas Freehill, Marc R. Safran

KEY FEATURES

- Adaptive structural changes occur in the throwing shoulder. These changes permit the shoulder to perform effective overhead athletic motion; however, they come at the expense of normal glenohumeral joint kinematics.
- Most shoulder injuries in the overhead athlete are the result of overuse and cumulative microtrauma.
- Non-surgical therapies are often effective and should be attempted before surgical intervention.
- Advances in diagnostic and minimally invasive surgical techniques have improved the management of overhead athletic injuries.

INTRODUCTION

The overhead throwing motion requires strength, flexibility, coordination, and neuromuscular control. In the overhead throwing motion, tremendous demands and stresses are borne by both the soft tissues and the osseous structures of the glenohumeral joint. Adaptive structural changes occur permitting the shoulder to perform effective overhead athletic motions, but this could be at the expense of normal kinematics at the glenohumeral joint. The musculoskeletal adaptive characteristics could potentially result in altered glenohumeral motion which has been reported in numerous sports including baseball (Myers et al. 2006), tennis (Kibler et al. 1996), volleyball (Wang and Cochrane 2001), and swimming (Rupp et al. 1995). Furthermore, numerous authors have postulated that abnormal kinematics with the addition of altered motion could result in internal impingement with subsequent injury at the shoulder (Burkhart et al. 2003a; Myers et al. 2006).

Most of the common pathologies seen at the shoulder of the overhead athlete are encompassed under the umbrella of internal impingement. These include superior labral anteroposterior (SLAP) lesions, partial-thickness, articular-sided rotator cuff tears, biceps tendon pathology, and capsular laxity. Other pathological processes include posterior glenoid lesions (Bennett's), tendonitis or bursitis of the rotator cuff, and scapular dyskinesia. In this chapter we discuss the anatomy and biomechanics of the overhead athlete, describe the pathophysiological process of internal impingement and rotator cuff overload, and review the most common injuries sustained at the shoulder of the overhead athlete.

SPORTS

The athlete must accelerate the arm and ball or racket from a stationary position until ball release or contact, converting stored or potential energy into kinetic energy, resulting in throwing a ball up to 100 miles/h or serving a ball up to 150 mph (240 kph). After ball contact or release, this energy must be safely dissipated. The athlete who participates in overhead sports must possess the ability to effectively decelerate the arm countless times to avoid injury. After a throw, the accelerated arm must be abruptly decelerated through an eccentric contraction. The large muscles create incredible internal rotational velocity, which allows the ball, racquet, or club to move at the highest possible velocity. These muscles include pectoralis major and minor, triceps, latissimus dorsi, and anterior deltoid. The muscles principally responsible for deceleration of the throwing arm are the smaller rotator cuff muscles: supraspinatus, infraspinatus, and teres minor. This is accomplished by the eccentric muscle action of contraction with simultaneous lengthening. With eccentric contraction, fewer muscle fibers are contracting more strongly than concentric contraction, placing the fibers at greater risk of injury.

There are many sports involving overhead motion that place the shoulder at risk. Generally, injury is the result of countless repetitions and the cumulative pathological processes that may be triggered, often referred to as microtrauma. Most injuries evaluated and treated in sports medicine result from throwing or striking from the overhead position.

The highest velocities of arm rotation in sports, as well as the largest portion of injuries in this population of athletes, are among baseball pitchers. However, other overhead sports are also responsible for a considerable number of injuries and amount of rotator cuff pathology. Some of these sports include softball, swimming, handball, javelin throwing, and volleyball.

BIOMECHANICS

In overhead sports, the shoulder requires a balance of muscular tension, proprioceptive muscular control, and ligamentous and osseous support. The thrower's shoulder needs to be loose enough to create high rotational velocities with maximum energy imparted at ball release, while remaining stable enough to avoid injury.

Angular velocities reach 7.250°/s during the acceleration phase of the baseball pitch and represent the fastest human movement recorded (Fleisig et al. 1995). During the pitching motion, anterior translation forces reach half body weight in late cocking and a distraction force equal to the body weight during the deceleration phase (Fleisig et al. 1999). Velocity can be improved by increasing the arc of rotation. The throwing shoulder, in its attempt to gain a larger arc at 90° abduction in the late cocking phase of throwing, develops several unique glenohumeral characteristics. These include increased external rotation which may be the result of increased glenoid and humeral head retroversion as well as anterior capsular laxity. The coordination and synchronicity between the dynamic and static stabilizers of the shoulder afford enough laxity and stability to deliver the ball at high speeds, yet with enough tension to maintain the humeral head in the center of the glenoid fossa. In these athletes, more motion allows enhanced function (increased arc to accelerate the ball or racquet). However, excessive motion comes at the expense of decreased stability. Altchek and Dines (1995) suggest that failure of this balance may lead to combination injuries such as partial-thickness rotator cuff tears and capsulolabral pathology.

Glenohumeral stability

Glenohumeral biomechanical stability is provided by numerous structures within two types of anatomical restraints: static and dynamic. The static restraints refer to bone, cartilaginous, ligamentous, and capsular structures. The dynamic restraints include all the musculature around the shoulder, the negative intra-articular pressure within the joint, and the property of adhesion–cohesion. These two groups of restraints work together to maintain glenohumeral stability by compressive forces directing the humeral head to the glenoid.

Damage or fatigue to any static or dynamic structure can hinder the physiological biomechanics, making overhead athletic maneuvers difficult or impossible. Limitation of abnormal motion or translation of the humeral head on the glenoid is therefore limited by synchronized muscle firing, stable glenohumeral ligaments, and a competent labrum (O'Brien et al. 1990). The dynamic nature of the repetitive throwing motion places extraordinary stresses on the shoulder, capsuloligamentous complex, and rotator cuff (Altchek and Dines 1995; Mazoué and Andrews 2006). Thus, maintenance of strength and integrity at the glenohumeral joint is paramount to the success of the overhead athlete.

ARTICULAR SURFACES

The articular surfaces of the humeral head and the glenoid oppose each other, but are not a true ball and socket. This can be likened to a golf ball on a tee on its side. The benefit of such a configuration is the tremendous range of motion allowed with the degree of freedom afforded at the glenohumeral joint. The disadvantage is dependence of the forces required by other structures of the glenohumeral joint to sustain biomechanical stability throughout the range of motion. Articular stability during motion is also aided by scapular mobility.

Labrum

The glenoid labrum is a triangular fibrocartilaginous ring around the glenoid rim, which serves to deepen the glenohumeral socket. Cadaveric models have demonstrated that 50% of the glenoid depth is provided by the labrum (Howell and Galinat 1989). The labrum is more tightly adhered to the inferior portion of the glenoid rim and more loosely attached to the superior portion. This property is pertinent for multiple reasons (**Fig. 9.1**).

First, the immobile inferior half encounters high translation forces, especially in traumatic situations, which could result in tearing from the glenoid rim. This is the classic Bankart lesion and is defined as detachment of the anteroinferior labrum and inferior glenohumeral ligament complex from the glenoid rim. The long head of biceps inserts at the supraglenoid tubercle of the labral complex, and the labrum also serves as the attachment site for the glenohumeral ligaments and capsule. Although the more mobile capabilities of the superior labrum is protective and more dynamic for overhead sports, this chapter presents instances where the tensile forces produced either at a single event or as the result of an cumulative damage from repetitions can lead to SLAP lesions.

Capsuloligamentous complex

The glenohumeral capsuloligamentous complex is made up of the capsule and the glenohumeral ligaments (GHLs). The capsule can show significant variability; however, it is usually composed of predominantly type I collagen and is less than 5 mm thick. The capsule has a primary role of maintaining negative intra-articular pressure at the glenohumeral joint.

The GHLs are thickenings of the capsule and consist of superior, middle, inferior complex, and coracohumeral ligaments. The GHLs act both to reinforce the capsule and to limit translation of the humeral head at different degrees of shoulder motion, by constraining and stabilizing as they tighten (Turkel et al. 1981). The shoulder joint is a circular capsuloligamentous complex and therefore injury or repair in one region can adversely affect the function of another region.

Rotator interval

The rotator cuff interval is the primary restraint limiting inferior translation with the arm in an adducted position, and provides no

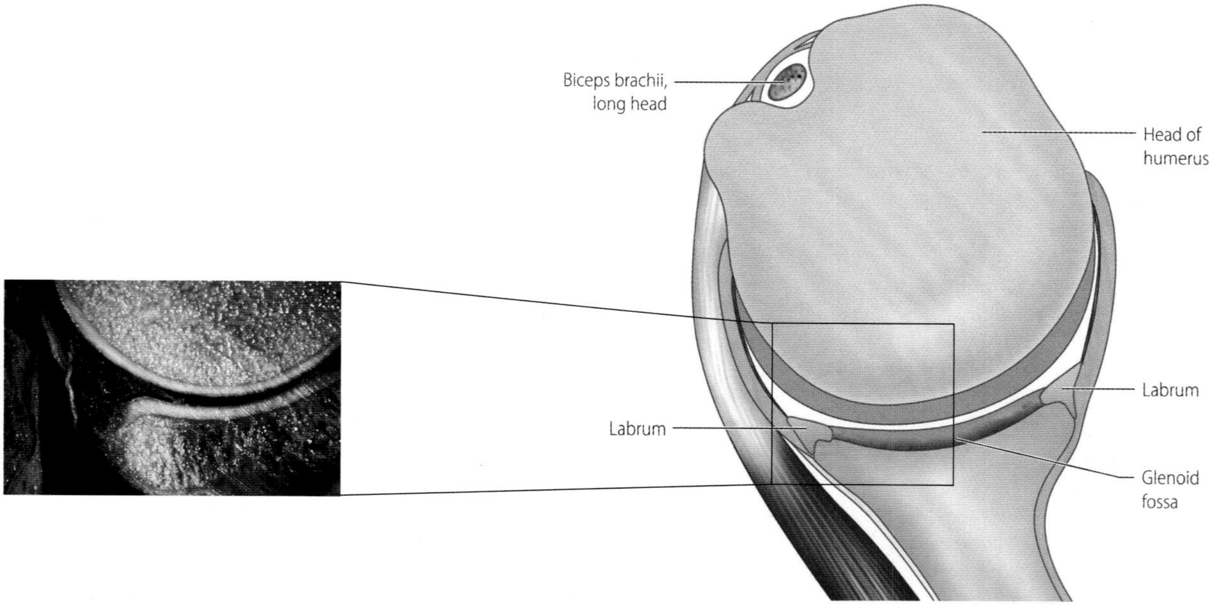

Figure 9.1 The glenoid labrum. Cross-section of glenohumeral joint. Humeral head above, glenoid below, with labrum (see inset for detail) helping to increase contact area between the two surfaces. (Redrawn based on Rockwood CA, Matsen FA, Wirth MA, Lippitt SB. The Shoulder, 4th edn. Philadelphia, PA: Saunders Elsevier, 2009: 15.)

mechanical stability in 90° of abduction because the ligaments are slack at that point. The interval consists of the coracohumeral ligament (CHL) and the superior glenohumeral ligament (SGHL) and serves as a bridge between the supraspinatus and subscapularis musculotendinous complexes. The SGHL serves as the floor in the bicipital groove over which the biceps tendon travels. The CHL originates on the lateral process of the coracoid and inserts over both the greater and the lesser tuberosities, coursing over the bicipital groove. Closure of the rotator interval results in a decrease in external rotation with the arm in the adducted position to 56.4% of normal motion, as reported by Gerber et al. (2003).

Middle glenohumeral ligament

The middle GHL demonstrates variability with regard to its size and attachment. The middle GHL is less well understood; however, if absent, the shoulder may be at a higher risk for anterior glenohumeral instability. It has been shown to be absent in 27% of shoulders (O'Brien et al. 1990). Although the ligament resists inferior translation in the midranges of abduction, it also works as an accessory stabilizer with the arm in 90° abduction when there is damage to the anteroinferior GHL (O'Brien et al. 1995).

Inferior glenohumeral ligament complex

The inferior GHL is the most important portion of the overall capsuloligamentous complex because it is the critical structure that prevents inferior translation and dislocation with the arm in the abducted position. The overhead athlete has the arm in this susceptible position frequently and therefore its function is essential in these individuals. The inferior GHL is a complex because it consists of an anterior band, a posterior band, and a pouch between the two bands. This entire complex forms an axillary pouch and is reported to function as a hammock, supporting the humeral head from below with varying degrees of rotation (**Fig. 9.2**).

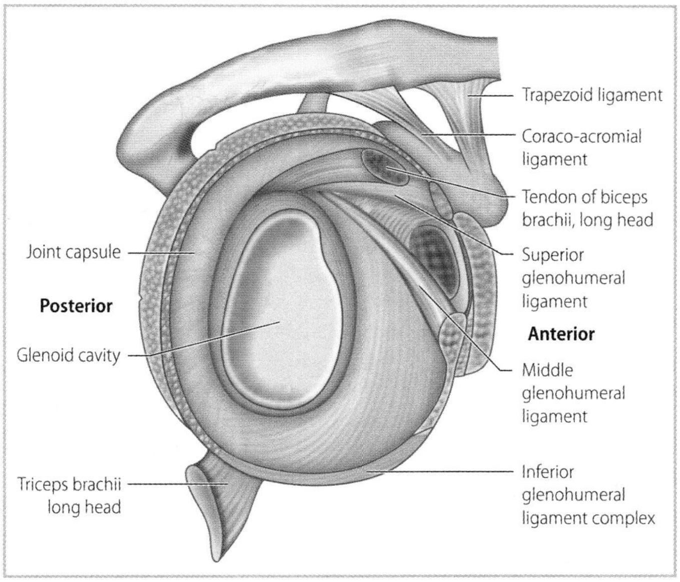

Figure 9.2 The glenohumeral ligament complex. The glenohumeral ligaments (GHLs) are thickenings of the capsule and consist of a superior, middle, and inferior complex, and coracohumeral ligament. The GHLs act to both reinforce the capsule and limit translation of the humeral head at different degrees of shoulder motion by constraining and stabilizing as they tighten. (Adapted from O'Brien SJ, Neves MC, Arnoczky SP, et al. The anatomy and histology of the inferior glenohumeral ligament complex of the shoulder. Am J Sports Med 1990;18:451.)

Rotator cuff

The dynamic stabilizers of the glenohumeral joint consist of the rotator cuff musculature and the larger muscles: pectoralis major, latissimus dorsi, and deltoid. Deltoid actually acts as a destabilizer secondary to its proximal pull, translating the humeral head proximally toward the acromion. The rotator cuff functions as a coupled unit, pulling the humeral head toward the glenoid, and is most important in the midranges of motion. This is critical, because the capsuloligamentous structures, by virtue of their passive nature, function only in the endranges of motion. The forces that these muscles impart to the humeral head provide stability via the "concavity-compression" mechanism, which acts to compress the humeral head into the concavity of the glenoid (**Fig. 9.3**).

The effect of the rotator cuff is not just concavity–compression forcing the humeral head into the glenoid; it also produces a passive barrier to superior, anterior, and posterior translation. However, the dynamic stabilizers decrease the amount of stress on the capsuloligamentous structures seen at the extremes of motion, by limiting the ultimate range at these positions. The dynamic stabilizers are also responsible for initiation of movement at the shoulder and the forces of creating acceleration and accomplishing deceleration during overhand motion in sports. When the larger deltoid overpowers a fatigued rotator cuff, superior translation of the humeral head could result in dynamic impingement of the cuff itself.

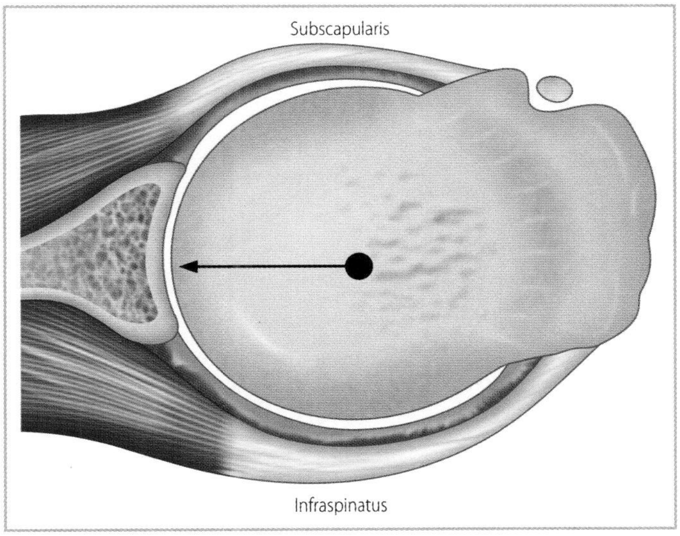

Figure 9.3 Concavity–compression. Subscapularis (anterior) and infraspinatus (posterior) compress the humeral head into the glenoid, helping glenohumeral stability. (Redrawn based on Matsen FA III, Lippitt SB, Sidles JA, et al. Practical Evaluation and Management of the Shoulder. Philadelphia, PA: WB Saunders, 1994: 71.)

Significant changes in glenohumeral motion can occur if a deficiency or injury disrupts the transverse force couple among subscapularis, infraspinatus, and teres minor. Evidence for this was demonstrated by Gibb et al. (1991) who simulated supraspinatus paralysis without disrupted glenohumeral kinematics. This suggests that the remaining rotator cuff muscles are adequate to provide a stable fulcrum for concentric compression of the glenohumeral joint during abduction.

However, a significant extension of a rotator cuff tear into the infraspinatus tendon disrupts the transverse force couple, and the stable fulcrum for glenohumeral abduction is lost. Therefore, if the transverse force couple remains functionally intact, there is sufficient force to maintain concentric reduction of the humeral head on the glenoid, and normal kinematics are preserved. Concavity–compression is more efficient in neutral or 0° abduction than with the elbow away from the body (abduction). Not surprisingly, most subluxation or dislocation episodes are seen with the arm in abduction and external rotation.

Maintained integrity and strength of the rotator cuff muscles are essential to neutralize superior directed forces of the deltoid muscle. Rotator cuff weakness, fatigue, dysfunction, inflammation, or massive tear cannot resist the pull of the humeral head by deltoid superiorly. The humeral head in this circumstance would be "overloaded" subacromially and damage to the rotator cuff could result from an extra-articular insult. This mechanism is sometimes called secondary impingement (**Fig. 9.4**).

External rotation of the humerus is controlled by infraspinatus and teres minor, and reduces strain on the anteroinferior capsuloligamentous structures. Subscapularis is of primary importance in stabilizing the glenohumeral joint anteriorly with the arm in abduction and neutral rotation, but becomes less important with external rotation, where the posterior cuff muscles reduce anterior strain. Subscapularis likewise resists anterior translation by a bulk effect of the muscle itself anteriorly and, when contracting, pushes the head posteriorly. The transverse force couple provides stability throughout the midranges of motion formed by the coordinated activity of both subscapularis and infraspinatus. Electromyography has shown that subscapularis and infraspinatus both contract to stabilize the glenohumeral joint in abduction from 60° to 150° (DePalma et al. 1967). In baseball pitchers, researchers have shown that, during late cocking, as the glenohumeral joint reaches extreme external rotation, subscapularis has the most activity, followed by infraspinatus and teres minor. Supraspinatus has the least activity, and infraspinatus and teres minor work hard to decelerate the arm after ball release and may be subjected to overload and injury. Repetitive insult could result in scarring of the tendon and adherent capsule causing tightness, which may be seen clinically as reduced glenohumeral internal rotation (glenohumeral internal rotation deficit – GIRD).

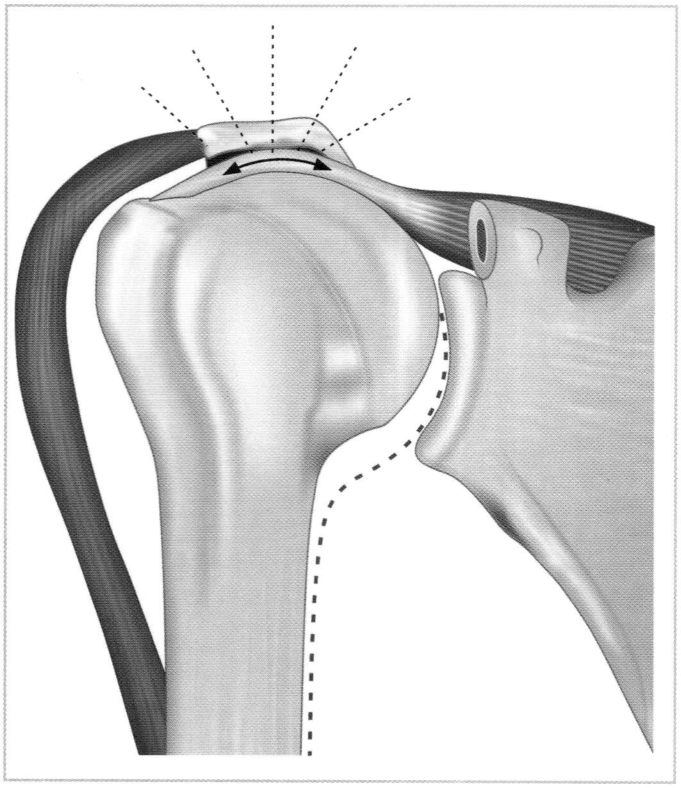

Figure 9.4 Secondary impingement. Weakness of the rotator cuff can result in a superior migration of the humeral head and the creation of a "secondary impingement" of the glenohumeral joint. (Redrawn based on Matsen FA III, Lippitt SB, Sidles JA, et al. Practical Evaluation and Management of the Shoulder. Philadelphia, PA: WB Saunders, 1994: 71.)

Biceps tendon

The long head of biceps tendon inserts into the superior glenoid tubercle and labrum after traversing superiorly through the bicipital groove of the proximal humeral head. Its structure is important as a dynamic restraint to external rotation in the abducted shoulder. Extreme rotation excessively loads the biceps tendon and could predispose to injury at the biceps–labrum complex (SLAP). Itoi and colleagues (1994) have suggested that the long head of biceps takes on a more important role than the rotator cuff in anterior stabilization when the stability of the capsuloligamentous structures has been compromised.

PITCHING MOTION

It is important to review the throwing motion to better understand the pathoetiology of shoulder pain in the overhead athlete. The pitching motion has been broken down into six phases, which are defined by the position and action of the arm and shoulder during the pitching cycle (**Figs 9.5a** to **f**).

A kinetic chain of energy begins in the lower extremities (starting with the foot against the ground), is transferred through the pelvis and trunk, and ultimately released through the upper extremity with release of the ball. The throwing cycle is initiated with the wind-up, when the player moves from a stand-still position until the hands spread apart (ball leaves the glove), and potential energy is generated with the center of gravity above the mound with minimal muscular activity or stresses seen at the shoulder. The next phase is the cocking phase, which can be subdivided into the early (first 75% of the phase) and late cocking phases (last 25%). The early cocking phase is defined by the ball leaving the glove, with the ball and throwing arm moving back away from its eventual destination. The phase ends when the stride (lead) foot contacts the ground. In the early cocking phase, the shoulder moves into 90° of abduction and there is early deltoid activation and late activation of supraspinatus, infraspinatus, and teres minor (Meister et al. 2000). In the late-cocking phase, both feet are planted, but the arm is still moving back while the body momentum begins moving forward. In the late cocking phase, maximum glenohumeral external rotation (ER) at 90° abduction is achieved via scapular retraction, which allows the shoulder to reach the hyperexternal rotation position. Deltoid begins decreasing its activity and supraspinatus, infraspinatus, and teres minor reach their peak activity. Stride foot touch down and the endpoint of the phase are reached when the torso starts to open, initiating the firing of subscapularis. Clinically, this phase ends when the ball starts to move forward.

The acceleration phase, which starts with the ball moving forward and ends at ball release, is also subdivided into two phases: early (first 25%) and late (last 75%). This phase is initiated by scapular protraction and the anterior muscles – pectoralis major, latissimus dorsi, serratus

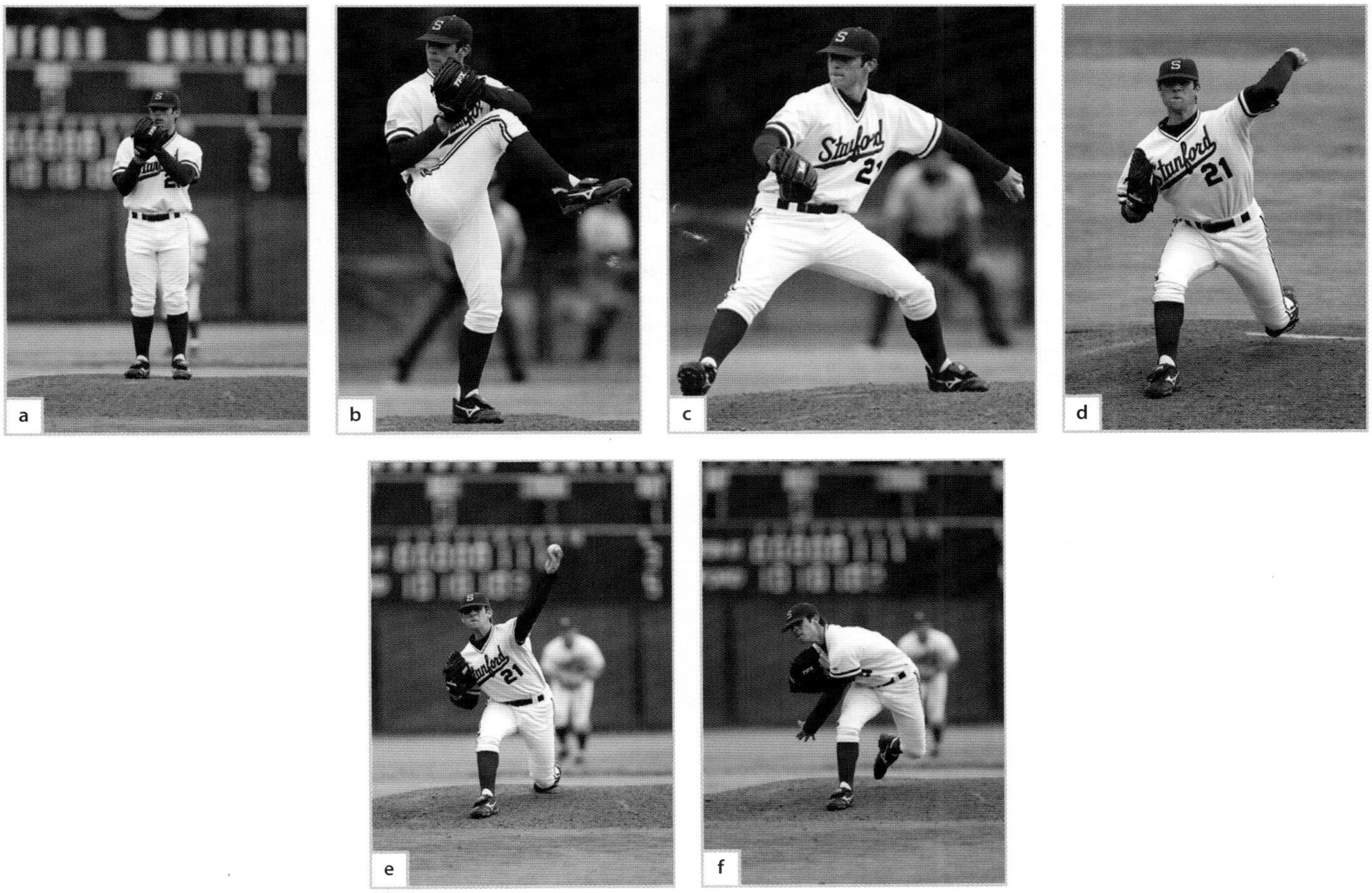

Figure 9.5 The phases of pitching. (a) Ready position; (b) wind-up; (c) early cocking; (d) late cocking; (e) acceleration; and (f) follow-through.

anterior, subscapularis – converting from eccentric to concentric contractions, while the posterior muscles –supraspinatus, infraspinatus, teres minor – convert their function from concentric to eccentric contraction (Pappas et al. 1985). The last phase is the follow-through or deceleration phase, which begins just after ball release until the player comes to a stop, dissipating the remaining stored energy. The deceleration phase is recognized as the most violent phase of the throwing cycle and is essentially a reversal of the first three phases, with any remaining energy that is not imparted to the ball dissipated through the shoulder. The powerful dissipation force is provided by the posterior musculature. Teres minor demonstrates the highest activity, but subscapularis is also active, helping to maintain the humeral head position and preventing subluxation. Finally, the follow-through is marked by all muscle activity returning to resting levels and the body proprioceptively rebalancing. It is at the point of transition between late cocking and early acceleration that Walch et al. (1991) first described internal impingement. This type of impingement is defined as contact between the articular side of the supraspinatus/infraspinatus tendon at the posterosuperior humeral head and the posterosuperior rim of the glenoid.

As kinetic energy is transferred from the lower extremity through the smaller motion segments of the upper extremity and release of the ball, structures at the shoulder experience tremendous biomechanical stresses. Joint loads are the highest in the deceleration phase with posterior shear forces reaching 400 N, inferior shear forces >300 N, and compressive forces >1000 N (Jobe et al. 1984; Dillman et al. 1993; Fleisig et al. 1995). These incredibly high forces in a repetitive motion are considered to be primary factors in tensile rotator cuff failure and other injuries at the shoulder. Likewise, the late-cocking and early acceleration phases are also considered injurious to the thrower because the anterior shear forces are greatest at that point.

Range of motion

It is well accepted and reported in the literature that the overhand throwing athlete develops and possesses unique glenohumeral range of motion characteristics of the throwing shoulder. Generally speaking, these include an increase in external rotation and a decrease in internal rotation at 90° abduction in the throwing shoulder whereas external rotation in adduction is usually unaffected. Despite these disparities, there is an overall retention of the total range of motion (ROM) comparatively between the two shoulders. This phenomenon can be thought of as a shift in the position of the rotational arc at the throwing shoulder. The passive ROM characteristics of 879 professional baseball players were reported by Wilk (2008) and included means of external rotation (136.9° ± 14.7°) and an internal rotation of 40.1° ± 9.6° at 90° abduction. The external rotation was approximately 9° greater in the throwing versus the non-throwing shoulder and the internal rotation was 8.5° less in the throwing shoulder in the pitchers. Total motion is generally retained because the loss in internal rotation is offset by the gain in external rotation.

With ball release occurring in a similar position of slight forward elevation, the increase in ER at the glenohumeral joint allows more time over which to accelerate the arm (and ball or racquet), allowing for increased velocities at which the arm, and hence the ball, can be propelled. Humeral and glenoid retroversion likewise appear to be necessary changes in the natural history of the thrower's shoulder. In this sense it could be reasoned that the athlete self-selects whether these changes occur and whether or not he or she can throw successfully. What remains unclear is at what point expected physiological changes progress to pathological processes.

It has been proposed that, if the loss of IR at the throwing shoulder is equal to the gain in ER, this is due to an osseous physiological process that developed secondary to the stresses of repetitive throwing at an early age (Lintner et al. 2007). However, when the loss in IR exceeds the adaptive gains in ER, this could represent a pathological process and is likely secondary to changes seen in the soft tissues (Lintner et al. 2007). This phenomenon of loss of IR in the throwing shoulder has been termed "glenohumeral internal rotation deficit" (GIRD) (**Figs 9.6a** and **b**).

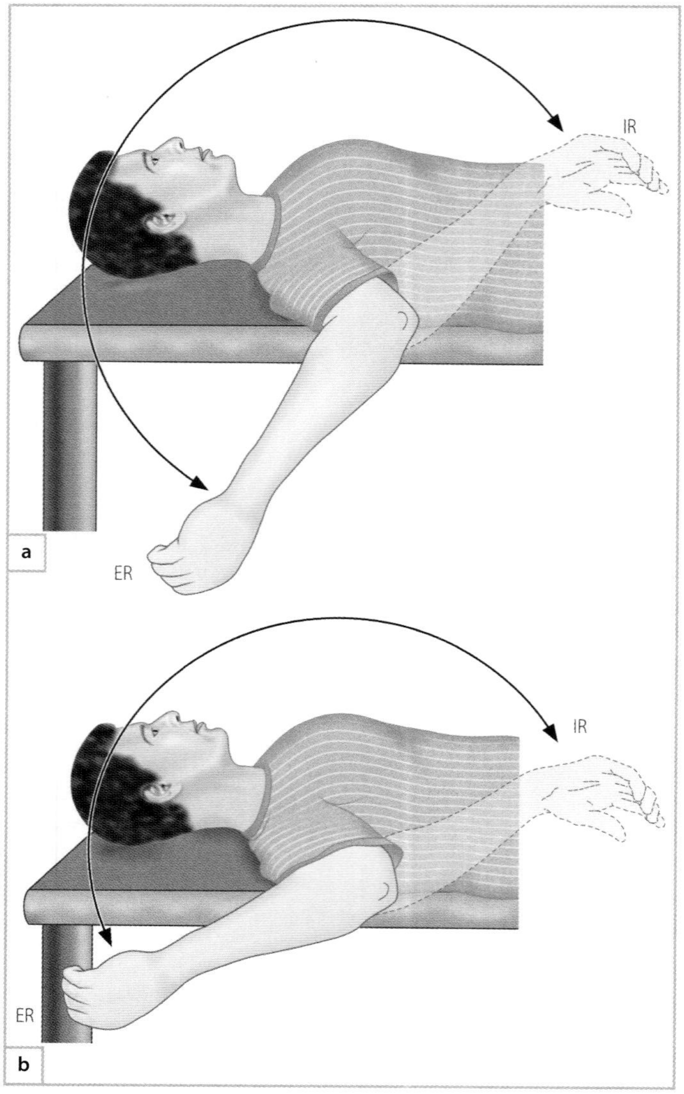

Figure 9.6 Glenohumeral range of motion in throwers. In the throwing (dominant) shoulder, (a) a gain in external rotation (ER) and loss of internal rotation (IR) are present compared with the non-throwing (non-dominant arm) (b). Total motion (ER + IR) is retained bilaterally. (Adapted from Wilk KE, Reinold MM, Andrews JR. The Athlete's Shoulder, 2nd edn. New York: Churchill Livingstone, 2009: 125.)

GIRD can progress over time in overhead athletes; however, the clinical significance of this process remains uncertain. GIRD is calculated by subtracting the IR of the throwing shoulder from the IR of the non-throwing shoulder. The original report on GIRD presented a threshold value of 25° as increased risk of injury (Burkhart et al. 2003a): 25° was selected because 124 baseball pitchers treated arthroscopically by the lead author for symptomatic type 2 SLAP lesions all possessed a GIRD >25° (mean 53°). Other authors have reported different thresholds of asymmetry as remarkable – 11° (Myers et al. 2005) and 18° (Morgan et al. 1998), associated with shoulder injury, mainly labral tears. The supraphysiological rotation obtained by overhand athletes can be achieved because of these glenohumeral adaptations.

Two mechanisms are responsible for the characteristic motion pattern in throwers. It has been reported that osseous and soft-tissue changes occur and are responsible. An incredible distraction force of 750 N has been reported to be absorbed by the posteroinferior aspect of the capsule during the follow-through phase of the throwing motion (Levitz et al. 2001). These stresses posteriorly can cause remodeling resulting in contracture and subsequent GIRD. Alternatively, the eccentric forces to decelerate the arm, as well as prevent distraction, may result in microscopic injury to the rotator cuff external rotators (teres minor and infraspinatus). This repetitive microscopic injury may result in scarring and contracture of the muscle–tendon unit. The tendons for these muscles are confluent with the posterior glenohumeral capsule and, thus, inflammation and contracture of the tendon may also occur in the capsule, resulting in GIRD. The development of GIRD remains a major concern for throwing athletes, trainers, and orthopedic surgeons because of these reported associations with injury due to abnormal glenohumeral mechanics, and the uncertainty that still surrounds this topic. Although it is accepted that both processes may exist, debate continues as to whether soft-tissue changes, bony alterations, or a combination of these is ultimately responsible for the development of pathological GIRD.

Osseous adaptations

Significantly increased humeral head retroversion, glenoid retroversion, and ER in the throwing shoulder compared with the non-throwing shoulder were reported by Crockett et al. (2002). They also found that IR was significantly less in the throwing shoulder than in the non-throwing shoulder. No significant differences were found between shoulders for total ROM, anterior or posterior glenohumeral laxity, or the sulcus sign. Probably, loss of IR is the normal adaptive process in the overhead thrower and should be considered abnormal or concerning only when there is loss of the total ROM secondary to increased losses of IR. Furthermore, the osseous adaptation allowing greater ER, and hence a greater arc for throwing, could be viewed as a process that protects the shoulder from internal impingement. Increased humeral retroversion likely occurs at a young age and has been theorized not to worsen, but to result from the throwing arm not undergoing a physiological derotation process during growth (Yamamoto et al. 2006).

Posterior capsular tightness

The literature is limited with regard to glenohumeral range of motion changes reported in a prospective fashion. Freehill et al. (2010) looked at a cohort of major league baseball pitchers to examine the changes in glenohumeral motion that occur over the course of a season. No statistically significant changes in ROM over the course of a full season were found in all pitchers as a group; however, significant differences were found when the starting and relief pitcher subgroups were closely examined. Interestingly, starting pitchers showed significantly improved IR and total ROM, whereas relief pitchers experienced a significant worsening of GIRD. The authors concluded that this was evidence of soft-tissue changes over the course of a season.

In addition, Lintner et al. (2007) demonstrated that a stretching program can result in protective, measurable changes in ROM. The muscles responsible for the ER during late cocking of the throwing motion also demonstrate high eccentric muscle activity during the follow-through phase, and are responsible for the deceleration of the arm crossing at this incredible velocity (Jobe et al. 1984). Eccentric muscle contraction has been shown to result in increased passive muscular tension and loss of joint ROM (Proske et al. 2001). Other studies have demonstrated that repetitive eccentric contractions produce a subsequent loss of joint ROM in the upper and lower extremities (Reisman et al. 2005).

MUSCLE STRENGTH AND BALANCE

Scapular

Appropriate movement and stability of the scapulothoracic musculature are vital in asymptomatic glenohumeral functioning. These larger muscles work in a coordinated and synchronized fashion, with the rotator cuff muscles and static stabilizers, to achieve stability at the glenohumeral joint, as well as rotating the acromion to allow overhead motion without impingement, and retracting and posterior tilting to reduce internal impingement. In addition, proper position of the scapula itself is important for effective glenohumeral motion in overhead athletics. Alterations in the position of the scapula during motion is called "scapular dyskinesia" and is discussed later. Wilk et al. (1999) reported, in 112 professional baseball players, significantly stronger depressor muscles on the throwing shoulder compared with the non-throwing side. Also, pitchers and catchers exhibited significantly stronger protractor and elevator muscles of the scapula compared with position players.

Rotator cuff

As previously described, the rotator cuff muscles play a critical role in glenohumeral stability during the throwing motion. A balance must be retained between the agonist and antagonist muscle groups for optimal glenohumeral function and strength in overhead throwers. It has been reported that the ER strength in the throwing shoulders of professional pitchers is significantly less (6%) than in the non-throwing shoulder. Conversely, the IR and adduction strength in the throwing shoulder were found to be significantly stronger (3% and 9–10%, respectively) than in the non-throwing shoulder and optimal external-to-internal rotator muscle strength should be 66–75% (Wilk et al. 1995). Supraspinatus in the throwing shoulder of professional pitchers has been reported to be significantly weaker than in the non-throwing shoulder as measured by a handheld dynamometer (Magnusson et al. 1994).

PATHOLOGICAL PROCESSES

Internal impingement

A spectrum of pathological conditions falls under the umbrella of internal impingement. These include partial-thickness, articular-sided rotator cuff tears, full-thickness rotator cuff tears, labral tears, biceps lesions, scapular dysfunction, glenoid and humeral head chondromalacia, capsular injury, and Bennett's lesion. The possible pathophysiological insults responsible for internal impingement have been suggested as anterior instability, posterior capsular contracture, and GIRD.

Internal impingement was differentiated from the original description by Neer (1972) who described contact of the bursal side of the rotator cuff with the coracoacromial arch during abduction. Internal impingement describes a pathological contact of the posterosuperior margin of the glenoid and the articular side of the rotator cuff and greater tuberosity. In the late-cocking position, the posterosuperior labrum and undersurface of supraspinatus and infraspinatus will impinge on each other, causing damage to these respective structures or cystic changes of the greater tuberosity, or even notching of the proximal portion of the humerus. This is the most common problem seen in the shoulder of the pitcher. This concept was initially described by Walch and colleagues (1992) in a cohort of tennis players. The authors provided clinical arthroscopic evidence from 17 patients who had debridement of partial-thickness, articular-sided rotator cuff tears.

It has been demonstrated that glenohumeral adaptations in the overhead athlete allow asymptomatic contact of the glenoid, labrum, and undersurface rotator cuff. An MRI study in 10 asymptomatic baseball pitchers demonstrated this abutment in the throwing shoulder, but not in the non-throwing shoulder (Halbrecht et al. 1999). Valadie et al. (2000) demonstrated, in cadaveric specimens, that the articular surface of the rotator cuff tendons and the anterosuperior glenoid are in contact in Neer and Hawkins' provocative testing positions. Although these positions show contact in the anterosuperior versus the posterosuperior portion of the rim seen in ER in throwers, it suggests that abutment between these structures is normal and not independently suggestive of pathology (Jobe and Sidles 1993). Thus, in the overhead throwing population, we can view internal impingement as a normal phenomenon; however, it potentially could become a pathological process when another insult such as anterior laxity, GIRD, or scapular dyskinesia is present. Anatomical differences of the shoulders exist such as humeral retroversion, anterior laxity, glenoid version changes, posterior capsular tightness, or a combination of these factors. Controversy remains about the primary etiology for internal impingement. It has been postulated that there are four critical components of internal impingement (see **Fig. 5.15**): excessive horizontal extension, over-rotation, increased glenohumeral translation, and GIRD.

PATHOMECHANICS

As asymptomatic throwers and normal cadavers (Jobe and Sidles 1993) demonstrate the described contact of internal impingement, another trigger or entity must occur to predispose to a pathological development. The repetitive nature coupled with the extreme forces produced by the overhead athlete likely predispose them to injury. A disturbance in the coordination of muscles, fatigue, or poor technique could be the initiating factor, causing an alteration in mechanics and subsequent injury to the rotator cuff, biceps tendon, posterior labrum, capsule, or glenoid.

Anterior capsular laxity

Anterior laxity leading to "microinstability" is one proposed mechanism responsible for internal impingement. During late cocking and early acceleration, the anterior translational forces result in significant stresses at the anterior shoulder. Jobe et al. (1989) originally proposed repetitive strain as a cause of anterior capsular laxity over time in the overhead athlete. The most common cause of this laxity is insufficiency of the anterior capsuloligamentous structures. There is controversy as to whether this anterior laxity leads to hyperexternal rotation or vice versa. Schneider et al. (2005) reported an 18° increase in ER with an increase in capsular elasticity of 30%. Mihata et al. (2004) demonstrated, in a cadaveric model, that the anterior band of the inferior GHL elongates with excessive external rotation. The late-cocking position of abduction and ER would therefore cause the humeral head to translate anteriorly. The impingement of the articular side of the rotator cuff, in this instance, would be a tensile draping over the posterosuperior glenoid rim during deceleration. The microinstability secondary to anterior capsular laxity would contribute to the inability to control the humeral head during deceleration, and could lead to an abrasive degeneration of the articular side of the rotator cuff on the posterosuperior glenoid. It has been postulated in this scenario that the repetitive motion can cause a progressive delamination (Andrews et al. 1985a) (**Fig. 9.7**).

Posterior capsular contracture

The next proposed mechanism responsible for internal impingement is contracture of the posterior capsule. It is believed that the chronic exposure to stresses posteriorly at the shoulder, secondary to eccentric loads exerted during the follow-through phase of throwing, results in a thickening of the posterior inferior GHL (Burkhart et al. 2003a). Burkhart et al. (2003b) believe that the posterior capsular contracture causes a functional lengthening of the anterior capsule or a "pseudolaxity," and not true instability. They proposed that the contracted posterior capsule results in GIRD, and that a posterior and superior translation of the humeral head occurs in abduction and ER when GIRD exists. This would result in hyperexternal rotation with increased "peel-back" forces. It has been shown that the contracted posteroinferior GHL causes a shift in the humeral head to a more posterosuperior position on the glenoid during abduction and ER.

Grossman and colleagues (2005) found a significant decrease in IR (8.8°) after the creation of a posterior capsular contracture in a cadaveric model. They also found that the humeral head translated to a more postero*inferior* position when the arm was brought from neutral to a late-cocking position and the addition of anterior capsular laxity of 30% did not significantly change this finding. However, the addition of the posterior capsular contracture caused an increased trend toward a more posterosuperior position of the humeral head when the arm was rotated into maximum ER, although not significant. Huffman and colleagues (2006) created a more physiological cadaveric model with regard to the scapular alignment during testing, and found that posterior capsular contracture shifts the humeral head significantly posteriorly in late cocking. The authors also reported that, during deceleration and follow-through, the humeral head shifted significantly anteriorly and inferiorly. Of note, the cadaveric models all had rotator cuff and overlying muscles removed and therefore the dynamic stabilization of the glenohumeral joint was not included in the model. The lack of dynamic contribution brings into question the true humeral head translation during throwing, because these models may not truly replicate the throwing shoulder adequately. However, an increased twisting mechanism occurring at the biceps tendon repetitively with large shear stresses, as seen with throwing, could cause eventual failure of both biceps insertion to the labrum and the rotator cuff.

Microinstability and over-rotation

If microinstability and/or over-rotation occurs in addition to the expected bony and soft-tissue adaptations characteristic of the throwing shoulder, internal impingement could result in a pathological consequences. Microinstability is abnormal rotational or directional laxity of the humeral head on the glenoid, which leads to altered mechanics without frank dislocation. Hyperexternal rotation, beyond the expected physiological adaptation, or over-rotation coupled with increased abnormal directional shifts of the humeral head, could result in internal impingement causing tearing of the labrum, fraying of the articular side of the rotator cuff, and further capsular changes or damage. Rizio and colleagues (2007) studied the effects of instability on the superior labrum. Using cadaveric models, lesions were produced in the inferior GHL to create anterior instability. Labral strain was measured with the shoulders in the late-cocking position. They found that the posterosuperior labral strain was increased 160% in unstable shoulders. Their results demonstrate that the addition of instability disrupts the delicate balance that exists in the overhead athlete's shoulder.

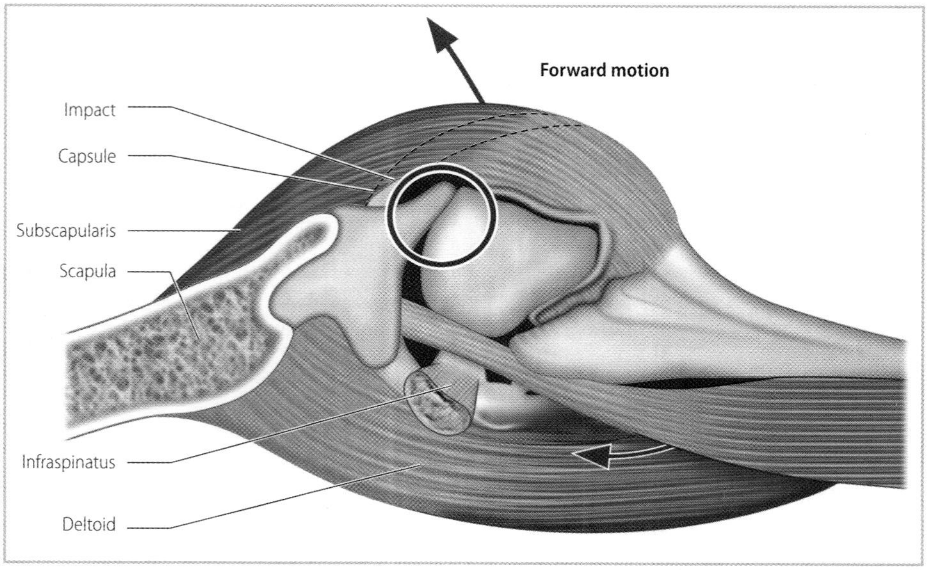

Figure 9.7 Anterior capsular laxity. Repetitive strain of the throwing motion can result in anterior capsuloligamentous laxity. During the late-cocking phase (abduction and external rotation), the humeral head translates anteriorly (Redrawn with permission from Jobe FW. Operative Techiques in Upper Extremity Sports Injuries. Philadelphia: Mosby, 1995).

Rotator cuff overload/tensile failure

The pathological process of rotator cuff tearing can occur through several different mechanisms. Intrinsic changes in the tendon related to vascularity and aging are seen more often in the older population. Subacromial impingement can cause extrinsic insult to the bursal side of the rotator cuff tendon and subsequent tearing. Lastly, traumatic tearing secondary to an excessive tensile load can occur either as a single traumatic event or secondary to accumulated microtrauma. This traumatic type is most often seen in overhead athletes. As previously discussed, the rotator cuff muscles are exposed to incredible stresses as they eccentrically contract in the deceleration of the throwing arm. The overhead athlete attempts to impart tremendous energy to the ball at release from the hand, club, or racquet. This is successfully accomplished by hyperexternal rotation followed by the ability to produce incredible internal rotational velocities. The rotator cuff is subsequently forced to decelerate the arm after ball release, resisting horizontal adduction, IR, anterior translation, and distracting forces, in an effort to simultaneously stabilize the humeral head to the glenoid. The eccentric tensile forces with repetitions of throwing can fatigue the rotator cuff which can become overwhelmed. Microtraumatic injuries can accumulate at the undersurface of the posterior half of supraspinatus and superior portion of infraspinatus, and develop articular-sided, partial-thickness tears.

Therefore, the impact of internal impingement coupled with associated fatigue of the rotator cuff can lead to greater anterior laxity. This, in turn, will result in greater anterior shear forces and translation which could wear down the anterior labrum and cause subsequent tearing. In addition, the rotator cuff could then be stressed further in its attempt to maintain the humeral head on the glenoid during late cocking and early acceleration, and the continuum could lead to cuff overload. Furthermore, a dysfunctional rotator cuff cannot resist the pull of deltoid superiorly, with the resultant secondary impingement against the acromion.

INJURIES IN THE OVERHEAD ATHLETE

Narrowing down the broad spectrum of differential diagnoses is critical for medical practitioners when taking care of these athletes. The presentation of pathology can be pain, ineffective performance, or decreased ROM. It is critical to determine the correct diagnosis because this will help formulate the most effective treatment protocol. Advanced imaging modalities have been tremendously beneficial, but one must be careful to correlate these studies with the symptoms of the overhead athlete. The importance of this is borne out in the report by Andrews and colleagues (2010) who evaluated 31 asymptomatic professional pitchers with MRI. Abnormal labrums were detected in 90%, changes within the rotator cuff in 87%, and cystic changes of the humeral head in 39%. The abduction–external rotation (ABER) view with MRI or MR arthrography allows excellent visualization of the glenohumeral joint and associated pathologies. The undersurface of the cuff, labrum, and humeral head shifting with stressing can all be appropriately evaluated. It is useful in the evaluation of undersurface rotator cuff tears because visualization of delamination can be appreciated.

Rotator cuff

Partial thickness

The relative frequency of partial-thickness rotator cuff tears in baseball players is much more than full-thickness tears. There may be many reasons for this, particularly that the natural history of partial-thickness rotator cuff tears in overhead athletes likely progresses to full-thickness tears. However, the reason is probably that it is the rare individual who can participate at high-level overhead sports with a full-thickness rotator cuff tear – thus, athletes retire with near full-thickness, or full-thickness tears, and thus such as tear is less common in throwing athletes. The etiology of tears in these individuals is not one of intrinsic attritional changes in the tendon from the aging process and at-risk vascularity zones, but secondary to the repetitive nature of the thrower's motion and extreme stresses at the shoulder. This places the rotator cuff muscles at risk for fatigue which could result in tensile failure or accumulated microtrauma, causing delamination over time.

Accumulative microtauma can lead to intratendinous, partial-thickness tearing of the rotator cuff. The rotator cuff is composed of five layers: layers two and three are most often affected at the undersurface of posterior supraspinatus and superior infraspinatus. These are the so-called "PASTA" (partial articular-sided tendon avulsion) lesions. If there is underlying instability, the risk of injury increases more as the cuff is forced to work harder to stabilize the joint during throwing. The overhead athlete with a symptomatic partial-thickness tear may complain of pain during late cocking or deceleration, and experience a loss of velocity, control, or poor recovery.

Treatment is initially non-surgical, consisting of physical therapy (stretching of the posterior shoulder capsule, as well as strengthening of the rotator cuff and scapular stabilizers), followed by an interval throwing program. A corticosteroid injection may be administered before this rehabilitation to help reduce the symptoms adequately to allow for rehabilitation. Failure of at least two courses of rehabilitation may warrant arthroscopic surgical intervention as definitive treatment. Again we emphasize the importance of evaluating for coexisting lesions. Undersurface tears of the rotator cuff should be debrided with a shaver. In the overhead athlete, the rule of tears greater than 50% being repaired should be abandoned secondary to poor results in this population. Some surgeons will opt to repair if the thickness of the tear is 75%, but again controversy exists.

Full thickness

Full-thickness rotator cuff tears in the overhead thrower are uncommon. These tears, as in partial-thickness tears, likely result from repetitive motion and occur over time. This mechanism is in contrast with the contact athlete in whom a single high-energy trauma can cause the tear. The region of the rotator cuff usually affected is the undersurface of posterior supraspinatus and the superior portion of infraspinatus. Associated injuries should be sought, such as SLAP lesions. On physical examination, pain, weakness, and rotator cuff inflammation signs are generally positive. Plain radiographs are often unremarkable. MRI is the advanced imaging modality of choice; however, if labral or biceps pathology is suspected, then an MR arthrogram should be obtained. Restoration of the anatomical footprint is the primary goal in surgical repair because this will optimize the contact area and thus the healing environment, while producing the best attempt at mechanical restoration of the throwing shoulder. Techniques described include open, mini-open, arthroscopic, transosseous, suture anchors, and single- versus double-row repairs. The surgeon must avoid repairing infraspinatus to the articular margin because this is not its normal anatomical attachment site.

Mazoué and Andrews (2006) reported the results of 16 professional baseball players with full-thickness rotator cuff tears who underwent repair using a mini-open repair, 12 of whom were pitchers. Of the 12 pitchers, 1 (8%) was able to return to a high competitive level. Nine of the twelve underwent a concurrent procedure, including a third who received thermal capsulorraphy, so the sample size of only full-thickness rotator cuff tears was small. Nevertheless, of the three with only rotator cuff tears and no concurrent diagnosis or procedure performed, none returned to a high competitive level.

Labrum

SLAP lesions refer to injury at the complex of the biceps tendon–superior labral attachment. Although Andrews et al. (1985b) were the first to describe this lesion, Snyder et al. (1990) first classified the various injuries to this complex. They referred to the injury as superior labrum anterior and posterior lesions and coined the term "SLAP" lesion. The internal impingement position of the throwing motion can lead to excessive traction and "peeling back" of the biceps tendon from the labrum, resulting in a type II lesion. Assorted points of view have been theorized as to the "peel-back" mechanism versus a deceleration traction avulsion injury to the labral complex, but perhaps the suggestion that the biceps tendon in the throwing motion is undergoing a "weed-pulling" phenomenon allows both theories to be entertained. The diagnosis can be difficult because symptoms can mimic rotator cuff pathology or instability and the sensitivity and specificity of physical examination tests for SLAP lesions are poor.

In treating patients, it must be determined whether the labral damage has destabilized the capsular ligaments or whether alteration of the biceps tendon has occurred. The ABER view on the MR image or arthrogram is critical to help diagnosis, but definitive diagnosis can be made only with arthroscopy. Although successful non-surgical treatment for SLAP lesions resulting in improved pain and function has been reported, return to overhead sports at the pre-injury level was only 66% (Edwards et al. 2010). Technical points in SLAP repairs in overhead athletes include restoration of the anatomical meniscoid position of the labrum on the glenoid, avoiding suture knots because the rotator cuff would abut after repair, and care not to over-constrain the biceps tendon because this will result in a loss of ER. Some surgeons advocate not placing sutures or anchors anterior to the biceps tendon in throwers because this may also affect ability to achieve ER by capturing the biceps tendon.

Biceps tendon

Questions still remain as to the exact function of the biceps tendon and its importance in the throwing action across the proximal shoulder. It likewise remains unknown whether biceps tendon tendinitis or dysfunction is isolated or exists as part of a spectrum of shoulder pathology. The clinician must evaluate and search for a coexisting diagnosis such as rotator cuff pathology, labral tears, or instability. The insertion into the superior glenoid tubercle–superior labral complex, implicates this structure with SLAP lesions. Although most SLAP lesions in the thrower are type II, intratendinous advancement may be present and needs to be evaluated on a case-by-case basis. Most biceps tendon pathology is in the form of tendinitis and therefore non-surgical modalities should initially be used.

Posterior glenoid exostosis (Bennett's lesion)

Bennett's lesion is an extra-articular ossification of the posteroinferior glenoid. This was first described in 1941 as an ossification of the posterior capsule of the throwing shoulder (Bennett 1941). It was hypothesized that these lesions occurred secondary to the pull of the posterior capsule and triceps during the throwing motion. Local irritation of the joint capsule and synovial membrane arising from the presence of these calcifications can result in posterior shoulder pain. The repetitive trauma of the throwing motion to the posterior capsule could lead to a secondary ossification. It has been associated with athletes having GIRD. The clinical significance of this lesion has been questioned because it is a relatively common finding in the throwing population. Wright and Paletta (2004) reported that 22% of asymptomatic professional baseball pitchers in their cohort of 55 demonstrated this lesion. However, in the symptomatic shoulder of the throwing athlete, a posterior exostosis could be considered a marker of internal impingement. The lesion could signify the presence of undersurface tearing of the rotator cuff as well as damage to the posterior labrum.

For athletes with thrower's exostosis who have symptomatic stable shoulders, arthroscopic debridement of the rotator cuff and labral lesions is indicated. Arthroscopic excision of the exostosis is recommended if the patient has a prominent lesion associated with posterior shoulder pain, particularly in the late-cocking phases of throwing, and if evocable tenderness in the region of the posterior glenoid rim and capsule is present (Meister et al. 1999) (**Fig. 9.8**).

Instability/Laxity

Overhead throwers possess increased anterior laxity. As previously described, this laxity allows the supraphysiological ER to increase rotational velocities through a greater arc of rotation, and impart greater energy to the ball when released or struck. Jobe and Pink (1994) postulated that repetitive microtrauma will cause capsular laxity and could ultimately be responsible for secondary pathologies such as labral or rotator cuff injuries. A certain degree of anterior laxity needs to be acquired to perform effectively in overhead athletics. However, a threshold is likely surpassed that predisposes to pain and potential injury. Thermal capsulorraphy has been largely abandoned in throwers secondary to concerns over loss of ER and chondrolysis of the glenohumeral joint. Arthroscopic plication of the capsule alone or with some labrum has been performed, but

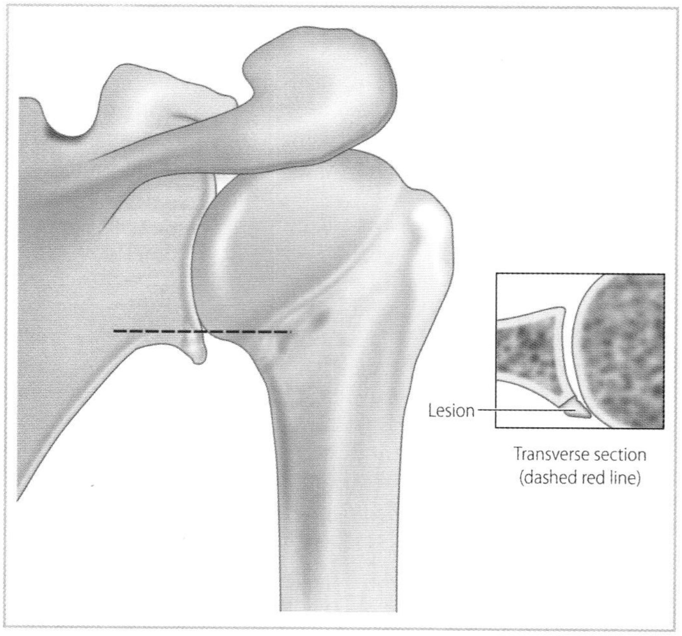

Figure 9.8 Bennett's lesion. Posterior glenoid exostosis (mineralization) can be a source of pain in the overhead athlete.

again loss of ROM and inability to perform overhead sports remain a question.

Scapular dyskinesia

Alterations in scapular positioning can create protraction and increased glenoid ante-tilting. The result is the scapula moving into IR as the humerus moves into ER. At rest, the position of the scapula is altered and has been termed "SICK" scapula. This stands for **s**capular malposition, **i**nferior medial border prominence, **c**oracoid pain, dyskinesis (Burkhart et al. 2003b). The "SICK" scapula position combined with altered motion is termed "scapular dyskinesis." Inflexibility or imbalance of muscles, as well as loss of muscle activation and coordination, results in an abnormal position of excessive protraction at rest and an inability to appropriately retract during motion. During throwing, the late-cocking and early acceleration phases produce a greater internal impingement, with excessive posterior compression and anterior tension secondary to inability to retract to accommodate the hyperexternal rotation of throwing. In this setting, labral tears, undersurface rotator cuff tears, and capsular injury could take place.

Front-line treatment for scapular dyskinesia is non-surgical modalities. Closed chain exercises are performed to address protraction, retraction, elevation with protraction and retraction, elevation and internal rotation, and external rotation and depression. Open chain exercises can be instituted after improvement in muscle balance, flexibility, and strength. Tenderness around the coracoid in this setting is secondary to a tight pectoralis minor tendon. This can be stretched by placing a rolled towel between the shoulder blades while laying in the supine position.

Subcoracoid impingement

Subcoracoid impingement is a diagnosis of exclusion. It presents as a dull anterior shoulder pain. Neer's testing is negative with this diagnosis, but pain relief is with an anesthetic injection at the coracoid. Although this impingement of subscapularis between the lesser tuberosity and the coracoid is often associated with an elongated coracoid, it may also be associated with anterior shoulder instability and can be seen in throwing athletes. Treatment generally is non-surgical but, in recalcitrant cases, an arthroscopic coracoidplasty may be beneficial. However, there are no studies in throwing athletes.

CONCLUSION

It has been well established that overhead athletes develop unique adaptive changes at their glenohumeral joints, allowing them to compete effectively in their respective sports. The repetitive nature of these motions and the stresses produced at the shoulder in these athletes place them at risk for potential dysfunction and structural injury. Understanding and distinguishing a pathological process from the throwing shoulder's physiological adaptive response is a difficult yet critical skill in treating these individuals. Initial efforts at non-surgical therapies should be exhausted before surgical intervention. Advancing diagnostics and surgical capabilities are improving the chances of returning overhead athletes to their preinjury level. Further research on the overhead athlete, internal impingement and its associated pathologies, and continued advancing techniques for surgical intervention, should remain at the forefront of this challenging population.

REFERENCES

Altchek DW, Dines DM. Shoulder injuries in the throwing athlete. J Am Acad Orthop Surg 1995;3:159–165.

Andrews JR, Broussard TS, Carson WG. Arthroscopy of the shoulder in the management of partial tears of the rotator cuff: a preliminary report. Arthroscopy 1985a;1:117–222.

Andrews JR, Carson WG, Jr, McCleod WD. Glenoid labrum tears related to the long head of the biceps. Am J Sports Med 1985b;13:337–41.

Andrews JR, Wilk KE, Reed J, et al. Spring Training 2000. Presented on VuMedi: Shoulder Injuries in Throwers. Webinar. August 16, 2010.

Bennett GE. Shoulder and elbow lesions of the professional baseball pitcher. JAMA 1941;117:510–554.

Burkhart SS, Morgan CD, Kibler WB. The disabled throwing shoulder: spectrum of pathology Part I: pathoanatomy and biomechanics. Arthroscopy 2003a;19:404–420.

Burkhart SS, Morgan CD, Kibler WB. The disabled throwing shoulder: spectrum of pathology Part III: The SICK scapula, scapular dyskinesis, the kinetic chain, and rehabilitation. Arthroscopy 2003b;19:641–661.

Crockett HC, Gross LB, Wilk KE, et al. Osseous adaptation and range of motion at the glenohumeral joint in professional baseball pitchers. Am J Sports Med 2002;30:20–26.

DePalma AF, Coker AJ, Probhaker M. The role of the subscapularis in recurrent anterior dislocation of the shoulder. Clin Orthop 1967;54:35–49.

Dillman CJ, Fleisig GS, Andrews JR. Biomechanics of pitching with emphasis upon shoulder kinematics. J Orthop Sports Phys Ther 1993;18:402–408.

Edwards SL, Lee JA, Bell JE, et al. Nonoperative treatment of superior labrum anterior posterior tears: Improvements in pain, function, and quality of life. Am J Sports Med 2010;38:1456–1461.

Fleisig GS, Andrews JR, Dillman CJ, Escamilla RF. Kinetics of baseball pitching with implications about injury mechanisms. Am J Sports Med 1995;23:233–239.

Fleisig GS, Barrentine SW, Zheng N, et al. Kinematic and kinetic comparison of baseball pitching among various levels of development. J Biomech 1999;32:1371–1375.

Freehill MT, Ebel B, Archer KR, et al. Glenohumeral range of motion in major league pitchers: changes over the playing season. Sports Health 2010;in press 2011;3:97–104.

Gerber C, Werner CM, Macy JC, et al. Effect of selective capsulorraphy on the passive range of motion of the glenohumeral joint. J Bone Joint Surg Am 2003;85:48–55.

Gibb TD, Sidles JA, Harryman DT, et al. The effect of the capsular venting on glenohumeral laxity. Clin Orthop 1991;268:120–127.

Grossman MG, Tibone JE, McGarry MH, et al. A cadaveric model of the throwing shoulder: a possible etiology of superior labrum anterior-to-posterior lesions. J Bone Joint Surg Am 2005;87:824–831.

Halbrecht JL, Tirman P, Atkin D. Internal impingement of the shoulder: comparison of findings between the throwing and nonthrowing shoulders of college baseball players. Arthroscopy 1999;15:253–258.

Howell SM, Galinat BJ. The glenoid-labral socket: A constrained articular surface. Clin Orthop Relat Res 1989;243:123–124.

Huffman GR, Tibone JE, McGarry MH, et al. Path of glenohumeral articulation throughout the rotational range of motion in a thrower's shoulder model. Am J Sports Med 2006;34:1662–1669.

Itoi E, Newman SR, Kuechle DK, et al. Dynamic anterior stabilizers of the shoulder with the arm in abduction. J Bone Joint Surg Br 1994;76:834–836.

Jobe CM, Sidles J. Evidence for a superior glenoid impingement upon the rotator cuff [abstract]. J Shoulder Elbow Surg 1993;2(suppl):S19.

Jobe FW, Pink M. The athlete's shoulder. J Hand Ther 1994;7:107–110.

Jobe FW, Moynes DR, Tibone JE, Perry J. An EMG analysis of the shoulder in pitching. A second report. Am J Sports Med 1984;12:218–220.

Jobe FW, Kvitne RS, Giangarra CE. Shoulder pain in the overhand or throwing athlete. The relationship of anterior instability and rotator cuff impingement. Orthop Rev 1989;18:963–975.

Kibler WB, Chandler TJ, Livingston BP, et al. Shoulder range of motion in elite tennis players. Effect of age and years of tournament play. Am J Sports Med 1996;24:279–285.

Levitz CL, Dugas J, Andrews JR. The use of arthroscopic thermal capsulorraphy to treat internal impingement in baseball players. Arthroscopy 2001;17:573–577.

Lintner D, Mayol M, Uzodinma O, et al. Glenohumeral internal rotation deficits in professional pitchers enrolled in an internal rotation stretching program. Am J Sports Med 2007;35:617–621.

Magnusson SP, Gleim GW, Nicholas JA. Shoulder weakness in professional baseball pitchers. Med Sci Sports Sci 1994;26:5–9.

Mazoué CG, Andrews JR. Repair of full-thickness rotator cuff tears in professional baseball players. Am J Sports Med 2006;34:182–189.

Meister K, Andrews JR, Batts J, et al. Symptomatic thrower's exostosis. Arthroscopic evaluation and treatment. Am J Sports Med 1999;27:133–136.

Mihata T, Lee Y, McGarry MH, et al. Excessive humeral external rotation results in increased shoulder laxity. Am J Sports Med 2004;32:1278–1285.

Morgan CD, Burkhart SS, Palmeri M, et al. Type II SLAP lesions: three subtypes and their relationships to superior instability and rotator cuff tears. Arthroscopy 1998;14:553–565.

Myers TH, Zemanovic JR, Andrews JR. The resisted supination external rotation test: a new test for the dignosis of superior labral anterior posterior lesions. Am J Sports Med 2005;33:1315–1320.

Myers JB, Laudner KG, Pasquale MR, et al. Glenohumeral range of motion deficits and posterior shoulder tightness in throwers with pathologic internal impingement. Am J Sports Med 2006;34:385–391.

Neer CS. Anterior acromioplasty for chronic impingement syndrome. J Bone Joint Surg Am 1972;54:41–50.

O'Brien SJ, Neves MC, Arnoczky SP, et al. The anatomy and histology of the inferior glenohumeral ligament complex of the shoulder. Am J Sports Med. 1990;18:449–456.

O'Brien SJ, Schwartz RS, Warren RF, Torzilli PA. Capsular restraints to anterior–posterior motion of the abducted shoulder. A biomechanical study. J Shoulder Elbow Surg 1995;4:298–308.

Pappas AM, Zawacki RM, Sullivan TJ. Biomechanics of baseball pitching: a preliminary report. Am J Sports Med 1985;13:216–22.

Proske U, Morgan DL. Muscle damage from eccentric exercise: mechanism, mechanical signs, adaptation and clinical applications. J Physiol 2001;537(pt 2):333–345.

Reisman S, Walsh LD, Proske U. Warm-up stretches reduce sensations of stiffness and soreness after eccentric exercise. Med Sci Sports Exer 2005;37:929–936.

Rizio L, Garcia J, Renard R, Got C. Orthopedics 2007;30:544–550.

Rupp S, Berninger K, Hopf T. Shoulder problems in high school level swimmers-impingement, anterior instability, muscular imbalance? Int J Sports Med 1995;16:557–562.

Schneider DJ, Tibone JE, McGarry MH, et al. Biomechanical evaluation after five- and ten-millimeter anterior glenohumeral capsulorraphy using a novel shoulder model of increased laxity. J Shoulder Elbow Surg 2005;14:318–423.

Snyder SJ, Karzel RP, Del Pizzo W, et al. SLAP lesions of the shoulder. Arthroscopy 1990;6:274–279.

Turkel SJ, Panio MW, Marshall JL, Girgis FG. Stabilizing mechanisms preventing anterior dislocation of the glenohumeral joint. J Bone Joint Surg Am 1981;63:1208–1217.

Valadie AL 3rd, Jobe CM, Pink MM, et al. Anatomy of provocative tests for impingement syndromes of the shoulder. J Shoulder Elbow Surg 2000;9:36–46.

Walch G, Liotard JP, Boileau P, Noel E. Posterosuperior glenoid impingement. Another shoulder impingement. Rev Chir Orthop Reparatrice Appar Mot 1991;77:571–574.

Walch G, Boileau P, Noel E, Donell ST. Impingement of the deep surface of the supraspinatus tenon on the posterosuperior glenoid rim: an arthroscopic study. J Shoulder Elbow Surg 1992;1:238–1245.

Wang HK, Cochrane T. Mobility impairment, muscle imbalance, muscle weakness, scapular asymmetry and shoulder injury in elite volleyball athletes. J Sports Med Phys Fitness 2001;41:403–410.

Wilk KE, Andrews JR, Arrigo CA. The abductor and adductor strength characteristics professional baseball pitchers. Am J Sports Med 1995;23:778.

Wilk KE, Suarez K, Reed J. Scapular muscular strength values in professional baseball players. Phys Ther 1999;79:S81–S82.

Wilk KE, Macrina L, Porterfield R, Harker P, McMichael CS, Andrews JR. Podium presentation: Loss of internal rotation and the correlation of shoulder injuries in professional baseball pitchers. Academy of Orthopaedic Surgeons Sports Medicine. Annual Meeting. July 10, 2008. Orlando, Florida.

Wright RW, Paletta GA Jr. Prevalence of the Bennett lesion of the shoulder in major league pitchers. Am J Sports Med 2004;32:121–124.

Yamamoto N, Itoi E, Minagawa H, et al. Why is the humeral retroversion of throwing athletes greater in dominant shoulders than in nondominant shoulders? J Shoulder Elbow Surg 2006;15:571–575.

Chapter 10 SLAP lesions and tendinopathy of the long head of biceps

Neema Pourtaheri, Anthony James Scillia, Jeffrey S. Abrams

KEY FEATURES

- Pathology in the long head of biceps and the superior labrum can be responsible for marked shoulder pain and loss of function. Management is controversial and multiple options are available.
- Treatment options range from benign neglect, to arthroscopic repair, to biceps tenodesis.
- SLAP lesions and biceps pathology are usually associated with concomitant shoulder disorders such as paralabral cysts.
- Management of paralabral and spinoglenoid cycsts is controversial, and multiple options are available.
- The choice among biceps tenodesis, tenotomy, and SLAP lesion repair is based on the patient's activity demands, anticipated return to sport or work, and the ability of the shoulder to accommodate additional constraint..

INTRODUCTION

Pathology in the long head of biceps and the superior labrum can be responsible for marked shoulder pain and loss of function. Superior labral tears can result from a single hyperextension injury or from repetitive strenuous motions such as throwing a baseball. Management is controversial, because there are now multiple options available to address injuries to the proximal component of the tendon of the long head of biceps, ranging from benign neglect, to arthroscopic repair, to biceps tenodesis. Recent reports have identified an increase in the number of arthroscopic repairs from fellowship-trained sports medicine physicians (Weber et al. 2010). This may be due to inconsistencies in diagnosis, patient selection, and treatment strategy which may affect the incidence of complications. Although traditional shoulder scoring systems have demonstrated improvement with repairs, a disturbing number of throwing athletes have not been able to return to their previous level (Brockmeier et al. 2009). This chapter reviews the management options for bicipital–labral pathology. Interventions intended to maximize the chance of recovery to full, unrestricted activity are considered.

Andrews et al. (1985) first described superior labral lesions as an injury to the anterosuperior labrum near the origin of the long head of biceps in overhead throwing athletes. He believed that these injuries occurred in high frequency in the throwing athlete because of the deceleration forces imparted by the biceps tendon during the follow-through phase.

Snyder et al. (1990) coined the term "SLAP" (superior labrum anterior and posterior) lesion when he described an injury to the superior labrum at the origin of the long head of biceps tendon. In the original article on SLAP lesions, Snyder et al. (1995) described four types of lesions involving the superior labrum and biceps tendon. In his referral practice, approximately 6% of operated patients had SLAP tears. Type I was characterized by degenerative fraying of the labrum but with the peripheral edge remaining firmly attached. The attachment of the biceps tendon to the labrum was also intact. Type II lesions had similar fraying; however, the superior labrum and attached biceps had been stripped off the underlying glenoid, resulting in an unstable bicipital-labral anchor. A type III lesion has a bucket-handle tear in the superior labrum. The central portion is displaced into the joint, whereas the peripheral labrum remains firmly attached to the underlying glenoid and the intact biceps tendon. A type IV lesion demonstrates a bucket-handle tear that extends into the biceps tendon.

Snyder's original classification has been expanded to include SLAP lesions associated with shoulder instability. Maffet et al. (1995) described three additional types: a type V lesion is an anteroinferior Bankart lesion that extends proximally to the biceps attachment; a type VI lesion is an anterior or posterior labral flap with a concomitant type II SLAP lesion; and a type VII lesion is a biceps attachment separation that extends into the middle glenohumeral ligament.

Nord and Ryu (Powell et al. 2004) further expanded the classification: a type VIII lesion is a type II SLAP lesion with posterior labral extension; a type IX lesion is a type II lesion with circumferential labral tearing; and a type X lesion is a type II lesion with posteroinferior labral separation.

Symptomatic SLAP lesions are generally treated surgically. Many options are available. With improvement in technology, nearly all of the currently popular surgical procedures are being performed arthroscopically.

It is important to recognize, however, that not all SLAP lesions need to be treated. Indeed, a SLAP lesion that occurs in the setting of other shoulder pathology may not be primarily responsible for the patient's symptoms. As an example, a SLAP lesion identified in a patient aged >40, or in patients with other pathology such as glenohumeral osteoarthritis or rotator cuff tears, may be a lesion best left alone because surgical repair can lead to poor outcomes (Franceschi et al. 2008; Abbot et al. 2009).

Unfortunately, complications after surgery for a bicipital–labral disorder are not infrequent. To avoid problems, surgical repairs should be anatomical and must be performed on appropriately selected patients. Postoperative stiffness is a well-recognized complication of patients undergoing SLAP repairs. There have been reports of broken or dislodged, bioabsorbable, poly-L-lactic acid tacks causing pain, symptomatic hardware that produces either mechanical symptoms or chondral injury, and failed SLAP lesion healing (Sassmannshausen et al. 2006). Metal suture anchors, in particular, have been implicated in a significant number of chondral injuries to the humeral head (Kaar et al. 2001). Other complications include formation of suture granuloma, iatrogenic impingement after arthroscopic SLAP repair, and foreign body reaction to bioabsorbable devices (Burkhart et al. 2000; Ifesanya et al. 2008). Given the potential serious complications and compromised results that can follow SLAP repair, attention to detail is paramount.

ANATOMY OF SUPERIOR LABRUM AND LONG HEAD OF BICEPS

The glenoid labrum is composed of dense fibrous tissue that is attached to the glenoid via fibrocartilage adjacent to the articular cartilage of the glenoid. The glenoid labrum surrounds the glenoid peripherally and deepens the socket. Perry (1983) showed that the humeral head contact area increased by 75% vertically and 67% horizontally when the labrum was intact. This deepening helps stabilize the glenohumeral joint. In addition, the labrum serves as the attachment of supporting shoulder ligaments (Cooper et al. 1992).

The biceps anchor originates from both the glenoid and the labrum (Cooper et al. 1992; Vangsness et al. 1994). Half of the attachment arises from a discrete point 5 mm medial to the superior rim of the glenoid at the supraglenoid tubercle (Vangsness et al. 1994). The labrum serves as the remaining attachment with four variations in morphology (Vangsness et al. 1994). The vascularity is derived from the capsule and periosteum. The superior and anterosuperior parts of the labrum have less vascularity than the posterosuperior and inferior parts.

Williams et al. (1994) described a normal variant, the "Buford complex," in which the middle glenohumeral ligament (GHL) inserts into the base of biceps and the anterosuperior labrum is absent (**Fig. 10.1**). This variant was seen in 1.5% of the patients studied. Williams et al. (1994) reported that attempted fixation of this normal variant would result in painful restriction of external rotation.

The long head of biceps tendon (LHBT) travels through the glenohumeral joint space from its origin and turns anteriorly to enter the intertubercular groove of the humerus at an angle of 35°. The LHBT is intra-articular and intracapsular, but extrasynovial. The intertubercular groove provides the bony constraint for the LHBT pulley system. The biceps glides in the groove and is constrained by a soft-tissue pulley system. The transverse humeral ligament, made from a confluence of fibers from supraspinatus and subscapularis, forms a roof over biceps and stabilizes its distal part in the groove (Gleason et al. 2006). The proximal portion of the groove is stabilized by an additional pulley from the superior GHL, coracohumeral ligament, subscapularis tendon, and supraspinatus tendon. The vascular supply of the proximal biceps tendon comes from the terminal branch of the anterior humeral circumflex artery, and is innervated by the sensory sympathetic fibers of the musculocutaneous nerve (Rathbun and McNab 1970; Alpantaki et al. 2005).

PATHOGENESIS/PATHOLOGY

SLAP lesions

Isolated SLAP tears are uncommon and usually found in combination with some other shoulder pathology (**Fig. 10.2**). Stetson and Templin (2002) showed that 81% of patients with SLAP tears had some other shoulder pathology. Snyder et al. (1995) showed that 43% of patients who had a SLAP lesion also had an associated partial or complete rotator cuff tear. Maffet et al. (1995) reported that 48% of patients with a SLAP lesion had some form of rotator cuff pathology and 20% had a lesion consistent with dinstability. Franceschi et al. (2008) demonstrated no advantage to repair of type II SLAP lesions when associated with rotator cuff repair in patients aged >50 years.

The prevalence of SLAP lesions is age dependent. Pfahler et al. (2003) analyzed 32 normal cadaveric shoulders and found age-related changes in the glenoid labrum. In patients aged 30–50 years, there were tears and defects of the superior and anterosuperior labrum. In patients aged >60, the labrum had variable lesions along the whole circumference.

Biceps pathology

Although less common than injuries to the rotator cuff, primary biceps pathology is a not infrequent common cause of anterior shoulder pain. The next section summarizes some of the important aspects of inflammatory, traumatic, instability, and space-occupying components of primary biceps pathology.

Inflammatory biceps pathology

Primary bicipital tenosynovitis is a condition limited to the tendon without evidence of associated shoulder pathology. Individuals who participate in sports that require repeated overhead motions are at risk. Narrowing of the biceps groove, which can occur when bony anatomy is altered after fracture, glenohumeral joint arthritis, and grove anoma-

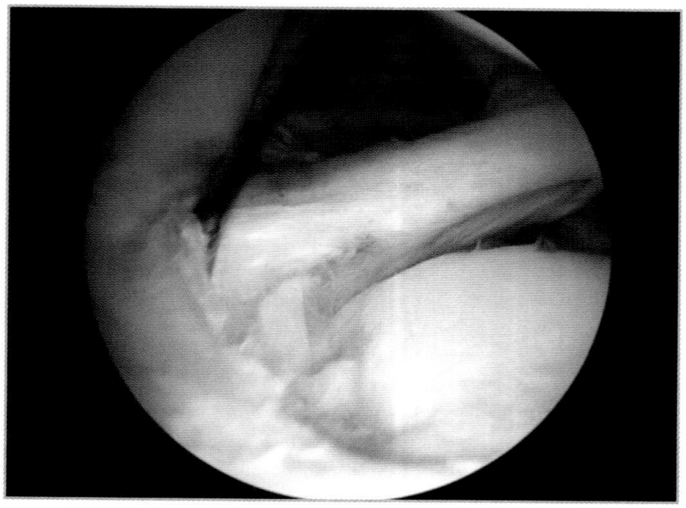

Figure 10.1 A Buford complex anatomical variant with absent anterior labrum and a mobile middle glenohumeral ligament attached to the base of biceps with superior glenoid disruption.

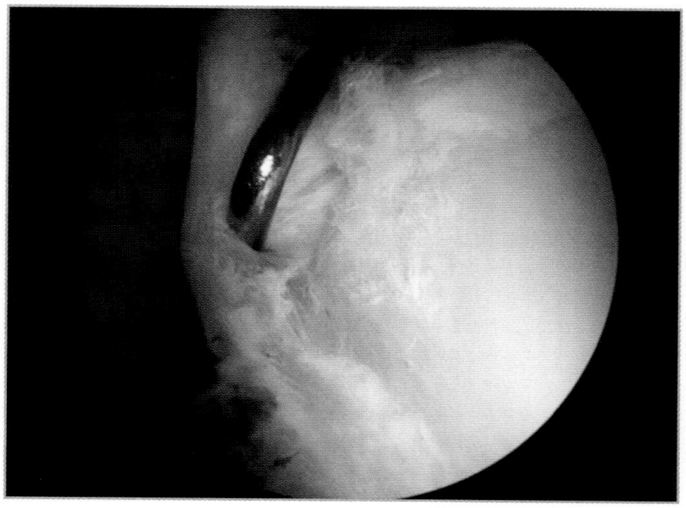

Figure 10.2 SLAP (superior labrum anterior and posterior) tear demonstrating abnormal glenoid articular rim and undersurface of the labrum.

lies, can all exacerbate biceps tenosynovitis (Davidson and Rivenburgh 2004 ; Neer and Horwitz 1965). The repetitive overhead motion, over time, can result in an inflammatory response as the tendon glides in the bicipital grove.

Inflammation of the LHBT and the surrounding synovial tissue within the groove can generate pain. In the early stages, the tendon appears dull, swollen, and discolored, but it is mobile. With disease progression, the surrounding soft tissues become thickened and fibrotic, and the blood supply becomes diminished through the surrounding viniculae. As the tendon becomes swollen through hypertrophy, an hourglass deformity where the tendon becomes entrapped may occur (Boileau et al. 2004).

Traumatic biceps pathology

Traumatic rupture of the LHBT is relatively common. The injury may occur after a fall, direct trauma, repetitive overuse, or after a sudden longitudinal force is applied to the arm.

When the biceps tendon ruptures it often retracts, resulting in a visible loss of contour or "Popeye" deformity. In thin or well-defined patients, the deformity is obvious; in obese individuals or individuals with poorly defined musculature, the deformity is more subtle (Osbar et al. 2002).

From a functional standpoint, the injury is well tolerated. Patients with spontaneous biceps tendon rupture may have some elbow and forearm weakness, and perhaps some cramping with repetitive forearm rotation, but shoulder weakness has not been demonstrated (Mariani et al. 1988).

Instability-related biceps pathology

Biceps instability is primarily the result of failure of the pulley system (Lafosse et al. 2007). Any trauma that disrupts the pulley restraints can lead to excessive biceps motion and ultimately instability. Common causes of pulley rupture include fractures, shoulder dislocations, and repetitive overuse.

Instability patterns are well recognized. Anterior inferior subluxation of the tendon results from a tear in the SGHL (superior glenohumeral ligament) insertion. Tears of the SGHL allow the biceps tendon to sublux anteroinferiorly toward the upper portion of the subscapularis tendon insertion. Biceps dislocation often frequently occurs together with a tear of subscapularis. When the superior border of the subscapularis tendon is disrupted, biceps may slide out of its grove and under the subscapularis tendon. Many clinicians treat this injury with biceps tenotomy or tenodesis to spare the subscapularis tendon from further injury.

Posterior instability of the biceps tendon has also been observed but is less common. Posterior instability occurs after a tear of the roof of the CHL (coracohumeral ligament). This injury allows the tendon to sublux superiorly and posteriorly and is associated with tears of supraspinatus (Lafosse et al. 2007).

Paralabral ganglion cysts

Paralabral ganglion and spinoglenoid notch cysts (SGNCs) often occur in close association with SLAP and labral pathology (Post and Mayer 1987; Moore et al. 1997) (**Figs 10.3a and b**). Although the exact mechanism of formation of these space-occupying lesions is unknown, cyst formation probably results from injury of the labrum or capsule. The torn labrum and capsule can allow a one-way valve mechanism to form where synovial fluid leaves the glenohumeral joint and accumulates medial to the labrum (Westerheide and Karzel 2003).

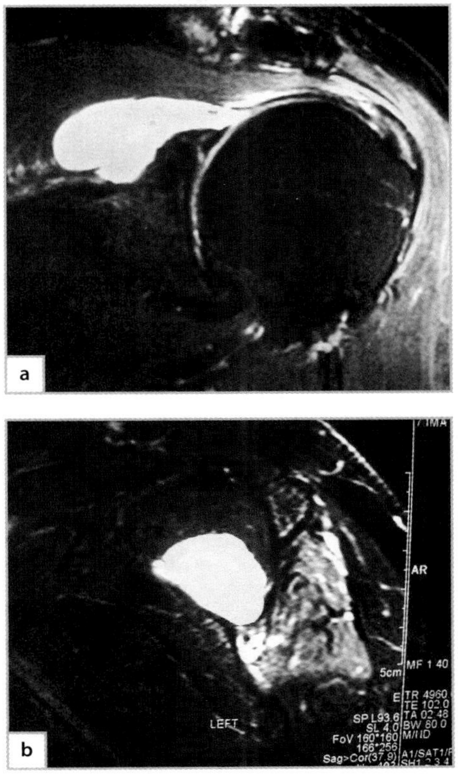

Figure 10.3 **A large paralabral cyst on MRI (two views).**

Clinically, paralabral cysts and SGNCs produce a mass effect on surrounding structures. The suprascapular nerve runs through the spinoglenoid notch and innervates infraspinatus. As the nerve exits the spinoglenoid notch, it is on average just 1.8 cm from the posterior glenoid rim, easily susceptible to compression (Moore et al. 1997). Not all patients with SGNCs are symptomatic, and those who are typically complain of posterior shoulder pain radiating into the neck or down the arm.

The clinical work-up for the patient who presents with posterior shoulder pain often includes magnetic resonance imaging (MRI) with or without an electromyography (EMG) study. The MR scan is very sensitive in detecting the fluid-filled cyst. EMG can be used to confirm or rule out an associated compressive neuropathy.

Many cysts are asymptomatic or minimally symptomatic and can be managed non-surgically with rehabilitation or observation. Symptomatic cysts can be managed with CT- or ultrasound-guided aspiration. This technique has, however, a recurrence rate between 48% and 75% (Post and Mayer 1987; Tung et al. 2000).

Open and arthroscopic techniques have been used to treat the cysts and repair associated labral tears. Open surgery requires a large incision, and it is often difficult to repair a SLAP tear through an open approach. Arthroscopy is minimally invasive and allows better visualization of the SLAP tear. For this reason, most clinicians favor an arthroscopic approach.

The optimal arthroscopic procedure to address the pathology remains unclear. If the patient has a compressive neuropathy and the cyst cannot be seen on arthroscopy, some advocate the repair of SLAP and leave the cyst alone (Post and Mayer 1987). If the cyst is seen, some advocate cyst decompression. Piatt et al. (2002) showed a higher satisfaction with labral repair and cyst excision as opposed to labral repair alone. In contrast, Youms et al. (2006) reported resolution of superior glenoid cysts in 8 of 10 patients with labral repair alone.

CLINICAL PRESENTATION OF SLAP LESIONS AND LONG HEAD OF BICEPS PROBLEMS

Signs and symptoms

The most common complaint of patients with a SLAP lesion is pain (Maffet et al. 1995). Patients can experience mechanical symptoms when the arm is externally rotated and abducted. The anterior shoulder pain is most intense in the biceps groove and can radiate down the arm. Patients with biceps instability may complain of clicking and snapping at the extremes of rotation, especially with the arm elevated (Neviaser 1980). Provocative positions of extension or a throwing position may also reproduce patient complaints.

Mechanism

The mechanism of injury to the superior labral complex has traditionally been seen as either compressive or related to traction. Traction injuries include trying to break a fall with the arm overhead or with the arm held below the shoulder, and suddenly catching a heavy object (Maffet et al. 1995). These injuries produce a tensile overload on the biceps anchor. Compression injuries produce a superiorly directed force on the humerus, which drives the head into the superior anchor. This occurs during a fall on an outstretched hand and a direct blow to the shoulder (Maffet et al. 1995).

A "peel-back" mechanism of injury also has been proposed. Peel-back lesions are typically seen in overhead throwing athletes. This injury occurs from a torsional load applied to biceps that "peels back" biceps and the posterior labrum from the glenoid, as the shoulder goes into extreme abduction and external rotation during the cocking phase of throwing. During the cocking position, the torsional forces applied to biceps cause progressive failure of the biceps anchor and posterior labrum (Burkhart and Morgan 1998). The load to the anchor is highest during the late-cocking phase of throwing motion (Kuhn et al. 2003). When throwing, the torso moves forward to produce further torsional stresses. Internal impingement of the posterosuperior labrum occurs and leads to tissue failure.

Physical examination

The findings at physical examination for SLAP lesions are often confounded by other shoulder pathology. Approximately 72% of SLAP lesions have associated shoulder pathology. Stetson and Templin (2002) showed that, with isolated SLAP tears, 52% of patients had positive impingement sign, 43% had a pop/snap with motion, 39% had anterior apprehension, and 35% had positive biceps tension sign.

There are numerous tests to diagnosis SLAP tears, including the compression rotation test, crank test, O'Brien's test, pain provocation test, and biceps load test. Most of these tests attempt to elicit pain by bringing the arm into the overhead throwing position and stressing the biceps anchor. In isolation, none of these tests is completely reliable. For this reason, many believe that clinical exam alone cannot be relied on to diagnose SLAP tears (McFarland et al. 2002; Parentis et al. 2006).

Patients with pathology of the LHBT most commonly have tenderness in the intertubercular groove (Sethi et al. 1999). The groove should be palpated at neutral, and then at internal and external rotation. The greater and lesser tuberosities should be felt rolling under the examiner's fingers. This can be difficult in patients with a well-developed deltoid muscle.

O'Brien's test positions the arm at 10° adduction, 90° forward flexion, and maximal internal rotation (O'Brien et al. 1998). With the forearm fully pronated, the examiner resists forward flexion by pushing down on the wrist. Next, with patient's hand in full supination, the examiner again pushes down on the hand. The experience of pain when the arm is fully pronated and relief when supinated are considered a positive test.

With a positive Speed's test, pain is produced at the anterior bicipital grove by resisted forward flexion with the shoulder flexed at 90° and the forearm fully supinated. This test can also be positive because of bicipital tendinopathy.

The crank test is performed in the upright or supine position with the shoulder elevated to 160° in the scapular plane. In this position, an axial load is applied by the examiner while the humerus is internally and externally rotated. Pain elicited particularly by external rotation is considered a positive test.

Stetson and Templin (2002) showed that O'Brien's and the crank test had just a 31% and 56% specificity, respectively. The results of the tests were frequently positive for patients with other shoulder conditions, including impingement and rotator cuff tears.

Speed's and Yergason's tests can also be used to examine for LHBT pathology. These tests have low sensitivity and moderate specificity (Holtby and Razmjou 2004). The test is positive if it elicits pain. With Yergason's test, the elbow is flexed to 90° with the arm at the patient's side. In this position, the patient attempts to forcefully supinate and externally rotate against the examiner's hand. Pain referred to the anterior shoulder in the region of the bicipital groove constitutes a positive test.

Imaging

Plain radiographs should be taken to evaluate for other shoulder pathology such as glenohumeral osteoarthritis. MR arthrography is the primary non-surgical means for confirming a SLAP lesion with sensitivity >90% (Jee et al. 2001). The addition of intra-articular gadolinium increases the sensitivity in discerning labral pathology (Reuss et al. 2006). Anatomical variations in the superior labrum can confound the diagnostic accuracy of MRI. A normal sublabral separation from the glenoid surface is common, varying from a slight crease to a sulcus measuring 1–2 mm. These variations are not pathological, and may be seen on MR arthrography (Jin et al. 2006). However, the presence of a ganglion or sublabral cyst, sometimes associated with suprascapular nerve compression, suggests the presence of SLAP lesion (Westerheide and Karzel 2003).

Radiographs can be used to evaluate fractures or deformities that affect the biceps pulley system. A biceps groove view, a view parallel to the long axis of the groove, can also be taken to evaluate the architecture of the groove. MRI is useful to evaluate the soft-tissue pulley system and the bony architecture of the groove. MRI has high sensitivity and specificity for rotator cuff tears involving the pulley system, but it is low to moderate for other biceps tendon pathologies (Beall et al. 2003; Mohtadi et al. 2004). This specificity is somewhat improved with MR arthrography. Intra-articular ultrasonography is only moderately sensitive and specific for most tendon pathology (Armstrong et al. 2006). However, for complete ruptures of the LHBT, ultrasonography and MRI are more highly sensitive and specific (Armstrong et al. 2006; Zanetti et al. 1998).

DIAGNOSIS

Although history, physical examination, and imaging studies suggest the presence of SLAP tears and tendinopathy of the LHBT, only an arthroscopic examination can confirm the diagnosis. In an anatomical study of 105 shoulders, the LHBT originated from the superior glenoid labrum in about half the cadaveric specimens and from the supraglenoid tubercle in the other 40–60% (Vangsness et al. 1994). This should be considered when diagnosing and classifying SLAP tears.

During diagnostic arthroscopy, a portion of the LHBT in the intertubercular groove can be visualized as well. This is accomplished by placing the probe in the anterior portal, and pushing the tendon into the articular viewing space. Approximately 1.5–2 cm of the LHBT can be visualized in the joint. Pathology of the LHBT was classified by Castagna and colleagues (Castagna et al. 2007):

- Normal LHBT with intact synovial sheath.
- Hyperemic LHBT in the intra-articular portion, without signs of tendinopathy.
- Hyperemic LHBT with tendon imprinting on the anterosuperior humeral head cartilage, evidence of weakening of the synovial sheath at the entrance of the bicipital groove.
- Flattened and enlarged LHBT showing anatomoarthroscopic signs of medial subluxation. Humeral chondropathy is observed. Evidence of weakening and macroscopic degeneration of the synovial sheath.
- Medial dislocation of the tendon with pathological adhesions involving subscapularis.
- Prerupture of the LHBT, macroscopic signs of tendon pathology visible as partial tears from fraying of the tendon accompanied by laceration and widespread weakening of the synovial sheath.

SLAP tears and LHB tendinopathy are diagnosed and classified during arthroscopic examination. With the arthroscope in the posterior portal, the superior labrum can be visualized and probed through the anterior portal. The glenohumeral ligaments should be visualized, and a positive drive-through sign may be present if anterior and inferior advancement of the arthroscope is done with ease. This may indicate either capsular laxity or labral instability. With the arthroscope in the posterior portal and the probe in the anterior portal, the superior labrum is evaluated for pathological lesions and then classified. A posterior SLAP lesion may be revealed to the examiner by the "peel-back mechanism" described by Burkhart and Morgan (1998). Abduction and external rotation of the shoulder place the LHBT at a vertical posterior angle, producing a torsional force that may separate the posterior superior labrum from the glenoid rim (Burkhart and Morgan 1998).

Normal variations should be considered when diagnosing biceps and superior labral pathology, along with the degenerative changes that occur during aging. Dynamic examination may help differentiate pathology from anatomical variations that, if not recognized, would flaw surgical decision-making. The Buford complex, sublabral foramen, rounded variants and meniscoid variants previously described may be misinterpreted as labral pathology.

Pfahler et al. (2003) demonstrated a histopathological difference in cadaveric specimens according to age, most notably in the 12 o'clock position. Fraying and compensatory laxity of the superior labrum of the glenoid occurs as a natural aging process (Pfahler et al. 2003). This will compensate for decreased motion at the glenohumeral joint which also occurs with aging. If the superior labrum is repaired and re-tensioned, shoulder stiffness is likely to result.

Franceschi et al. (2008) reported no advantage in repair of type II SLAP lesions in patients aged >50 years with rotator cuff tears. They demonstrated that there was a significant improvement in UCLA (university of California at Los Angeles) shoulder scores and ROM when comparing rotator cuff repair with biceps tenotomy versus rotator cuff repair with type II SLAP repair. Forsythe et al. (2010) showed similar outcomes in middle-aged patients with combined SLAP and rotator cuff repairs versus those who underwent cuff repair alone.

MANAGEMENT

Conservative management

The conservative management of SLAP tears includes the use of nonsteroidal anti-inflammatory drugs (NSAIDs), rest, cold therapy, and a short period of immobilization in the acute setting. Early ROM and stretching activities are initiated soon after the initial injury with a focus on stretching of the posterior capsule with a sleeper stretch. Once full ROM is obtained, therapy is advanced to a strengthening protocol of the shoulder girdle focusing on the rotator cuff musculature. As noted by Kibler and McMullen (2003), there is a high incidence of scapular dyskinesis, which can be addressed with core and thoracic spine strengthening as well as a "proximal-to-distal protocol," including exercises such as wall slides (Kibler and McMullen 2003). At 3 months, sports-specific therapy can be started. The patient may return to sport when full ROM and strength are equivalent to the contralateral shoulder. However, if at 3 months symptoms have not resolved, then surgical treatment should be considered.

Similarly, the initial treatment of tendinopathy of the LHBT is 3 months of conservative treatment. Avoidance of exacerbating activities, and NSAIDs as well as corticosteroid injections should be considered. Subacromial, intra-articular, and bicipital tendon sheath injections may be used, and should be chosen based on the presence of secondary pathology, e.g., in a patient with impingement syndrome and tendinopathy of the biceps tendon, a subacromial steroid injection would be ideal. Once symptoms ameliorate, ROM activities followed by strengthening should be initiated.

Surgical management of SLAP tears

The surgical management of SLAP tears is based on the classification of the lesion, associated injuries, and the patient's history and physical examination. The surgical management for type I SLAP tears would include debridement of the frayed or degenerative portion of the labrum with care to avoid injury to the articular cartilage.

The indications for surgical repair of a type II SLAP tear include 3 months of failed conservative management, including but not limited to use of NSAIDs, rest, activity modification and avoidance, ROM, strengthening, and physical therapy modalities. The tear must demonstrate a discontinuity of the superior labrum and biceps complex that can be displaced during diagnostic arthroscopy with a probe (see **Fig. 10.2**). There must be visible changes to the glenoid articular cartilage, as well as the undersurface of the labrum. Patient selection is extremely important and reserved for patients with shoulder instability, laxity, or in overhead-throwing athletes. Special caution to surgical repair of a type II SLAP tear includes an anatomical variation and degenerative joint disease. An anatomical variant such as a Buford complex, sublabral foramen, and meniscoid- and rounded-type labral variants may be misdiagnosed as a tear.

Repairing a type II SLAP tear aims to restore the anatomical attachment of the superior labrum and biceps anchor. Anterior, anterolateral (1 cm away from the anterolateral corner of the acromion), and posterior portals are produced. Alternative portals may be utilized including the Neviaser portal and the transrotator cuff portal, located lateral to the acromion at the muscle–tendon junction of supraspinatus.

With the arthroscope placed in the posterior or superior lateral portal, the superior labrum is probed and carefully inspected to mobilize the tear. The biceps–labrum complex should be visualized initially from two portals (**Fig. 10.4**). The frayed labral tissue is debrided, and a bed of bleeding bone is prepared with a shaver. Suture anchors should be placed on the glenoid neck at the edge of the articular cartilage at an angle of approximately 45° (**Fig. 10.5**).

Anterior placement can be introduced through the anterolateral portal, transrotator cuff, port of Wilmington (1 cm lateral and 2 cm anterior to the posterolateral aspect of the acromion), or Neviaser portal, depending on the tear, patient anatomy, and surgeon preference. With the transrotator cuff portal, no cannula is utilized, and a Kirschner wire is placed to make a starting hole for the anchor (O'Brien et al. 2002; Crockett et al. 2004). A single working portal, created within the rotator interval, permits suture hook translabral placement (Buess 2006)

SLAP fixation starts at the level of the anterior margin of the biceps and extends posteriorly. Anterior fixation is at risk of over-tensioning and unintended closure of a naturally occurring fovea. A double-loaded anchor or two suture anchors, one on either side of the biceps anchor, can be placed with a horizontal mattress-suturing pattern. The anchor at the posterior margin of biceps should be placed first, and the labrum is held in anatomical reduction when the sites are chosen for puncture with the tissue penetrator or curved spectrum hooks |(**Fig. 10.6**). A sliding knot with the posterior limb as the post is placed with a knot pusher, followed by half-hitches. Suture tails are cut short to avoid suture impingement. Non bulky knots are preferred, with fewer knots necessary with the use of ultra-high-molecular-weight polyethylene sutures. Ultimately, the repair should establish anatomical restoration of the biceps–labral complex and eliminate the drive-through sign and peel-back mechanism that can be simulated with a posterior directed and externally rotated force to the humerus (Barber et al. 2007; Morgan et al. 2008) (**Fig. 10.7**).

Type III SLAP tears are treated by debridement of the unstable bucket-handle labral tissue with a shaver or basket from the anterior portal. Care is taken to avoid disturbing the biceps anchor while ensuring removal of all non-viable tissue. Some type III tears may have characteristics of a type II detachment. Here, debridementof the loose

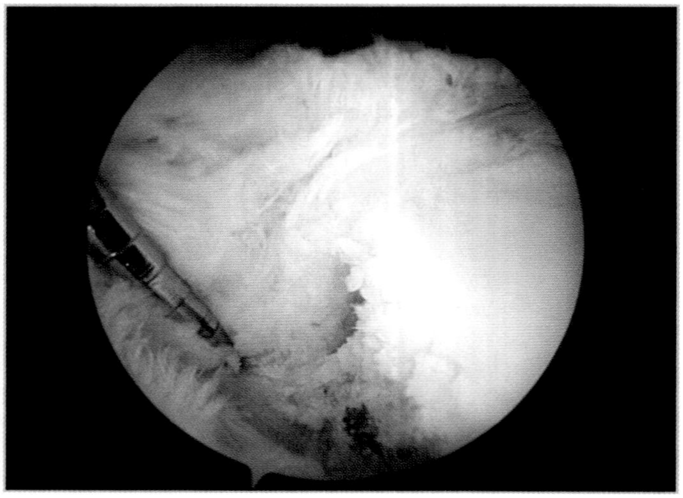

Figure 10.4 SLAP (superior labrum anterior and posterior) repair, preparing the glenoid neck and anchor hole for suture anchor reattachment.

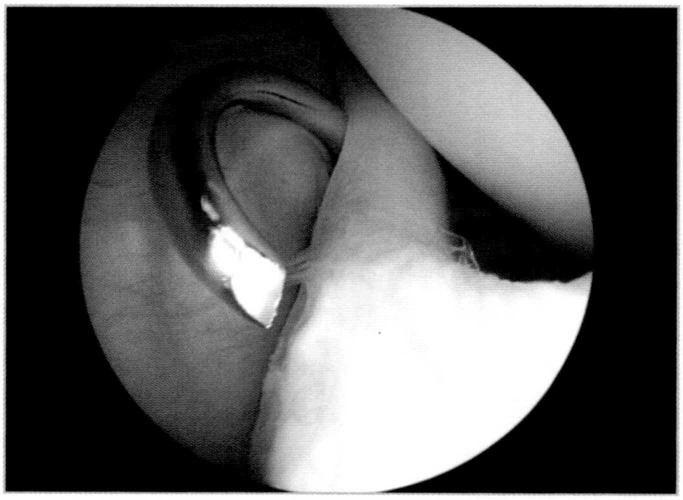

Figure 10.6 A curved suture hook enters the anterior portal and pierces the labrum posterior to the suture anchor.

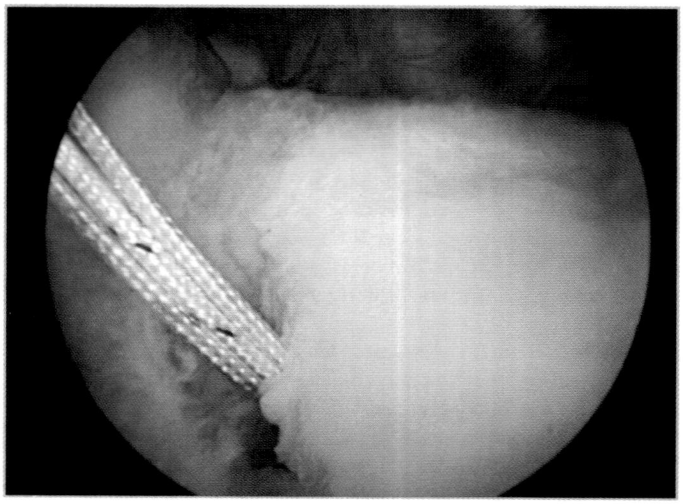

Figure 10.5 A suture anchor is inserted below the articular surface at a 45° angle.

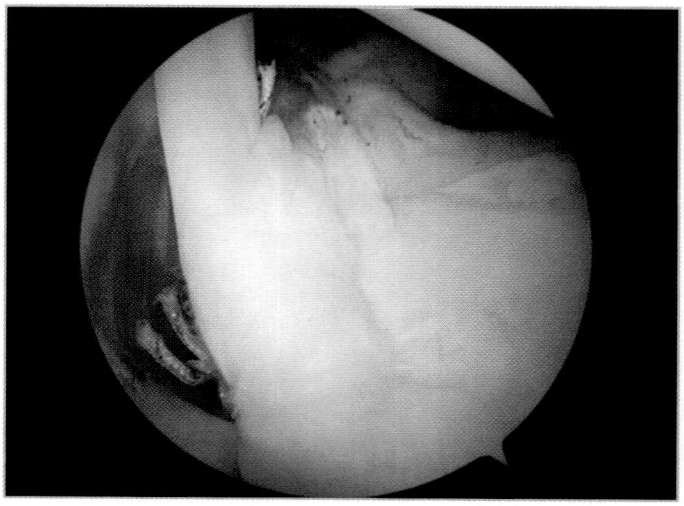

Figure 10.7 A completed superior labral repair and biceps anchor using mattress sutures.

portion may accompany a suture anchor repair of the unstable portion. Options for treatment of type IV SLAP tears include debridement, repair, biceps tenodesis, and biceps tenotomy. If the bucket-handle tear comprises a significant portion of the superior labrum, then an attempt at repair should be considered in cases of shoulder instability (Davila 2009) If the tear comprises greater than 50% of the biceps tendon, one may consider biceps tenodesis or tenotomy (Davila 2009). If the biceps tendon is split vertically, it may be repaired with a side-to-side suturing technique in select type IV lesions (Angelo et al. 2010) (**Figs 10.8a** and **b**).

If the SLAP tear is accompanied by a Bankart lesion, a type V SLAP tear, then both should be repaired when possible to correct the shoulder instability. A flap tear of the superior labrum with separation of the biceps anchor, a type VI SLAP tear, is treated surgically with arthroscopic debridement of the flap tear. After removal of the flap of labral tissue, the labrum and shoulder are assessed for stability. Both type III and IV tears may involve the middle glenohumeral ligament and should be evaluated and repaired. If there is separation of the biceps anchor that continues through the middle glenohumeral ligament, a type VII SLAP tear, arthroscopic repair should be performed. The three additional variations on type II SLAP tears include posterior, circumferential, and posteroinferior extension, named by Nord and Ryu as types VIII, IX, and X, respectively. These complex tears follow the same treatment algorithm described above with debridement of frayed tissue and repair when there is glenohumeral instability or hyperlaxity.

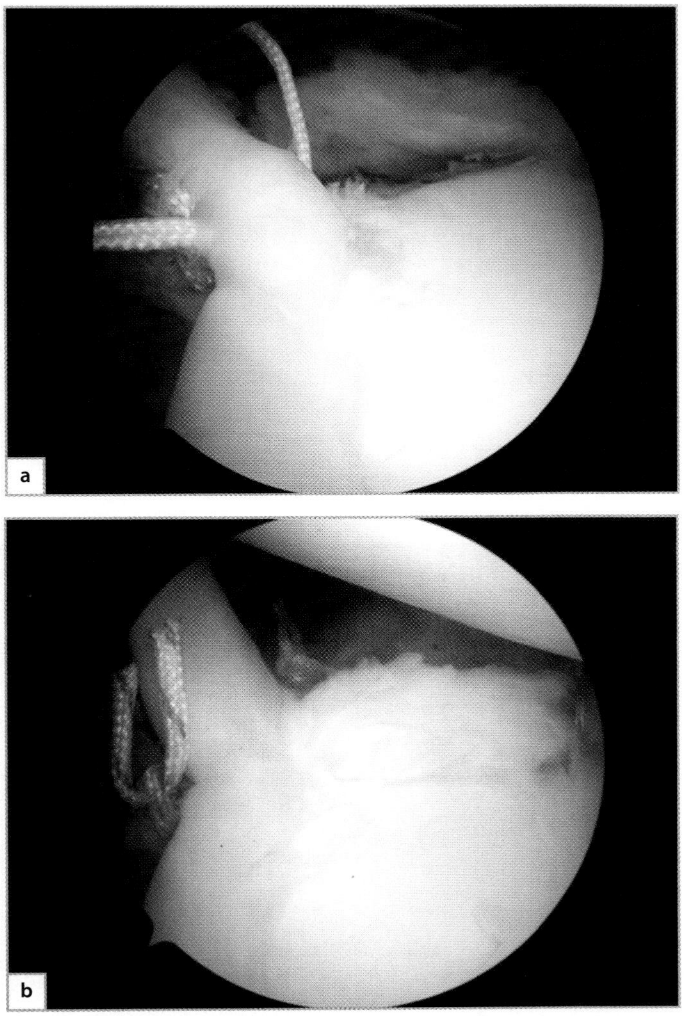

Figure 10.8 SLAP (superior labrum anterior and posterior) tear extending through the anterior labrum. Suture anchor with multiple sutures to repair complex tear. Repair of the unstable labrum and biceps.

SURGICAL MANAGEMENT OF LONG HEAD OF BICEPS TENDINOPATHY

Surgical management of LHB tendinopathy is indicated for symptoms or instability despite conservative management. Temporary relief of symptoms with corticosteroid injection is a useful predictor of successful surgical treatment and accurate diagnosis. Procedures include debridement, tenotomy, and tenodesis. Concomitant shoulder pathology such as a rotator cuff tear, a SLAP tear, or impingement syndrome must be considered, and may influence which type of procedure should be performed. The patient's history, physical examination, and imaging studies should be influential in this process.

Debridement of the LHBT is indicated when degeneration or tearing involves less than 25% of the tendon (Barber et al. 2007). In a very low-demand patient, this can be considered in pathology involving up to 50% of the tendon (Barber et al. 2007). In this technique, a shaver is utilized to remove the entire diseased portion of the tendon. Subacromial decompression as well as Mumford procedures should be performed when indicated.

LHBT tenotomy should be discussed with the patient before surgery, because the disadvantages of this procedure include the potential for retraction of biceps and the resultant "Popeye" deformity, cramping, and mild loss of forearm supination strength. Tenotomy is fast and simple and does not impart any restrictions in rehabilitation. Relative indications for tenotomy include age >60, obesity, and sedentary lifestyle, because this patient population is less likely to have a cosmetic deformity or functional weakness. The standard anterior and posterior arthroscopic portals are made and, using electrocautery or a basket, the tendon is removed from its origin with great care to protect the superior labrum.

Biceps tenodesis, where the LHBT is released from its origin and fixed proximally to humerus or soft tissue, has the advantages of eliminating the potential for a "Popeye" deformity and weakness in supination. The procedure is technically more involved and requires restrictions in postoperative rehabilitation. Therefore, tenodesis is indicated in a patient with a significant tendinopathy, instability, or torn LHBT in a younger, active patient willing to comply with a restricted rehabilitation protocol. Numerous techniques are described to perform tenodesis of the LHBT, including soft-tissue or bony reattachment, and reinsertion proximal or distal to the pectoralis major tendon. These techniques may be performed entirely arthroscopically or through an arthroscopically assisted approach.

Mazzocca and others (2005) described a technique of open subpectoral biceps tenodesis with an interference screw. With this technique, the standard anterior and posterior portals are established. After diagnostic arthroscopy, the LHBT is released and tagged with a suture through a spinal needle. The arm is then abducted and externally rotated. A 3-cm incision is made 1 cm above the inferior border of pectoralis major in the axilla. After incising the fascia of coracobrachialis and biceps, the LHBT is bluntly dissected and retrieved. With a non-absorbable suture using Krackow's technique, the proximal 1.5 cm of tendon is sutured. An 8-mm drill hole is made so that the musculotendinous junction should lie deep to the inferior border of the pectoralis major tendon after tenodesis. An 8-mm biotenodesis screw is then placed with appropriate tension on the LHBT.

Boileau et al. (2002) reported an arthroscopic technique of biceps tenodesis with an interference screw avoiding a mini-open portion of the procedure. Posterior, anteromedial, and anterolateral portals are established where the anteromedial portal is the working portal. These anterior portals are made 1.5 cm on either side of the bicipital groove, 3 cm from the acromion. Diagnostic arthroscopy is performed, and the LHBT is tagged with a spinal needle as it enters the bicipital groove. The tendon is then released from its origin, and the bicipital groove is opened using electrocautery. The LHBT is brought through the anteromedial portal with an arthroscopic grasper after removal of the spinal needle. With the elbow in flexion, 8 mm of the proximal extent of the tendon is doubled and whip stitched with non-absorbable suture. The tendon is brought outside the cannula, and the humerus is reamed at the appropriate size over a guidewire placed 10 mm distal to the most proximal portion of the bicipital groove. A Beath pin is then passed through the anteromedial portal perpendicular to the shaft of the humerus with sutures loaded through the eyelet 2 cm inferior and medial to the posterolateral edge of the acromion. Appropriate tension is then placed on the sutures, and an interference screw of an appropriate size is placed through the anteromedial portal while the elbow is maintained flexed at 90°.

Arthroscopic biceps tenodesis can be achieved with the use of suture anchors with and without the presence of a rotator cuff tear. Nord and colleagues (2005) described this technique with use of the subclavian portal, which is 1–2 cm medial to the acromioclavicular joint and above the coracoid, in addition to the standard anterior, lateral, and posterior portals. A suture anchor is placed via the subclavian portal through the LHBT proximal to the bicipital groove (**Fig. 10.9**). Sutures passed through the biceps tendon are then tied through the anterior portal unless there is a rotator cuff tear, in which case they are tied through the lateral portal and the cuff tear is addressed. Once tenodesis is complete, the LHBT is released from its origin using a basket punch.

Several authors described a percutaneous intra-articular transtendon technique for biceps tenodesis (Sekiya et al. 2003). The anterior and posterior arthoscopic portals are established, and a spinal needle is placed into the biceps tendon in the groove through the transverse humeral ligament. A suture is passed through the spinal needle and brought out through the anterior portal. This process is repeated with a second spinal needle and suture. A non-absorbable suture is then pulled through the tendon using one strand of the suture. The end of the non-absorbable stitch is brought back out through the anterior portal and passed with the other suture, forming a horizontal mattress. This is then repeated to form a second horizontal mattress suture, and the knots are tied through the anterior portal (**Fig. 10.10**). The LHBT is then released from its origin and the intra-articular portion is resected.

The LHBT may be transferred to the coracoid arthroscopically. Verma et al. (2005) described this procedure using the posterior and superolateral portals. The tendon is tagged with a suture, and the subdeltoid space is exposed. Additional portals are made to provide visualization of the subdeltoid space and coracoid including pectoralis, inferior, and conjoint portals. The LHBT is then sutured to the anterolateral aspect of the conjoint tendon to avoid the musculocutaneous nerve.

POSTOPERATIVE MANAGEMENT

For SLAP repairs, a sling with abduction pillow is utilized and removed when performing pendulum exercises, shoulder shrugs, elbow flexion, extension, and grip strengthening in the immediate postoperative time period. Passive shoulder external rotation is limited to 30°. Sutures are removed at 1 week after surgery, and after 3 weeks postoperatively external rotation is increased to 45°. Supine passive shoulder flexion is allowed to 145° at 4 weeks; 9 weeks postoperatively, terminal elevation of the shoulder is achieved, and external rotation is increased to 50°. Resisted strength training is initiated. At 12 weeks from surgery, sport-specific exercises are started, and at 16 weeks the patient is allowed to return to sport if their symptoms have resolved.

The postoperative management of patients after tenodesis of the LHBT is initiated on the first postoperative day with pendulum exercises out of the abduction sling, assisted elbow flexion, and grip and core strengthening. The dressing is removed and showers are allowed 3 days after surgery. Sutures are removed at 1 week. Arm elevation is allowed to 90°. Five weeks after surgery, active-assisted arm elevation is allowed to 150° along with external rotation to 30°. Core strengthening is continued. At 9 weeks after surgery, gentle resisted elbow flexion and full shoulder ROM is initiated. At 12 weeks, resisted strength training is encouraged and return to sport at 16 weeks.

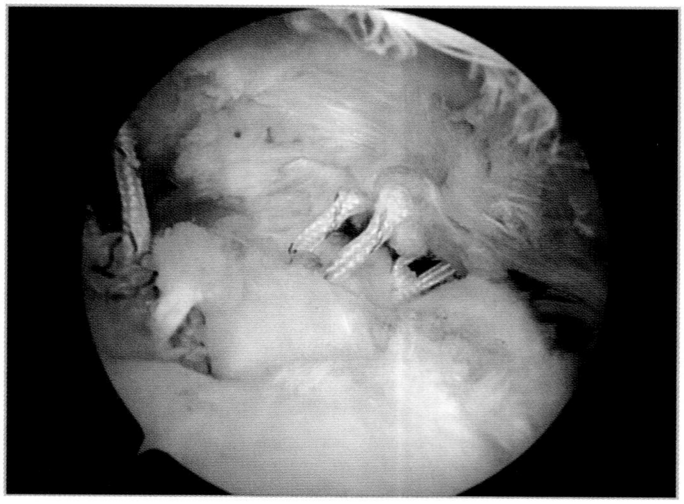

Figure 10.9 Suprapectoralis biceps tenodesis at the base of the groove using suture anchor technique.

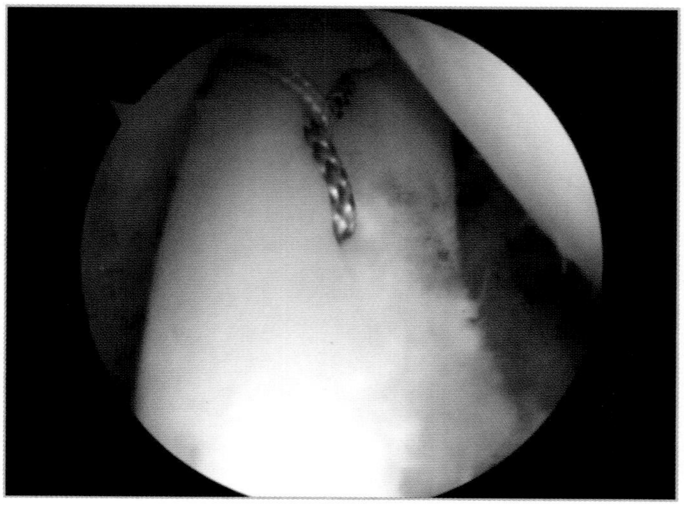

Figure 10.10 Biceps tenodesis using a soft-tissue tenodesis to the undersurface of the leading edge of supraspinatus.

RESULTS

SLAP tears

Tomlinson and Glousman (1995) performed a retrospective review of 46 overhead throwing athletes who had undergone debridement of glenoid labral tears. Of these tears, 35 were posterior, 9 anterosuperior, and 2 anteroinferior. At a minimum of 18 months of follow-up, 54% of patients had good or excellent results, and 26 had 1+ laxity. The authors concluded that debridement of labral lesions does not produce consistent results. In a retrospective study of 28 athletes who underwent arthroscopic labral tear resection with a minimum follow-up of 2 years, there was a statistically significant difference in functional outcome between patients with stable and those with unstable shoulders (Glasgo et al. 1992). There were 91% good or excellent outcomes in those with a stable joint, compared with 25% in those with instability. Of note, seven of the eight superior labral tears that were resected were in stable shoulders. Altcheck et al. (1992) demonstrated that at a minimum 2-year follow-up after arthroscopic labral tear debridement, only 7% of these athletes had significant relief of their symptoms. Cordasco et al. (1993) reported 78% excellent pain relief after arthroscopic debridement of SLAP tears which decreased to 63% at 2-year follow-up. In addition, the 52% of patients who had returned to previous level of performance at 1 year decreased to 44% at 2 years. Therefore, labral debridement alone is not adequate in the treatment of athletes with shoulder instability.

In 40 overhead athletes who underwent two anchor SLAP type II repairs, 90% of patients had satisfactory results, but only 75% returned to their level of activity before injury at a mean follow-up of 41 months (Ide et al. 2005). Brockmeier et al. (2009) demonstrated similar statistics in a prospective study on arthroscopic repair of SLAP tears, with 87% good or excellent results, but only 74% return to sport at pre-injury level at an average of 2.7 years. However, when isolating the athletes with a traumatic event, 92% of these patients returned to their pre-injury activity level after repair. Furthermore, four patients had severe shoulder stiffness after repair. Three of these patients had isolated atraumatic type II SLAP tears and eventually went on to regain ROM within 15° of pre-injury motion with non-surgical treatment. One patient with a history of diabetes mellitus and a traumatic type II SLAP tear with a bursal-sided rotator cuff injury required arthroscopic lysis of adhesions for postoperative adhesive capsulitis. This study highlights that patient selection is the key factor in successful outcomes for type II SLAP repairs. Patient selection should be focused on the presence of instability, laxity, and overhead athletic participation rather than by factors such as age. This is supported by Alpert et al. (2010) who found no statistical difference between patients aged >40 by shoulder scores in patients who underwent type II SLAP repairs when compared with patients aged <40.

Katz et al. (2009) reported 40 patients referred for poor outcome after type II SLAP repair at a mean time of 9 months with a range of 2–24 months. The mean age was 43 with range 16–58 years, with 21 isolated repairs and 19 combined with additional procedures. Patients were included with pain, stiffness, and/or mechanical symptoms after SLAP repair, and excluded if resurfacing was performed in conjunction with the repair. Twenty-eight were male and, in 25, the dominant arm was affected; 10% smoked tobacco, 7% were diabetic, 42.5% were traumatic, and 50% were workers' compensation. Seventy-five percent of the patients presented with pain and decreased ROM, with 71% dissatisfied with conservative management; 32% remained dissatisfied after revision surgery. Furthermore, the authors state that, in patients with complications after SLAP repair, the labral pathology may have represented normal aging, and the patients' symptoms may have been due to other causes of shoulder pain. This is supported by their revision surgery of 14% for rotator cuff repair and 71% for acromioplasty versus 19% for biceps tenodesis and 5% for revision SLAP repair (Katz et al. 2009). Therefore, the poor results that can be expected if SLAP repair is performed when not necessary are likely not to respond to postoperative rehabilitation and further conservative management, and may lead to revision surgery.

Tenotomy versus tenodesis

In a retrospective study, over 5 years 279 patients with either tenotomy or tenodesis of the LHBT were asked to complete a questionnaire about their anterior shoulder pain, cosmetic appearance of their biceps, and grade of muscle spasm (Osbahr et al. 2002). Tenotomy was performed in patients who were not manual laborers, aged >50 years, and not candidates for open rotator cuff repair. All other patients had a tenodesis performed. When these groups were compared, there was no significant difference between them. Wolf et al. (2005) performed cyclic loading of 10 cadaveric shoulders after LHB tenotomy and tenodesis. There was a 40% retraction rate with LHB tenotomy and 0% in the LHB tenodesis group. The researchers concluded that there is a significant risk of LHBT retraction with tenotomy compared with tenodesis. As the loads used on the specimens are consistent with gentle active ROM, cosmetic deformity is a significant risk in biceps tenotomy. In a literature review by Frost et al. (2009), they were unable to demonstrate a difference in complications between tenotomy and tenodesis of the LHBT other than the presence of "Popeye" deformity, and state that they have similar success rates. Therefore, tenodesis is preferred in patients who would prefer to avoid a "Popeye" deformity and will comply with postoperative rehabilitation protocols.

Biceps tenodesis and transfer

Mazzocca et al. (2005) reported no failure of hardware, loss of function, or continued pain with their technique of open subpectoral biceps tenodesis. Boileau et al. (2002) reported the results of arthroscopic biceps tenodesis in 43 patients with at least 1 year of follow-up; there were significant improvements in Constant scores, and these patients had 90% of the strength of the contralateral shoulder. The two patients that had tenodesis failures had 7-mm diameter screws placed and had friable biceps tendons.. Nord et al. (2005) reported 90% good and excellent results on the UCLA scale and 100% satisfaction with cosmesis in 10 patients who underwent tenodesis with suture anchors through the subclavian portal. Drakos et al. (2008) reported arthroscopic transfer of the LHBT in 40 shoulders with 3 traumatic failures and 80% self-reported good-to-excellent results.

Ozalay et al. (2005) performed a load-to-failure biomechanical study on sheep shoulders using tunnel, interference screw, anchor, and keyhole techniques. In this study, the strongest construct was the interference screw followed by the tunnel, anchor, and keyhole procedures. Kilicoglu and colleagues (2005) studied the tenodesis screw, suture sling, and suture anchor techniques, which were tested to failure at four time points 0, 3, 6, and 9 weeks, also in a sheep model. There was a significant increase in load to failure in the tenodesis screw group from 0 to 3 weeks and in the suture sling and suture anchor groups from 0 to 6 weeks. However, this study did not demonstrate a statistically significant failure load among these three groups at each time point. In 20 fresh frozen cadaveric shoulders, the open subpectoral bone tunnel, open subpectoral interference screw, arthroscopic suture anchor, and arthroscopic interference screw techniques were compared with cyclic load to failures (Mazzocca et al. 2005). The investigators did not demonstrate a statistically significant difference in failure strength, but a significantly greater cyclic displacement in the open subpectoral bone tunnel technique.

CONCLUSION

SLAP tears and tendinopathy of the LHBT comprises a diverse group of pathologies that are treated appropriately by different means depending on the patient population and etiology of the injury. There appears to be an increased interest in repairing these articular tears. However, there has been a noteworthy increase in the number of complications as well as failures of athletes to return to their previous level of function. Surgical decision-making must not be based on the imaging or arthroscopic appearance alone. The primary cause for considering surgery is failure of a non-surgical program, shoulder instability, hyperlaxity, or persistent biceps symptoms. The decision between LHB tenodesis, tenotomy, or SLAP repair should be influenced by the activity demands, anticipated return to sport or work, and the ability of the shoulder to accommodate additional constraint. With the numerous options for surgical and non-surgical treatment of these entities, great care must be taken to optimize the patient's chance for successful recovery with a specific treatment strategy for each athlete.

REFERENCES

Abbot AE, Li X, Busconi BD. Arthroscopic treatment of concomitant superior labral anterior posterior (SLAP) lesions and rotator cuff tears in patients over the age of 45 years. Am J Sports Med 2009;37:1358–1362.

Alpantaki K, McLaughlin D, Karagogeos D, Hadjipavlou A, Kontakis G. Sympathetic and sensory neural elements in the tendon of the long head of the biceps. J Bone Joint Surg Am 2005;87:1580–1583.

Alpert JM, Wuerz TH, O'Donnell TF, et al. The effect of age on the outcomes of arthroscopic repair of type II superior labral anterior and posterior lesions. Am J Sports Med 2010;38:2299–2303.

Altchek DW, Warren RF, Wickiewicz TL, Ortiz G. Arthroscopic labral debridement. A three-year follow-up study. Am J Sports Med 1992;20:702–706.

Andrews JR, Carson WG Jr, McLeod WD. Glenoid labrum tears related to the long head of the biceps. Am J Sports Med 1985;13:337–341.

Angelo RL, Esch J, Ryu RK, eds. The Shoulder: Expert consult. Online, print and DVD. Philadelphia, PA: Saunders, 2010.

Armstrong A, Teefey SA, Wu T, et al. The efficacy of ultrasound in the diagnosis of long head of the biceps tendon pathology. J Shoulder Elbow Surg 2006;15:7–11.

Barber A, Field LD, Ryu R. Biceps tendon and superior labrum injuries: decision-marking. J Bone Joint Surg Am 2007;89:1844–1855.

Beall DP, Williamson EE, Ly JQ, et al. Association of biceps tendon tears of the anterior and superior portions of the rotator cuff. AJR Am J Roentgenol 2003;180:633–639.

Boileau P, Krishnan SG, Coste JS, Walch G. Arthroscopic biceps tenodesis: A new technique using bioabsorbable interference screw fixation. Arthroscopy 2002;18:1002–1012.

Boileau P, Ahrens PM, Hatzidakis AM. Entrapment of the long head of the biceps tendon: the hourglass biceps – a cause of pain and locking of the shoulder. J Shoulder Elbow Surg 2004;13:249–257.

Brockmeier SF, Voos JE, Williams RJ, 3rd, et al. Outcomes after arthroscopic repair of type-II SLAP lesions. J Bone Joint Surg Am 2009;91:1595–1603.

Buess E, Schneider C. Simplified single-portal V-shaped SLAP repair. Arthroscopy 2006;22:680,e1–4.

Burkart A, Imhoff AB, Roscher E. Foreign-body reaction to the bioabsorbable suretac device. Arthroscopy 2000;16:91–95.

Burkhart SS, Morgan CD. The peel-back mechanism: its role in producing and extending posterior type II SLAP lesions and its effect on SLAP repair rehabilitation. Arthroscopy 1998;14:637–640.

Castagna A, Garofalo R, Conti M, Naula VM. Biceps soft tissue tenodesis. In: Abrams JS, Bell RH (eds). Arthroscopic Rotator Cuff Surgery: a practical approach to management. New York: Springer Verlag, 2008: pp. 276–89.

Cooper DE, Arnoczky SP, O'Brien SJ, et al. Anatomy, histology, and vascularity of the glenoid labrum. An anatomical study. J Bone Joint Surg Am 1992;74:46–52.

Cordasco FA, Steinmann S, Flatow EL, Bigliani LU. Arthroscopic treatment of glenoid labral tears. Am J Sports Med 1993;21:425–430; discussion 430–431.

Crockett HC, Wright JM, Slawski DP, et al. Minimally invasive transrotator cuff approach for arthroscopic stabilization of the posterosuperior glenoid labrum. Arthroscopy 2004;20(suppl 2):94–99.

Davidson PA, Rivenburgh DW. Mobile superior glenoid labrum: a normal variant or pathologic condition? Am J Sports Med 2004;32:962–966.

Davila J. SLAP tears. In: Rockwood CA Jr, Matsen FA III, Wirth MA, Lippitt SB (eds). The Shoulder, 4th edn. Philadelphia, PA: Saunders Elsevier, 2009.

Drakos MC, Verma NN, Gulotta LV, et al. Arthroscopic transfer of the long head of the biceps tendon: functional outcome and clinical results. Arthroscopy 2008;24:217–223.

Forsythe B, Guss D, Anthony SG, Martin SD. Concomitant arthroscopic SLAP and rotator cuff repair. J Bone Joint Surg Am 2010;92:1362–1369.

Franceschi F, Longo UG, Ruzzini L, et al. No advantages in repairing a type II superior labrum anterior and posterior (SLAP) lesion when associated with rotator cuff repair in patients over age 50: A randomized controlled trial. Am J Sports Med 2008;3:6247–6253.

Frost A, Zafar MS, Maffulli N. Tenotomy versus tenodesis in the management of pathologic lesions of the tendon of the long head of the biceps brachii. Am J Sports Med 2009;37:828–833.

Gaunche CA, Jones DC. Clinical testing for tears of the glenoid labrum. Arthroscopy 2003;19:517–523.

Glasgow SG, Bruce RA, Yacobucci GN, Torg JS. Arthroscopic resection of glenoid labral tears in the athlete: a report of 29 cases. Arthroscopy 1992;8:48–54.

Gleason PD, Beall DP, Sanders TG, et al. The transverse humeral ligament: a separate anatomical structure or a continuation of the osseous attachment of the rotator cuff? Am J Sports Med 2006;34:72–77.

Holtby R, Razmjou H. Accuracy of the Speed's and Yergason's tests in detecting biceps pathology and SLAP lesions: Comparison with arthroscopic findings. Arthroscopy 2004;20:231–236.

Ide J, Maeda S, Takagi K. Sports activity after arthroscopic superior labral repair using suture anchors in overhead-throwing athletes. Am J Sports Med 2005;33:507–514.

Ifesanya A, Scheibel M. Posterosuperior suture granuloma impingement after arthroscopic SLAP repair using suture anchors: a case report. Knee Surg Sports Traumatol Arthrosc 2008;16:703–706.

Jee WH, McCauley TR, Katz LD, et al. Superior labral anterior posterior (SLAP) lesions of the glenoid labrum: reliability and accuracy of MR arthrography for diagnosis. Radiology 2001;218:127–132.

Jin W, Ryu KN, Kwon SH, Rhee YG, Yang DM. MR arthrography in the differential diagnosis of type II superior labral anteroposterior lesion and sublabral recess. AJR Am J Roentgenol 2006;187:887–893.

Kaar TK, Schenck RC Jr, Wirth MA, Rockwood CA Jr. Complications of metallic suture anchors in shoulder surgery: A report of 8 cases. Arthroscopy 2001;17:31–37.

Katz LM, Hsu S, Miller SL, et al. Poor outcomes after SLAP repair: descriptive analysis and prognosis. Arthroscopy 2009;25:849–855.

Kibler WB, McMullen J. Scapular dyskinesis and its relation to shoulder pain. J Am Acad Orthop Surg 2003;11:142–151.

Kilicoglu O, Koyuncu O, Demirhan M, et al. Time-dependent changes in failure loads of 3 biceps tenodesis techniques: in vivo study in a sheep model. Am J Sports Med 2005;33:1536–1544.

Kuhn JE, Lindholm SR, Huston LJ, Soslowsky LJ, Blasier RB. Failure of the biceps superior labral complex: a cadaveric biomechanical investigation comparing the late cocking and early deceleration positions of throwing. Arthroscopy 2003;19:373–379.

Lafosse L, Reiland Y, Baier GP, Toussaint B, Jost B. Anterior and posterior instability of the long head of the biceps tendon in rotator cuff tears: A new classification based on arthroscopic observations. Arthroscopy 2007;23:73–80.

McFarland EG, Kim TK, Savino RM. Clinical assessment of the three common tests for the superior labral anterior-posterior lesions. Am J Sports Med 2002;30:810–815.
Maffet MW, Gartsman GM, Moseley B. Superior labrum-biceps tendon complex lesions of the shoulder. Am J Sports Med 1995;23:93.
Mariani EM, Cofield RH, Askew LJ, Li G, Chao Eys. Rupture of the tendon of the long head of the biceps brachii. Surgical versus nonsurgical treatment. Clin Orthop 1988;228:233–239.
Mazzocca AD, Bicos J, Santangelo S, Romeo AA, Arciero RA. The biomechanical evaluation of four fixation techniques for proximal biceps tenodesis. Arthroscopy 2005;21:1296–306.
Mohtadi NG, Vellet AD, Clark ML, et al. A prospective, double-blind comparison of magnetic resonance imaging and arthroscopy in the evaluation of patients presenting with shoulder pain. J Shoulder Elbow Surg 2004;13:258–265.
Moore TP, Fritts HM, Quick DC, Buss DD. Suprascapular nerve entrapment caused by supraglenoid cyst compression. J Shoulder Elbow Surg 1997;6:455–462.
Morgan RJ, Kuremsky MA, Peindl RD, Fleischli JE. A biomechanical comparison of two suture anchor configurations for the repair of type II SLAP lesions subjected to a peel-back mechanism of failure. Arthroscopy 2008;24:383–388.
Neer CS, Horwitz BS. Fractures of the proximal humerus epiphyseal plate. Clin Orthop Relat Res 1965;41:24-31
Neviaser RJ. Tears of the rotator cuff. Orthop Clin North Am 1980;11:295–306.
Nord KD, Smith GB, Mauck BM. Arthroscopic biceps tenodesis using suture anchors through the subclavian portal. Arthroscopy 2005;21:248–252.
O'Brien SJ, Pagnani MJ, Fealy S, McGlynn SR, Wilson JB. The active compression test: A new and effective test for diagnosing labral tears and acromioclavicular joint abnormality. Am J Sports Med 1998;26:610–613.
O'Brien SJ, Allen AA, Coleman SH, Drakos MC. The trans-rotator cuff approach to SLAP lesions: technical aspects for repair and a clinical follow-up of 31 patients at a minimum of 2 years. Arthroscopy 2002;18:372–377.
Osbahr DC, Diamond AB, Speer KP. The cosmetic appearance of the biceps muscle after long-head tenotomy versus tenodesis. Arthroscopy 2002;18:483–487.
Ozalay M, Akpinar S, Karaeminogullari O, et al. Mechanical strength of four different biceps tenodesis techniques. Arthroscopy 2005;21:992–998.
Parentis MA, Glousman RE, Mohr KS, Yocum LA. An evaluation of the provocative tests for superior labral anterior posterior lesions. Am J Sports Med 2006;34:265–8.
Perry J. Anatomy and biomechanics of the shoulder in throwing, swimming, gymnastics, and tennis. Clin Sports Med 1983;2:247–270.
Pfahler M, Haraida S, Schulz C, et al. Age-related changes of the glenoid labrum in normal shoulders. J Shoulder Elbow Surg 2003;12:40–52.
Piatt BE, Hawkins RJ, Fritz RC, et al. Clinical evaluation and treatment of spinoglenoid notch ganglion cysts. J Shoulder Elbow Surg 2002;11:600–604.
Post M, Mayer J. Suprascapular nerve entrapment. Diagnosis and treatment. Clin Orthop Relat Res 1987;223:126–136.
Powell SE, Nord KD, Ryu RKN. The diagnosis, classification, and treatment of SLAP lesions. Oper Tech Sports Med 2004;12:99–110.
Rathbun JB, McNab I: The microvascular pattern of the rotator cuff. J Bone Joint Surg Br 1970;52:540–553.
Reuss BL, Schwartzberg R, Zlatkin MB, Cooperman A, Dixon JR. Magnetic resonance imaging accuracy for the diagnosis of superior labrum anterior-posterior lesions in the community setting: eighty-three arthroscopically confirmed cases. J Shoulder Elbow Surg 2006;15:580–585.
Sassmannshausen G, Sukay M, Mair SD. Broken or dislodged poly-L-lactic acid bioabsorbable tacks in patients after SLAP lesion surgery. Arthroscopy 2006;22:615–619.
Sekiya JK, Elkousy HA, Rodosky MW. Arthroscopic biceps tenodesis using the percutaneous intra-articular transtendon technique. Arthroscopy 2003;19:1137–1141.
Sethi N, Wright R, Yamaguchi K. Disorders of the long head of the biceps tendon. J Shoulder Elbow Surg 1999;8:644–654.
Snyder SJ, Karzel RP, Del Pizzo W, Ferkel RD, Friedman MJ. SLAP lesions of the shoulder. Arthroscopy 1990;6:274–279.
Snyder SJ, Banas MP, Karzel RP. An analysis of 140 injuries to the superior glenoid labrum. J Shoulder and Elbow Surg 1995;4:243–248.
Stetson WB, Templin K. The crank test, the O'Brien test, and routine magnetic resonance imaging scans in the diagnosis of labral tears. Am J Sports Med 2002;30:806–809.
Stoller DW. MR arthrography of the glenohumeral joint. Radiol Clin North Am 1997;35:97–116.
Tomlinson RJ Jr, Glousman RE. Arthroscopic debridement of glenoid labral tears in athletes. Arthroscopy 1995;11:42–51.
Tung GA, Entzian D, Stern JB, Green A. MR imaging and MR arthrography of paraglenoid labral cysts. AJR Am J Roentgenol 2000;174:1707–1715.
Vangsness CT, Jr, Jorgenson SS, Watson T, Johnson DL. The origin of the long head of the biceps from the scapula and glenoid labrum. An anatomical study of 100 shoulders. J Bone Joint Surg Br 1994;76:951–954.
Verma NN, Drakos M, O'Brien SJ. Arthroscopic transfer of the long head biceps to the conjoint tendon. Arthroscopy 2005;21:764.
Weber SC, Payvandi S, Martin DF, Harrast JJ. SLAP lesions of the shoulder: Incidence rates, complications, and outcomes as reported by ABOS part II candidates. Paper SS-19. Presented at the 2010 Annual Meeting of the Arthroscopy Association of North America, May 20–23. Hollywood, FL, 2010.
Westerheide KJ, Karzel RP. Ganglion cysts of the shoulder: technique of arthroscopic decompression and fixation of associated type II superior labral anterior to posterior lesions. Orthop Clin North Am 2003;34:521–528.
Williams MM, Snyder SJ, Buford D Jr. The Buford complex – the "cord-like" middle glenohumeral ligament and absent anterosuperior labrum complex: a normal anatomic capsulolabral variant. Arthroscopy 1994;10:241–247.
Wolf RS, Zheng N, Weichel D. Long head biceps tenotomy versus tenodesis: a cadaveric biomechanical analysis. Arthroscopy 2005;21:182–185.
Youm T, Matthews PV, El Attrache NS. Treatment of patients with spinoglenoid cysts associated with superior labral tears without cyst aspiration, debridement, or excision. Arthroscopy 2006;22:548–552.
Zanetti M, Weishaupt D, Gerber C, Hodler J. Tendinopathy and rupture of the tendon of the long head of the biceps brachii muscle: Evaluation with MR arthrography. AJR Am J Roentgenol 1998;170:1557–1561.

Chapter 11 Full-thickness rotator cuff tears

Leonardo Osti, Rocco Papalia, Nicola Maffulli, John Furia, Vincenzo Denaro

KEY FEATURES

- A full-thickness rotator cuff tear has little or no potential for spontaneous healing.
- Asymptomatic tears can become symptomatic over time.
- Non-surgical treatment with activity modification, steroid injection, and physical therapy may relieve symptoms and improve function.
- The goals of surgical treatment are to restore the rotator cuff force couplets.
- Arthroscopic rotator cuff repair offers the advantage of treating the associated intra-articular pathologies and is now considered the "gold standard" for treating this condition.

EPIDEMIOLOGY AND NATURAL HISTORY

Rotator cuff tears are common injuries that can impair upper extremity and overall health status (McKee and Yoo 2000; Osti et al. 2010a). Cadaveric studies reveal an incidence of 30% whereas ultrasound studies reveal even higher prevalence of this condition (Lehman et al. 1995; McKee and Yoo 2000; Mali et al. 2010; Osti et al. 2010a).

A full-thickness tear has no potential for spontaneous healing. Asymptomatic tears can become symptomatic over time. Yamaguchi et al. (2001), in a large series, found that in no case did tear size decrease and, over time, the chance of an asymptomatic tear becoming symptomatic was over 50%.

Patients with a tear on one side had a 35% chance of having a contralateral side tear. In patients with bilateral tears, the one with the smaller size could be the only one who is symptomatic (Yamaguchi et al. 2001).

Repair of the tendon does not reverse the process of muscle atrophy/degeneration. Progression of the lesion over the years can lead to irreparability, including static superior migration of the humeral head, a narrowed or absent acromiohumeral interval, and fatty muscle infiltration. Fatty degeneration can contribute to persistent shoulder disability, even after surgical rotator cuff repair, and does not reverse after the repair (Kibler et al. 2009; Yamaguchi and Tashjian 2008; Lin et al. 2010).

ETIOLOGY

The etiology of rotator cuff tears can be divided in two main categories: traumatic and non-traumatic/degenerative.

Chopp et al. (2011), in a recent biomechanical study, evaluated the subacromial impingement changes caused by applying muscle fatigue protocols. Statistically significant changes in scapular tilt and rotation occurred, suggesting that the rotator cuff muscles have more importance than the scapular stabilizers in preventing subacromial impingement (Kibler and Sciasia 2008, 2010).

Walch et al. (1992) studied the etiology of rotator cuff tears in overhead athletes. He identified impingement and partial tear of the posteriorly oriented supraspinatus and infraspinatus against the glenoid rim and the posterior capsule in these athletes. Halbrecht et al. (1999) used magnetic resonance imaging (MRI) data to confirm these findings.

Pharmacological agents

Recent investigations ruled out the role of pharmacological agents in affecting both the status of a rotator cuff tear and the biology of rotator cuff repair healing.

Non-steroidal anti-inflammatory drugs (NSAIDs) have been show to adversely affect the healing rate of repaired rotator cuff tear in animal (rabbit) model. The tendons that underwent NSAID treatment of the tendon tissue produced a more disorganized and weaker tissue response; however, these data have not been validated in a human model (Kibler et al. 2009; Esch and Leek 2010; Lin et al. 2010).

Smoking

Smoking has an adverse affect on tendon healing. Nicotine has been shown to delay healing of repaired tendon and prolongs the inflammatory response (Kibler et al. 2009; Esch and Leek 2010; Lin et al. 2010).

Steroids

Steroids also have a role in tendon healing, but they have been shown to impair this.

There are conflicting data about the role of anabolic steroids in tendon healing. Anabolic steroid usage has been reported to increase the incidence of tendon rupture. However, laboratory models reveal that steroid treatment also improved tendon remodeling (Kibler et al. 2009; Esch and Leek 2010; Lin et al. 2010).

DIAGNOSIS

The diagnosis of a rotator cuff tear begins with the history and physical examination. A history of pain with overhead activities, decreased upper extremity strength, and a painful arc of motion also suggest rotator cuff pathology.

Imaging

Plain radiographs can rule out possible fractures and arthritis. Radiographs should include anteroposterior, axillary lateral, and outlet views. The outlet view is particularly helpful in evaluating the acromion morphology as a possible cause of primary impingement.

Ultrasonography can be helpful: it can reveal partial- and full-thickness tearing of the rotator cuff, and subacromial bursitis and rotator cuff tendinopathy. However, the reliability depends on the examiner's experience (Ottenheijm et al. 2010).

MRI is probably the most reliable examination, and provides valuable information about tendon detail. It can effectively demonstrate tendon width, atrophy, fatty infiltration, and tearing. MRI can detect both full- and partial-thickness rotator cuff tears, but has higher sensitivity and specificity for full-thickness rotator cuff tears (Murray and Shaffer 2009).

MR arthrography studies can further enhance the reliability of this modality. MR arthrograms improve the sensitivity and specificity of the conventional MRI and are particularly useful for the detection of partial rotator cuff tears and labral tears, evaluating the possible laxity of glenohumeral ligaments (Murray and Shaffer 2009).

A final study, the arthrographic computed tomography (CT) scan, provides additional information about the three-dimensional structure of the lesion and the fatty infiltration of the muscle (Goutallier et al. 2003).

CLASSIFICATION

Several classification systems have been proposed. Ellmann et al. (1993) classified rotator cuff tears based on size. He describes tears as small (1–3 cm), large (3 cm), and massive (>5 cm). McLaughlin (1944) described lesions of the rotator cuff as transverse ruptures, vertical splits, and retracted tears.

Cofield et al. (2001) categorized the tear in four groups according to the length of the greatest diameter of the tear – small, medium, large, or massive (more than 5 cm) – whereas Harryman et al. (1991) characterized the status of the cuff based on the number of tendons torn.

Recently a geometric classification of rotator cuff tears was proposed. This system attempts to link tear pattern to both treatment and prognosis. The geometric classification is based on preoperative MR scans. According to this classification the tears are divided into three different subgroups: type 1, crescent-shaped tears reparable trough end to bone; type 2, longitudinal (L- or U-shaped) tears which can be repaired trough margin convergence; type 3, massive contracted tears with coronal and sagittal dimensions >2 × 2 cm, and can be repaired with interval slides or partial repair (Davidson and Burkhart 2010).

CLINICAL PRESENTATION

Patients with rotator cuff tears present with pain and loss of shoulder function. They typically have weakness with repetitive overhead activities. Sleeping at night is often difficult.

Examination reveals loss of shoulder strength, particularly external rotation. Often, but not always, there is loss of active motion, but preservation of passive motion. Standard provocative maneuvers for rotator cuff pathology are typically positive (Kibler et al. 2009; Di Giacomo et al. 2010; Lin et al. 2010).

TREATMENT

Conservative treatment

Conservative treatment has a role in management. Modification of activities, especially those involving overhead use, can lead to decreased symptoms (Rowe 1975; Tanaka et al. 2010). Steroid injections can also lead to decreased symptoms and improved function (Koester et al. 2007; Mikolyzk et al. 2009).

Physical therapy treatment goals include restoration of range of motion, strength, and function. To be effective, therapy should target both the rotator cuff and scapular muscles (Kibler et al. 2009; Bartolozzi et al. 1994; Ainsworth and Lewis 2007; Lin et al. 2010; Melis et al. 2010; Tucker et al. 2010).

Surgical treatment

The goals of surgical treatment are to restore the rotator cuff force couplets. Traditionally, this was performed through an open approach using transosseous sutures (Cofield 1985; Shaffer 2008).

In the last two decades, suture anchors were introduced, and suture anchor fixation has allowed the development of enhanced arthroscopic techniques. Mini-open and all arthroscopic techniques are now relatively widespread, and have yielded results equivalent to or better than traditional open techniques (Shaffer 2008; Osti et al. 2010b).

Arthroscopic rotator cuff repair offers the advantage of treating the associated articular pathologies. Associated pathologies such as chondral damage, SLAP tears, and biceps pathology/instability are much more easily treated with these newer techniques (Franceschi 2008; Kibler et al. 2009; Snyder 2003; Burkhart et al. 2006a,b; Lin et al. 2010).

Most surgeons perform subacromial arthroscopy and decompression before rotator cuff repair. Subacromial decompression can be carried out according to the shape of the acromion; however, level I evidence-based studies showed no benefits from subacromial arthroscopy in term of functional results, but consistent advantages for growth factor release have been reported after a limited acromioplasty (Milano et al. 2007; Randelli et al. 2009).

Tendon preparation is an important step, debriding the tissue adhesions and providing limited removal of the non-vital ends of the tendon tissue. A careful decortication of the footprint is recommended to obtain a regular plane/interface for the tendon–bone interface (Szabó et al. 2008).

The pattern of the tear should be carefully evaluated in order to plan the most appropriate repair (**Fig. 11.1**). Some common strategies are as discussed below.

The small tear pattern usually requires a simple tendon-to-bone reattachment and it can be carried out through anchors at the lateral side of the footprint (Bell 2010). **Figs 11.2–11.6** show a simplified sequence of the main steps of rotator cuff repair. For the larger tear with a longitudinal component, the first step is a side-to-side repair of the tendon, followed by a tendon-to-bone reattachment. The tendon mobility/retraction should be evaluated from multiple portals to evaluate the possible reduction and insertion site at the footprint.

In case of poor mobility of the tendons the interval slide technique has been recommended, performing a release of the coracohumeral ligament followed by mobilization and rotator cuff repair (Burkhart and Koo 2010).

Margin convergence techniques are recommended for large U-shaped and L-shaped tears, shifting the margins of the tendons and closing the gap via three to four side-to-side sutures. Once this is completed, the edge of the repaired tissue is reattached to the tuberosity (Franceschi et al. 2007a; Burkhart and Koo 2010).

Tendon-to-bone repair is typically performed using suture anchor fixation. The repair can be carried out via full arthroscopy or utilizing a mini-open technique, with similar results according to surgeons' specific experiences.

Before anchor insertion, the footprint should be prepared by removing the soft tissue and exposing the underlying cortical bone.

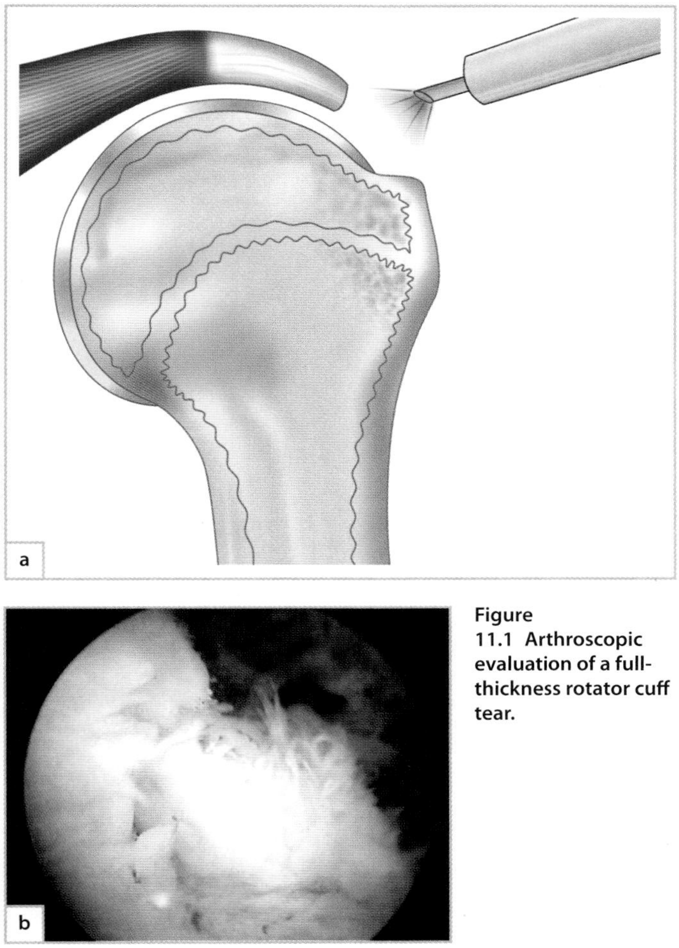

Figure 11.1 Arthroscopic evaluation of a full-thickness rotator cuff tear.

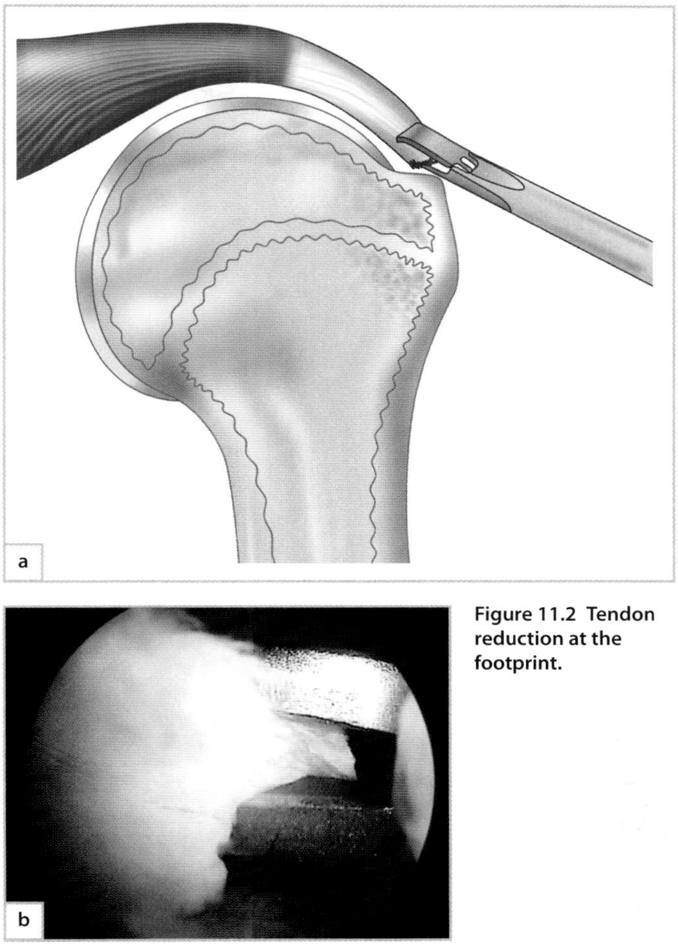

Figure 11.2 Tendon reduction at the footprint.

Microfractures can be performed at the footprint to stimulate the healing response at the bone–tendon interface (Osti et al. personal communication). The anchors are usually double loaded; metallic or bioadsorbable anchors offer comparable pull-out strength. The anchor should be inserted at an angle that minimizes the strain on the anchor. Bone cysts should be avoided (Snyder 2003; Burkhart et al. 2006a,b; Bell 2010; Burkhart and Koo 2010).

Single row anchor repair has been the standard technique for the last two decades. Recently, the double row technique, using two rows of suture anchors, has been advocated for a larger coverage of the footprint area (**Fig. 11.7**). However, this new technique offers minimal or no benefits when measured objectively in terms of functional results (Papalia 2011, Grasso 2009, Franceschi 2007).

Several alternative techniques to double row repair (e.g., Mason Allen, Modified Mason Alex, Roman Bridge techniques) have been proposed to increase and optimize the tendon–footprint contact area (Castagna 2008; Franceschi 2007a).

Tendon healing: biology of the repair

Tendon reattachment to bone initiates the healing process, which consists of three different phases:

1. Inflammatory phase
2. Fibroblastic phase
3. Remodeling phase.

In the first phase, platelets play an important role, producing important chemotactic agents such as insulin-like grow factor 1 (IGF-1), platelet-derived growth factors (PDGFs), and transforming growth factor β (TGF-β). These factors activate cells such as fibroblast and macrophages and initiate the healing cascade.

The second phase begins at day 2 and ends at 8 weeks. The so-called fibroblastic phase is fibroblast mediated, and this phase is characterized by the production of collagen.

In the third phase, the remodeling phase, there is decreased fibrobast activity and increased collagen remodeling. Sharp fibers are formed and repair strength is improved (Accousti and Flatow 2007; Zgonis et al. 2008; Esch and Leek 2010).

SHOULDER REHABILITATION

Rehabilitation stages can be summarized in three main phases: acute or protective stage; subacute or recovery stage; and functional or strengthening stage (Ticker and Egan 2008).

In the acute stage postoperative sling immobilization has been advocated to protect the repair and promote healing of the tendon in an organized fashion (Burkhart et al. 2006b; Ticker and Egan 2008). Gerber (2004) showed that the tendon immobilized for several weeks healed with a parallel array, whereas the tendon fibers showed a random alignment when undergoing early passive motion.

Burkhart suggested a mean time of sling use of 6 weeks after arthroscopic rotator cuff repair because of the decreased scarring tissue

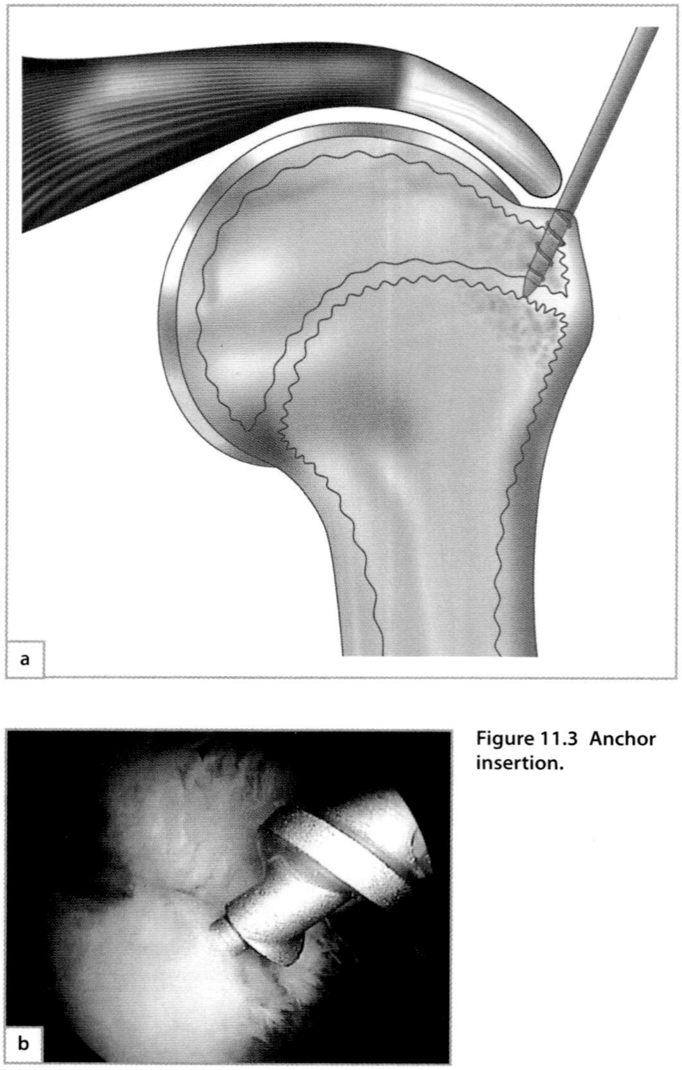

Figure 11.3 Anchor insertion.

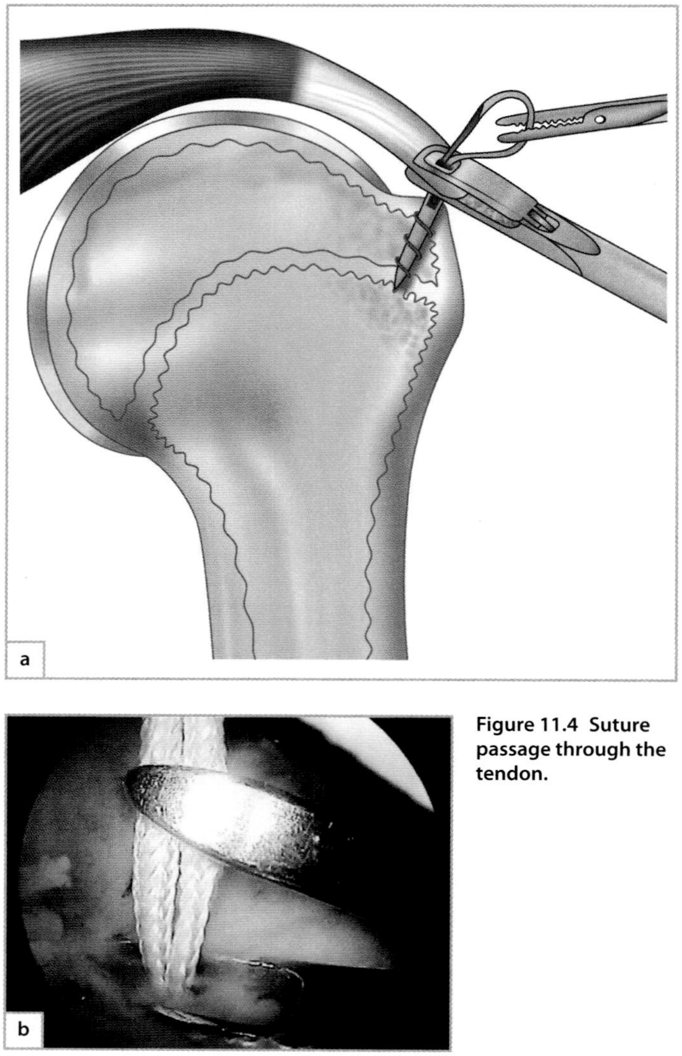

Figure 11.4 Suture passage through the tendon.

produced compared with that for open rotator cuff repair (Huberty et al. 2009).

Sling immobilization is not detrimental to the healing process. Gruson et al. (2009) confirmed, in a series of 43 patients undergoing rotator cuff repair, that the use of a postoperative sling for 6 weeks does not produce a long-term stiffness and decreased function.

Patients are typically limited to passive range of motion for several weeks after rotator cuff surgery. Active range of motion is then initiated (Galatz et al. 2009; Ghodadra et al. 2009; Koo et al. 2011).

Water rehabilitation can improve the speed of recovery and home rehabilitation can achieve similar results at final follow-up compared with the supervised approach (Osti et al. 2004, 2007; Clement et al. 2010).

COMPLICATIONS AND ROTATOR CUFF REPAIR FAILURES

The major complications related to rotator cuff repair are stiffness, infection, and failure of rotator cuff repair (Brislin et al. 2007; Trantalis and Lo 2009).

Stiffness, or postoperative capsulitis, is a common complication after arthroscopic rotator cuff repair. Postoperative stiffness has been shown to be greatly related to the preoperative passive range of motion (Hatch et al. 2006; Brislin et al. 2007; Trantalis and Lo 2009). Patients who are stiff preoperatively are more likely to be stiff postoperatively.

Treatment of adhesive capsulitis consists of modified and aggressive physical therapy.

Infection is an uncommon complication after rotator cuff tear repair. Infections are more prevalent with mini-open and open series. An early diagnosis and aggressive treatment are considered the key to eradicating the infection (Herrera et al. 2002; Kwon et al. 2005; Trantalis and Lo 2009).

Failure of the repair can be related to technical issues such as knot tying or patient factors such as advanced age, smoking, size of the tear, poor tendon quality, and lower expectations (Romeo et al. 1999; Snyder 2003; Harryman et al. 2003; Burkhart et al. 2006a,b).

Untreated or undertreated associated pathologies can also lead to repair failure. Concomitant disorders such as tears of tendon of the long head of biceps, SLAP tears, and labral tears can all lead to suboptimal results (Romeo et al. 1999; Pai and Larson 2001; Cho and Rhee 2009; Duquin et al. 2010).

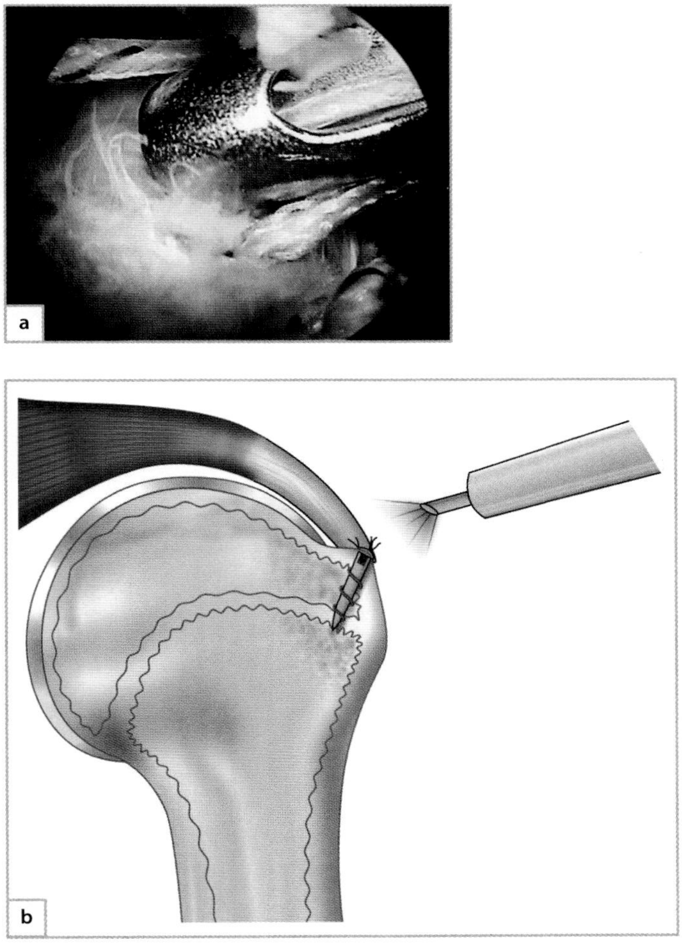

Figure 11.5 Intraoperative tensioning of the sutures and a single-row repair.

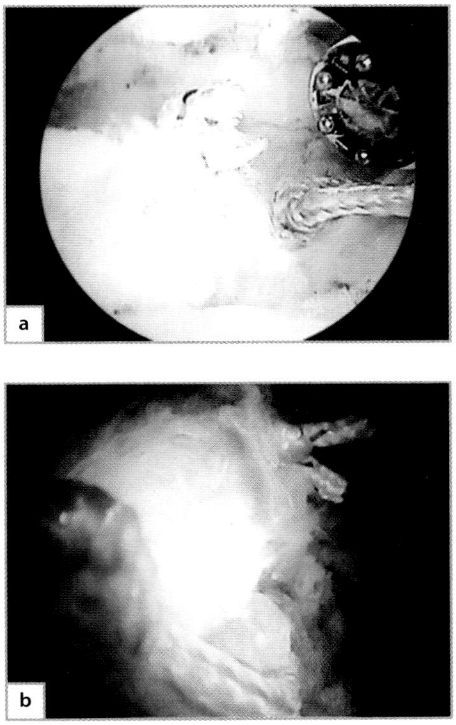

Figure 11.6 Rotator cuff tendons repaired at the footprint.

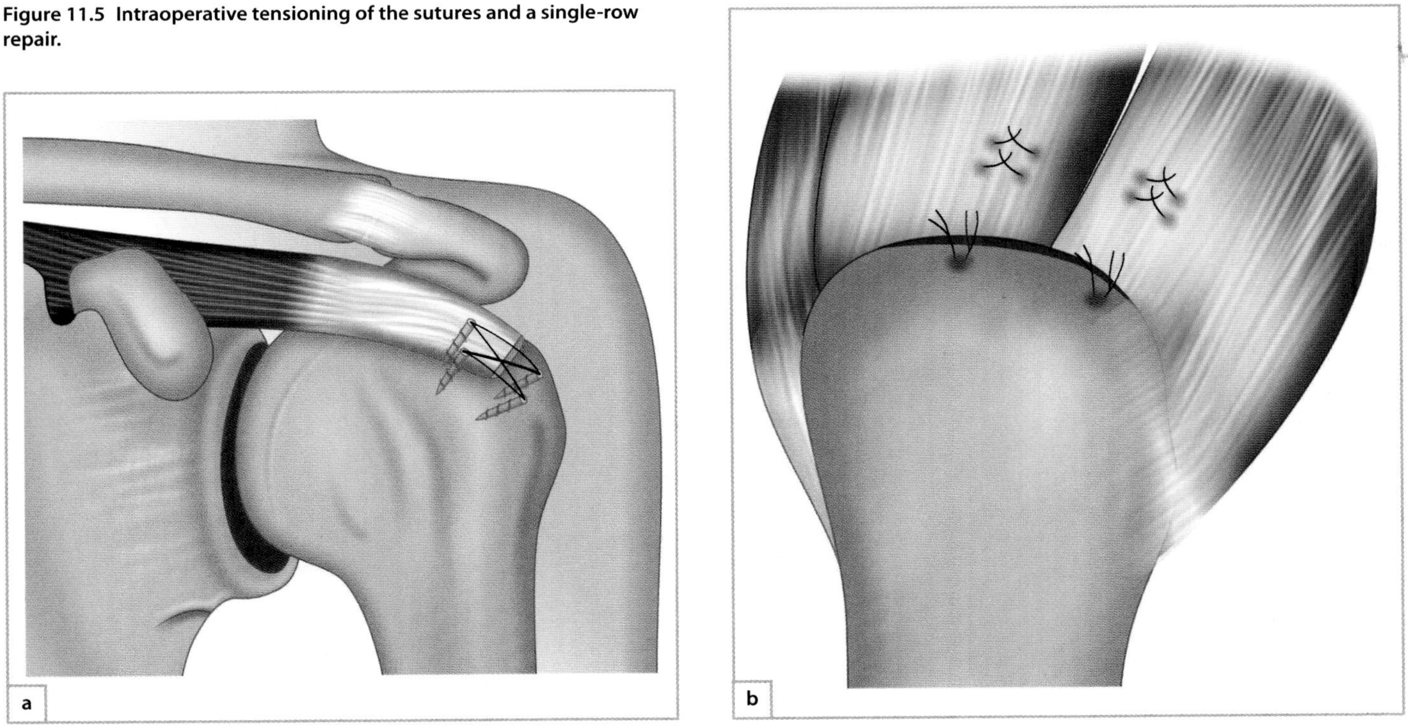

Figure 11.7 (a) Frontal and (b) lateral view of a double-row rotator cuff repair (Francheschi et al. 2007b; Grasso et al. 2009).

REFERENCES

Accousti KJ, Flatow EL.Technical pearls on how to maximize healing of the rotator cuff. Instr Course Lect 2007;56:3–12.

Ainsworth R, Lewis JS. Exercise therapy for the conservative management of full thickness tears of the rotator cuff: a systematic review. Br J Sports Med 2007;41:200–10.

Bartolozzi A, Andreychik D, Ahmad S. Determinants of outcome in the treatment of rotator cuff disease. Clin Orthop Relat Res 1994;308:90–97.

Bell R. Small to medium rotator cuff tear. In: Angelo RL, Esch JC, Ryu RKN (eds), AANA Advanced Arthroscopy. The shoulder. Philadelphia, PA: Saunders Elsevier, 2010: 199–207.

Brislin K, Field L, Savoie FIII. Complications after arthroscopic rotator cuff repair. Arthroscopy 2007;23:124–128.

Burkhart SS, Lo IKK, Brady PC, (eds), Rotator cuff tears pattern: repairing a tear the way it ought to be. In: A Cowboy's Guide to Advanced Shoulder Arthroscopy. Philadelphia, PA: Lippincott Williams & Wilkins, 2006a: 193–202.

Burkhart SS, Lo IKK, Brady PC. Rotator cuff. In: Burkhart SS, Lo IKK, Brady PC (eds), A Cowboy's Guide to Advanced Shoulder Arthroscopy. Philadelphia, PA: Lippincott Williams & Wilkins, 2006b: 249–288.

Burkhart S, Koo S. Large to massive RC tear. In: Angelo RL, Esch JC, Ryu RKN (eds), AANA Advanced Arthroscopy. The shoulder. Philadelphia, PA: Saunders Elsevier, 2010: 208–222.

Castagna A, Conti M, Markopoulos N, et al. Arthroscopic repair of rotator cuff tear with a modified Mason-Allen stitch: mid-term clinical and ultrasound outcomes. Knee Surg Sports Traumatol Arthrosc 2008;16:497–503.

Cho NS, Rhee YG. The factors affecting the clinical outcome and integrity of arthroscopically repaired rotator cuff tears of the shoulder. Clin Orthop Surg 2009;1:96–104.

Chopp JN, Fischer SL, Dickerson CR . The specificity of fatiguing protocols affects scapular orientation: Implications for subacromial impingement. Clin Biomech 2011;26:40–45.

Clement ND, Hallett A, MacDonald D, Howie C, McBirnie J. Does diabetes affect outcome after arthroscopic repair of the rotator cuff? J Bone Joint Surg Br 2010;92:1112–1117.

Cofield RH. Rotator cuff disease of the shoulder. J Bone Joint Surg Am 1985;67:974–979.

Cofield R, Parvizi J, Hoffmeyer P et al. Surgical repair of chronic rotator cuff tear. A prospective long term study. J Bone Joint Surg Am 2001;83:71–77.

Davidson J, Burkhart SS. The geometric classification of rotator cuff tears: a system linking tear pattern to treatment and prognosis. Arthroscopy 2010;26:417–424.

Di Giacomo G, Costantini A, De Vita A. Shoulder disorders: From disfunction to the lesion. In: Angelo RL, Esch JC, Ryu RKN (eds), AANA Advanced Arthroscopy. The shoulder. Philadelphia, PA: Saunders Elsevier, 2010: 14–23.

Duquin TR, Buyea C, Bisson LJ. Which method of rotator cuff repair leads to the highest rate of structural healing? A systematic review. Am J Sports Med 2010;38:835–841.

Ellman H, Kay SP, Wirth M. Arthroscopic treatment of full-thickness rotator cuff tears: 2- to 7-year follow-up study. Arthroscopy 1993;9:195–200.

Esch JC, Leek BT. Biology of healing and tissue repair. In: Angelo RL, Esch JC, Ryu RKN (eds), AANA Advanced Arthroscopy. The shoulder. New York: Saunders Elsevier, 2010: 2–15.

Franceschi F, Longo UG, Ruzzini L, et al.The Roman Bridge: a "double pulley–suture bridges" technique for rotator cuff repair. BMC Musculoskel Disord 2007a;8:123.

Franceschi F, Ruzzini L, Longo U, et al. Equivalent clinical results of arthroscopic single-row and double-row suture anchor repair for rotator cuff tears: a randomized controlled trial. Am J Sports Med 2007b;35:1254–1260.

Franceschi F, Longo UG, Ruzzini L, et al. No advantages in repairing a type II superior labrum anterior and posterior (SLAP) lesion when associated with rotator cuff repair in patients over age 50: a randomized controlled trial. Am J Sports Med 2008;36:247–253.

Galatz LM, Charlton N, Das R, et al. Complete removal of load is detrimental for rotator cuff healing . J Shoulder Elbow Surg 2009;18:669–75

Gerber C. Histologic findings in the healing rotator cuff repair. Presented at NICE Shoulder Course. London: NICE, 2004.

Ghodadra NS, Provencher MT, Verma NN, Wilk KE, Romeo AA. Open, mini-open and all arthroscopic rotator cuff repair surgery: indications and implications for rehabilitation. J Orthop Sports Phys Ther 2009;39:81–9.

Goutallier D, Postel JM, Gleyze P, et al. Influence of cuff muscle fatty degeneration on anatomic and functional outcomes after simple suture of full-thickness tears. J Shoulder Elbow Surg 2003;12:550–554.

Grasso A, Milano G, Salvatore M, et al. Single-row versus double-row arthroscopic rotator cuff repair: a prospective randomized clinical study. Arthroscopy 2009;25:4–12.

Gruson KI, Chen DD, Harrison AK, Gladstone J, Flatow EL. Does slower rehabilitation after arthroscopic rotator cuff repair lead to long-term stiffness? Clin Rehabil 2009;23:622–638.

Halbrecht JL, Tirman P, Atkin D. Internal impinegement of the shoulder. Comparison between the trowing and non trowing shoulders of College baseball players. Atrhroscopy 1999;15:253–258.

Harryman DT 2nd, Mack LA, Wang KY, et al. Repairs of the rotator cuff. Correlation of functional results with integrity of the cuff. J Bone Joint Surg Am 1991;73:982–989.

Harryman DT 2nd, Hettrich CM, Smith KL, et al. A prospective multipractice investigation of patients with full-thickness rotator cuff tears: the importance of comorbidities, practice, and other covariables on self-assessed shoulder function and health status J Bone Joint Surg Am 2003;85:690.

Hatch RGF, Gobetzie R, Miller PJ. Stiffness after rotator cuff repair. In: Green A (ed.), Complications in Orthopaedics: Rotator cuff surgery. Rosemont, IL: American Academy of Orthopaedic Surgeons, 2006: 13–29.

Herrera M, Bauer G, Reynolds F, et al. Infections after mini-open rotatr cuff repair. J Shoulder Elbow Surg 2002;11:605–608.

Huberty DP, Schoolfield JD, Brady PC, et al. Incidence and treatment of postoperative stiffness following arthroscopic rotator cuff repair. Arthroscopy 2009;25:880–890.

Iannotti JP, et al. Accuracy of office-based ultrasonography of the shoulder for the diagnosis of rotator cuff tears. J Bone Joint Surg Am 2005;7:1305–1311.

Kibler BW, Sciascia A. What went wrong and what to do about it: pitfalls in the treatment of shoulder impingement. Instr Course Lect 2008;57:103–112.

Kibler WB, Sciascia A. Current concepts: scapular dyskinesis. Br J Sports Med 2010;44:300–305.

Kibler WBK, Sciascia A, Wolf BR, Warme B, Khun JE. Non acute shoulder injuries In: Kibler WBK (ed), Orthopaedic Knowledge Update 4: Sports Medicine. Rosemont, IL: American Academy of Orthopaedic Surgeons, 2009: 19-39.

Koester MC, Dunn WR, Khun JE, Spindler KP. The efficacy of subacromial cortison injections in the treatment of rotator cuff disease:a sistematic review. J Am Acad Orthop Surg 2007;15:3–11.

Koo SS, Parsley BK, Burkhart SS, Schoolfield JD. Reduction of post-operative stiffness after arthroscopic rotator cuff repair: results of a customized physical therapy regimen based on risk fators for stiffness. Arthroscopy 2011;27:155–160.

Kwon Y, Kalainov D, Rose H, et al. Management of deep infection after rotator cuff repair surgery. J Shoulder Elbow Surgery 2005;14:1–5.

Lehman C, Cuomo F, Kummer FJ, Zuckerman JD. The incidence of full thickness rotator cuff tears in a large cadaveric population. Bull Hosp Jt Dis 1995;54:30–31.

Lin KC , Krishan SG, Burkhead WZ. Rotator cuff. In: DeLee JC, Drez D, Miller MD (eds), DeLee and Drez's Orthopaedic Sports Medicine: Principles and Practice, Third Edition. Philadelphia, PA: Saunders Elsevier, 2010: 986–1015.

McKee MD, Yoo DJ. The effect of surgery for rotator cuff disease on general health status: results of a prospective trial. J Bone Joint Surg Am 2000;82:970–979.

McLaughlin HL. Lesions of the musculotendinous cuff of the shoulder. The exposure and treatment of tears with retraction. Clin Orthop Relat Res 1994;304:3–9.

Mall NA, Kim HM, Keener JD, et al. Symptomatic progression of asymptomatic rotator cuff tears: a prospective study of clinical and sonographic variables. J Bone Joint Surg Am 2010;92:2623–2633.

Melis B, Wall B, Walch G. Natural history of infraspinatus fatty infiltration in rotator cuff tears. J Shoulder Elbow Surg 2010;19:757–763.

Mikolyzk DK, Wei AS, Tonino P, et al. Effect of corticosteroids on the biomechanical strength of rat rotator cuff tendon. J Bone Joint Surg Am 2009;91:1172–1180.

Milano G, Grasso A, Salvatore M, et al. Arthroscopic rotator cuff repair with and without subacromial decompression: a prospective randomized study. Arthroscopy 2007;23:81–88.

Murray PJ, Shaffer BS.Clinical update: MR imaging of the shoulder. Sports Med Arthrosc 2009;17:40–48.

Osti L, Franci M, Chiarelli S, Sommazzi P. Water rehabilition following rotator cuff surgery: A prospective study. Abstract Book, 11th ESSKA Meeting, Athens, 2004: 92.
Osti L, Papalia R, Del Buono A, et al. Home rehabilitation vs supervised approach following arthroscopic rotator cuff repair surgery. A randomized control trial: Abstract Book. 14th ESSKA Congress, 2010: S72–S73.
Osti L, Papalia R, Del Buono A, Denaro V, Maffulli N. Comparison of arthroscopic rotator cuff reapairin healty patients over and under 65 years of age. Knee Surg Sports Traumatol Arthrosc 2010a;18:1700–1706.
Osti L, Papalia R, Paganelli M, Maffulli N, Del Buono A. Mini-open and all arthroscopic rotator cuff repair. Int Orthop 2010b;34:389–394.
Ottenheijm RP, Jansen MJ, Staal JB, et al. Accuracy of diagnostic ultrasound in patients with suspected subacromial disorders: a systematic review and metanalysis. Arch Phys Med Rehabil 2010;91:1616–1625.
Pai V, Larson D. Rotator cuff repair in a district hospital setting:outocmes and analysis of prognostic factors. J Shoulder Elbow 2001;10:236–241.
Randelli P, Margheritini F, Cabitza P, et al. Release of growth factors after arthroscopic acromioplasty. Knee Surg Sports Traumatol Arthrosc 2009;17:98–101.
Romeo A, Hang D, Bach B, et al. Repair of full tickness rotator cuff tears. Gender, age and other factors affecting outcome. Clin Orthop Rel Res 1999;367:243–255.
Rowe CR. Ruptures of rotator cuff: selection for conservative treatment. Surg Clin North Am 1975;43:1531–1540.
Shaffer B. Making the transition from mini-open to all arthroscopic repair. In: Abrams JS, Bell RH (eds), Arthroscopic Rotator Cuff Surgery. New York: Springer, 2008: 15–24.
Snyder SJ. Shoulder Arthroscopy. Basic techniques for arthroscopic shoulder reconstruction. Philadelphia, PA: Lippincott Williams & Wilkins, 2003:46–65.
Szabó I, Boileau P, Walch G. The proximal biceps as a pain generator and results of tenotomy. Sports Med Arthrosc 2008;16:180–186.
Tanaka M, Itoi E, Sato K, et al. Factors related to successful outcome of conservative treatment for rotator cuff tears. Ups J Med Sci 2010;115:193–200.
Ticker JB, Egan JJ. Post-operative rehabilitation following arthroscopic rotator cuff repair. In: Abhrams JF, Bell RH (eds), Arthroscopic Rotator cuff Surgery. New York: Springer, 2008: 348–362.
Trantalis J, Lo IKL. Avoiding and managing rotator cuff complications of arthroscopic rotator cuff tear. In: Meislin RJ, Albrecht J (eds), Complications of Knee and Shoulder Surgery. New York: Springer, 2009: 225–244.
Tucker WS, Armstrong CW, Gribble PA, Timmons MK, Yeasting RA. Scapular muscle activity in overhead athletes with symptoms of secondary shoulder impingement during closed chain exercises. Arch Phys Med Rehabil 2010;91:550–556.
Walch G, Boileau J, Noel E, et al. Impingement of the deep surface of the supraspinatus tendon in the posterior superior glenoid rim: an arthroscopic study. J Shoulder Elbow Surg 1992;1:238–243.
Yamaguchi K, Tashjian R. Surgical indications and reparability of rotator cuff tears. In: Abrams JS, Bell RH (eds), Arthroscopic Rotator Cuff Surgery. New York: Springer, 2008: 1–14.
Yamaguchi K, Tetro AM, Blam O, et al. Natural history of asymptomatic rotator cuff tears: a longitudinal analysis of asymptomatic tears detected sonographically. J Shoulder Elbow Surg 2001;10:199–203.
Zgonis MH, Andarawis NA, Soslowky LJ. Mechanics and healing of rotator cuff Injury. In: Abhrams JF, Bell RH (eds), Arthroscopic Rotator Cuff Surgery. New York: Springer 2008: 332–347.

Chapter 12 Subscapularis tears

Uma Srikumaran, James T. Monica, Ifedayo O. Kuye,
Jon J. P. Warner

KEY FEATURES

- Subscapularis is the largest rotator cuff tendon; it provides balanced compression and stabilization of the humeral head on to the glenoid surface.
- Tears of subscapularis are uncommon compared with tears of supraspinatus and infraspinatus.
- Subscapularis tendon tears present with vague anterior shoulder pain, weakness in internal rotation, and increased external rotation compared with the uninjured side.
- Arthroscopic studies have shown that the prevalence of subscapularis tears is higher than previously thought.
- Subscapularis tears are rarely isolated injuries.

INTRODUCTION

The subscapularis tendon makes up the anterior-most portion of the rotator cuff, functioning as a powerful internal rotator of the arm (**Fig. 12.1**). As part of the force couple, the subscapularis also provides balanced compression and stabilization of the humeral head on to the glenoid face (Ward et al. 2006). Compared with superior and posterosuperior cuff tears, pathology of the anterior rotator cuff has, until recently, been largely ignored in the literature (Gerber and Krushell 1991; Gerber et al. 1996; Warner et al. 2001). Tears of the subscapularis are uncommon compared with tears of the supraspinatus and infraspinatus (Codman 1934; Patten 1994; Deutsch et al. 1997; Sakurai et al. 1998; Li et al. 1999; Bennett 2001; Kim et al. 2005; Flury et al. 2006; Arai et al. 2008).

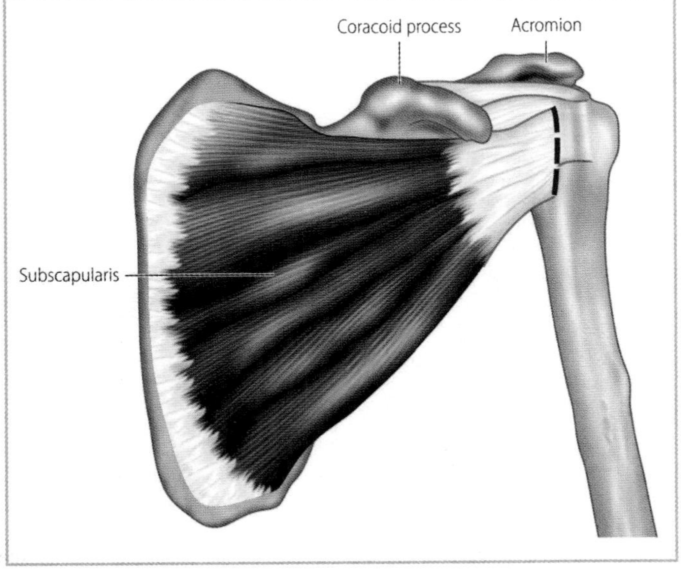

Figure 12.1 Muscular anatomy of subscapularis. The normal subscapularis muscle is very powerful with a small footprint of insertion (highlighted in red) on the lesser tuberosity and adjacent proximal humerus.

The exact prevalence of subscapularis tendon tears varies depending upon the methodology used to identify these injuries, the age of the individuals studied, and the type of population examined (**Table 12.1**). In a cadaveric study by Codman (1934), a 3.5% prevalence of combined subscapularis and supraspinatus tears was found in a population of 102 patients (200 shoulders). However, another cadaveric study by Sakurai et al. (1998) found a much higher prevalence of 37% of partial subscapularis tears in 46 shoulders. Magnetic resonance imaging (MRI) of patients with rotator cuff tears have found a prevalence of subscapularis tears that has ranged from 2% to 9.3% (Patten 1994; Sakurai et al. 1998; Li et al. 1999). Arthroscopic studies, which examine the prevalence of subscapularis tears among those undergoing arthroscopic procedures, have found a higher rate. The prevalence rate ranges from 7% to 29% (Bennett 2001; Barth et al. 2006; Arai et al. 2008). Despite the variance in the prevalence reported, these studies have consistently found the prevalence of isolated tears to be much lower than combined supraspinatus and subscapularis tears.

PATHOGENESIS AND PATHOLOGY

Anatomy

The subscapularis is the largest of the rotator cuff muscles. It arises from the anterior scapula and has multiple interspersed tendons that converge superiorly and laterally, running under the coracoid, to insert along the lesser tuberosity. A study by D'Addesi et al. (2006) showed the footprint formed by subscapularis insertion to have an average height of 25.8 mm and width of 18.1 mm. The insertion is broad proximally and tapered distally. The superior fibers of the subscapularis tendon interdigitate with the anterior fibers of the supraspinatus tendon to form a portion of the rotator cuff interval.

The superior and inferior aspects of subscapularis are innervated by the upper and lower subscapularis nerves respectively. The upper subscapular nerve originates from C5–6 whereas the lower subscapular nerve is from C5–7. The dual innervation may suggest that subscapularis functions as two independent muscle units (Kadaba et al. 1992). A common variation involves the lower subscapular nerve arising from the axillary nerve (Kasper et al. 2008). The axillary nerve runs just inferior to subscapularis as it travels from the posterior cord of the brachial plexus through the quadrangular space. The position of the axillary nerve changes with the position of the arm; in abduction the axillary nerve moves further away from the glenoid rim (Uno et al. 1999; Yoo et al. 2007). Anatomy of the subscapular and axillary nerves is relevant to both arthroscopic and open surgery because they are vulnerable at the base of the coracoid process if soft-tissue releases are performed in this region during surgery (Yung et al. 1996; Kasper et al. 2008). Identification and protection of the axillary nerve are needed to safely dissect the subscapularis for purposes of tendon mobilization during subscapularis repairs in isolation or during arthroplasty (Yung et al. 1996).

Table 12.1 Prevalence of isolated and combined subscapularis tears

Source	Method	Population	Prevalence of subscapularis tears
Codman (1934)	Cadaveric study	200 shoulders in 102 patients: 73% male, 27% female	3.5% had combined subscapularis and supraspinatus rotator cuff tears
Sakurai et al. (1998)	Cadaveric study	46 shoulders Average age – 76.3 years 65% male, 25% female	37% had partial tears of the subscapularis: 13% – isolated tears 24% – combined tears of the subscapularis and supraspinatus
Li et al. (1999)	MRI	2167 patients with rotator cuff tears	2% had tears of the subscapularis: 0.4% had isolated tears 1.6% had combined subscapularis and supraspinatus tears
Sakurai et al. (1998)	MRI	162 patients with rotator cuff tears	9.3% patients had a partial tear of the subscapularis combined with small or medium-sized tears of the supraspinatus
Patten (1994)	MRI	149 patients with rotator cuff tears	7% of patients had rotator cuff tears predominantly or exclusively involving the subscapularis
Bennett (2001)	Arthroscopic	165 patients treated for rotator tears and/or instability	27% of the patients had subscapularis tears: 6% were isolated tears 11% were combined subscapularis and supraspinatus tears 7% were combined subscapularis, supraspinatus, and infraspinatus tears
Barth et al. (2006)	Arthroscopic	68 patients undergoing arthroscopic procedures	29% of the patients had isolated or combined subscapularis tears
Arai et al. (2008)	Arthroscopic	435 patients undergoing arthroscopic rotator cuff repair: Average age – 49 years 59% women, 41% men	27% had subscapularis tendon tears: 0.6% had isolated tears 26.4% had combined tears (subscapularis, infraspinatus, and supraspinatus)
Kim et al. (2003)	Arthroscopic	314 patients undergoing shoulder arthroscopic surgery	19% had partial subscapularis tears
Deutsch et al. (1997)	MRI, arthroscopic	350 patients who had rotator cuff surgery	4% had subscapularis tears
Flury et al. (2006)	Not Stated	1345 patients who underwent rotator cuff repair	5.5% of the patients had isolated rupture or combined ruptures of the subscapularis and supraspinatus

The coracohumeral ligament and the superior glenohumeral ligament form the long head of biceps tendon "reflection pulley," which stabilizes the long head of biceps before it enters the intertubercular groove (Weishaupt et al. 1999). As the pulley is in direct contact with the uppermost insertion of the subscapularis tendon, this area likely supports the biceps tendon from behind the pulley (Arai et al. 2008). Tears of the upper aspect of the subscapularis tendon are often associated with subluxation or dislocation of the long head of the biceps tendon (Walch et al. 1998).

Etiology and mechanism of injury

Tears of the subscapularis tendon can result from either degeneration in older patients or trauma in younger patients (Morag et al. 2011). In an extensive study of subscapularis tears, Edwards et al. (2005) examined 84 patients with isolated tears of the subscapularis. They found that 57 tears had resulted from traumatic episodes and 27 had degenerative origins. Traumatic tears most often occur after injuries that result from hyperextension and external rotation of the arm (Deutsch et al. 1997). The greatest force exerted by the subscapularis occurs when a strong external rotation and abduction force is applied with the arm at maximum external rotation and about 60° abduction (Haas 1944). Deutsch et al. (1997) examined 14 patients with isolated tears of the subscapularis, 11 of which occurred due to traumatic hyperextension and external rotation. Gerber and Krushell (1991) described post-traumatic rupture of the subscapularis in 16 men; in 7, the ruptures resulted from a violent external rotation of the adducted arm, and in 6 they resulted from violent hyperextension, sustained during falls on the outstretched arm.

Although less common, tears of the subscapularis can also result from traumatic anterior dislocations (Gerber and Krushell 1991; Deutsch et al. 1997). While studying cadavers, Symeonides (1972) brought the arm to a position of abduction and lateral rotation and applied a force until dislocation resulted. He noticed ruptures in the fibers of subscapularis as the greater tuberosity overrode the posterior margin of the glenoid fossa. Subscapularis tears have also been associated with the development of recurrent dislocations after a traumatic onset (Hauser 1954; Neviaser and Neviaser 1995). Whether acute or chronic, a history of instability, particularly in the older patient, warrants a thorough evaluation of subscapularis by examination and imaging.

An association between both anterosuperior and subcoracoid impingement and the development of articular-side subscapularis wear has been described. Anterosuperior impingement is described as mechanical contact of the biceps tendon, pulley region, and anterosuperior labrum when the shoulder is placed at full internal rotation and forward flexion of between 80° and <120°. At forward flexion of less than 80° but more than 50°, mechanical contact occurs between the deep surface of subscapularis and the anterior glenoid rim. Gerber and Sebesta (2000) examined 16 patients with anterosuperior impingement and noted an articular-sided partial subscapularis tendon tear in 10 cases.

Subcoracoid impingement of the subscapularis tendon occurs between the coracoid process and the lesser tuberosity of the humerus (Ferrick 2000). Lo and Burkhart (2003) proposed that, in patients with subcoracoid impingement, the coracoid rolled against the subscapularis, which increased the tensile force on the undersurface of the subscapularis tendon and led to fiber failure on the articular surface of the subscapularis. Nové-Josserand et al. (1999), however, noted no difference in the size of the subcoracoid space in the CT scans of patients with isolated tears of the subscapularis and those without.

Clinical presentation

Patients with subscapularis tendon tears present with vague anterior shoulder pain, weakness in internal rotation, and increased external rotation compared with the uninjured side (Gerber and Krushell 1991; Gerberet al. 1996; Deutsch et al. 1997; Warner et al. 2001). Gerber and Krushell (1991) examined 16 patients with isolated subscapularis tears and found all reported anterior shoulder pain when the arm was used overhead or below the shoulder. Gerber et al. (1996) found that 13 of 16 patients with subscapularis tears experienced pain at night, whereas 15 of 16 patients noted discomfort in activities in which the hand was elevated above the shoulder. Of 16 patients 12 had weakness in tasks that required internal rotation, such as reaching behind their bodies or placing their hands in the back pockets (Gerber et al. 1996).

DIAGNOSIS

Clinical examination

Several tests are available to the clinician to suggest subscapularis pathology. The lift-off test (**Fig. 12.2**), described by Gerber and Krushell (1991), is positive for a tear when the patient is unable to lift a hand off the back. Gerber and Krushell (1991) found that the lift-off test was positive in 12 of 13 patients with isolated subscapularis tears. Gerber et al. (1996) described a variation in which the arm was first passively brought to maximum internal rotation behind the patient's back and then released. The patient is considered to have a lag if he or she is unable to maintain the elevated position. The lift-off test and its "internal rotation lag" variation are often difficult to perform due to pain. The test is also more sensitive to complete tears than to partial tears of subscapularis. Kreuz et al. (2005) found that the test was positive in all complete tears but only positive in 62% of the partial tears.

The belly press or Napoleon's sign can also be used to identify subscapularis tears. The patient is asked to press the abdomen with the hand flat while keeping the arm at maximum internal rotation. If the subscapularis is impaired, the elbow drops back (**Fig. 12.3**). Gerber et al. (1996) reported that the belly press test was positive in all eight patients with isolated subscapularis tears. Bukhart and Tehrany (2002) noted that the degree to which the subscapularis was torn was directly related to the degree to which the hand flexed during the test.

The bear hug test, described by Barth et al. (2006) involves placing the palm of the affected hand on the opposite shoulder. Inability to maintain the hand in this position while the examiner attempts to elevate the hand suggests subscapularis dysfunction (**Fig. 12.4**). The bear hug test has a greater sensitivity in diagnosing partial tears of the subscapularis (Barth et al. 2006).

The belly-off test was described by Scheibel et al. (2005). The arm of the patient is passively brought into flexion and maximum internal rotation with the elbow flexed at 90°. The elbow is supported by one of the examiner's hand and with the other hand he or she places the patient's palm on the patient's abdomen. The patient is then asked to maintain the position as the examiner releases the wrist (**Fig. 12.5**). The test is positive if the patient cannot maintain this position and the hand lifts off the abdomen. Scheibel et al. (2005) found that the belly-off sign was just as effective as Napoleon's sign and the lift-off test in diagnosing patients with complete subscapularis tears, and more effective in diagnosing patients with isolated partial tears of the rotator cuff. However, in patients with a partial tear of the subscapularis and a complete tear of external rotators, especially the infraspinatus, the belly-off sign was negative.

Electromyographic (EMG) analysis has shown that these tests effectively activate the subscapularis. Tokish et al. (2003) found that the lift-off and belly press tests were effective in isolating EMG activity of the subscapularis from the surrounding muscles. Upper subscapularis had greater EMG activity during the belly press test than the lift-off test, whereas the lower subscapularis had greater activity during the lift-off test. Chao et al. (2008) demonstrated that the examiner can target various parts of the subscapularis by varying the angle that the elbow is flexed during the bear hug test. At 45°, there was significant activation

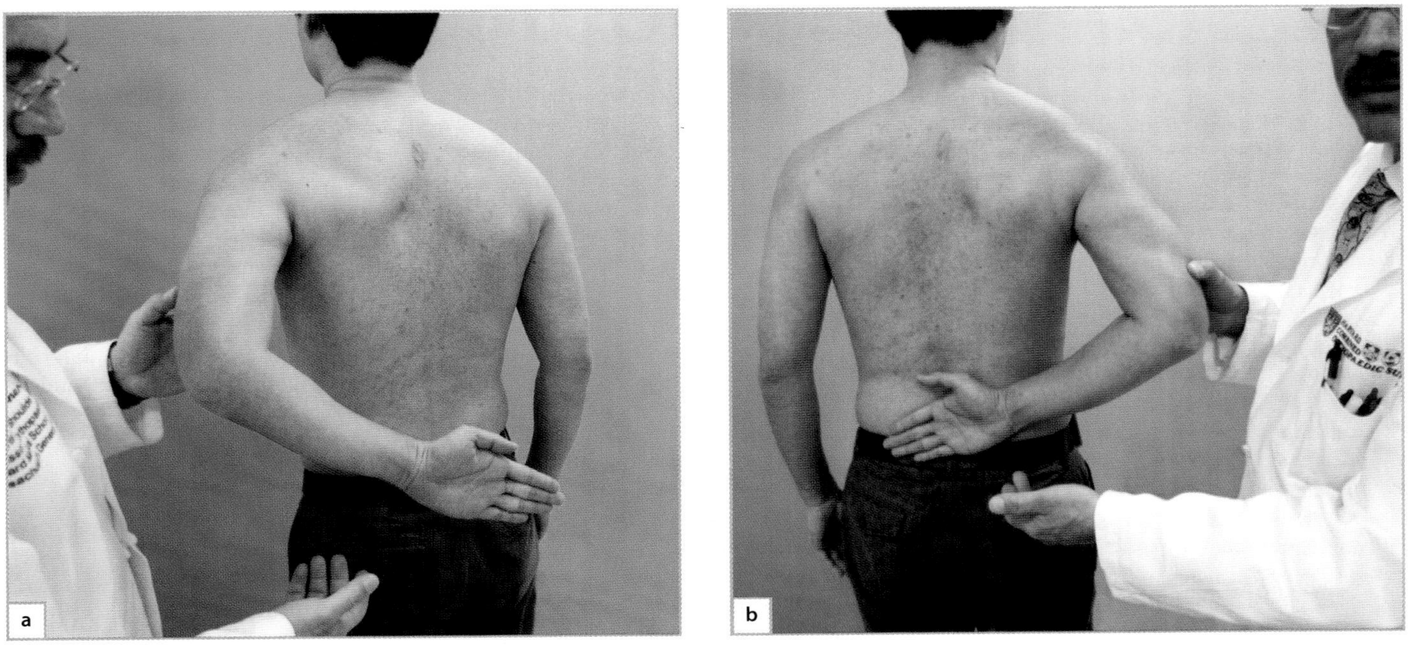

Figure 12.2 The lift-off test. The examiner asks the patient to lift the hand away from the back. (a) If the patient is able to do this and maintain this position, the test is negative. (b) If the patient is unable to maintain the position, the test is positive.

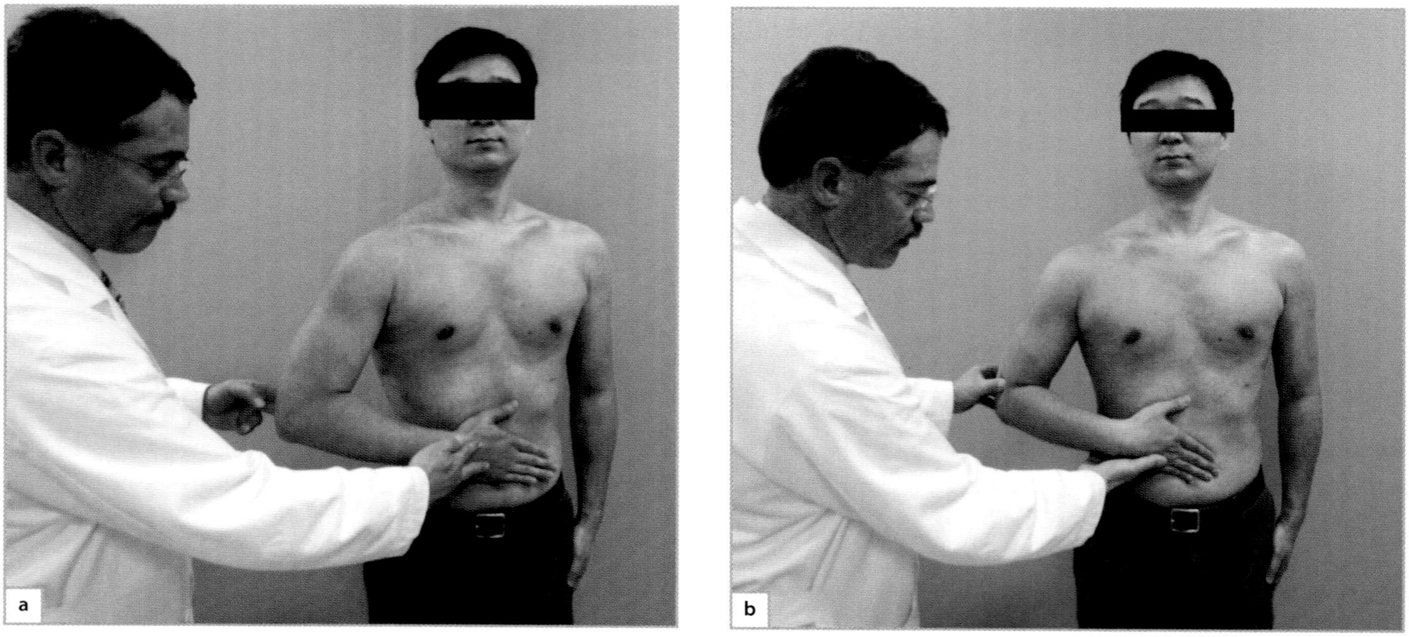

Figure 12.3 The belly press test. (a) The examiner asks the patient to press the palm of the hand against the belly with the wrist in neutral. (b) If the patient flexes the wrist and the elbow falls posteriorly, as in this example, the test is considered positive.

of both upper and lower subscapularis compared with pectoralis major and latissimus dorsi, and at 90° of elbow flexion lower subscapularis had significantly more activity than the surrounding muscles. The sensitivities and specificities of these various tests are listed in **Table 12.2**.

Imaging

Careful imaging interpretation is vital for the appropriate diagnosis of subscapularis tears because the clinical presentation and exam findings are often non-specific. Radiographs are of limited value for the direct assessment of subscapularis tears. However, associated pathology, such as avulsions of the lesser tuberosity or fractures of the glenoid rim related to traumatic instability, can appear on plain radiographs. In addition, the clinician can evaluate the position of bone anchors in cases of prior surgical treatment.

The most commonly used imaging modalities to evaluate for subscapularis pathology include MRI, MR arthrography, CT arthrography, and ultrasonography (**Figs 12.6** and **12.7**). These studies can provide details about the extent and location of the tear, as well as identify associated lesions involving the biceps pulley, biceps tendon, or rotator cuff interval.

MR arthrography is particularly suited to identify smaller full- or partial-thickness tears (Pfirrmann et al. 1999). Pfirrmann et al. (1999) demonstrated a sensitivity of 91% and a specificity of 86% in the identification of subscapularis tears, with the combined evaluation of transverse and parasagittal images; this level of accuracy is consistent with the accuracy of MR arthrography for evaluation of supraspinatus and infraspinatus tears. Besides tendon discontinuity, focal signal changes of the tendon, or tendon retraction, MRI indicators of subscapularis tears include an uncovered lesser tuberosity or contrast extension immediately above the tuberosity (Pfirrmann et al. 1999; Morag et al. 2011). Fatty infiltration of the subscapularis muscle belly, primarily its superior portion, and medial displacement of the biceps tendon are specific findings suggestive of subscapularis tears as well (Pfirrmann et al. 1999). Studler et al. (2008) also reported an association of cortical abnormalities and cysts of the lesser tuberosity with tears of the subscapularis tendon. A classification scheme listed in **Table 12.3** based on MR sagittal images and the craniocaudal extent of the tear has been described by Pfirrmann et al. (1999).

CT arthrography is particularly useful in the patient with metal anchors already in place, because the artifact generated with MRI limits its usefulness. Charousset et al. (2005) found a sensitivity of 65% and specificity of 98% for identification of subscapularis tears with this modality. Similar to MRI, CT arthrography is capable of assessing the extent of the tear, level of retraction, and degree of fatty infiltration (Goutallier et al. 1994; Charousset et al. 2005). As listed in **Table 12.4**, grading of fatty infiltration ranges from 0 (normal muscle) to 4 (>50% fatty replacement) using the classification of Goutallier et al. (1994).

Ultrasonography has largely been studied for the identification of superior and posterosuperior cuff tears, but is also capable of identifying subscapularis pathology. Although some studies suggest an equivalent accuracy rate between MRI and ultrasonography for identifying rotator cuff tears, results are dependent on investigator expertise with the modality (Teefey et al. 2004). For the specific evaluation of subscapularis tears, dynamic ultrasonography with the arm in external rotation can help determine the continuity of the tendon with the lesser tuberosity (Morag et al. 2011). Ultrasonography has also been found to accurately identify dislocated biceps tendons (Teefey et al. 2004). Despite its limitations, ultrasonography is less expensive and less invasive than MRI or CT, and can be quickly performed bilaterally, as well as in an office setting (Iannotti et al. 2005).

Arthroscopic and surgical evaluation

Diagnosis of subscapularis tears can be further refined during arthroscopic or open surgical evaluation. Preoperative imaging evaluation remains critical, because there are significant limitations of arthroscopic and surgical visualization. Arthroscopy is well suited to visualize the superolateral portion of the subscapularis tendon and

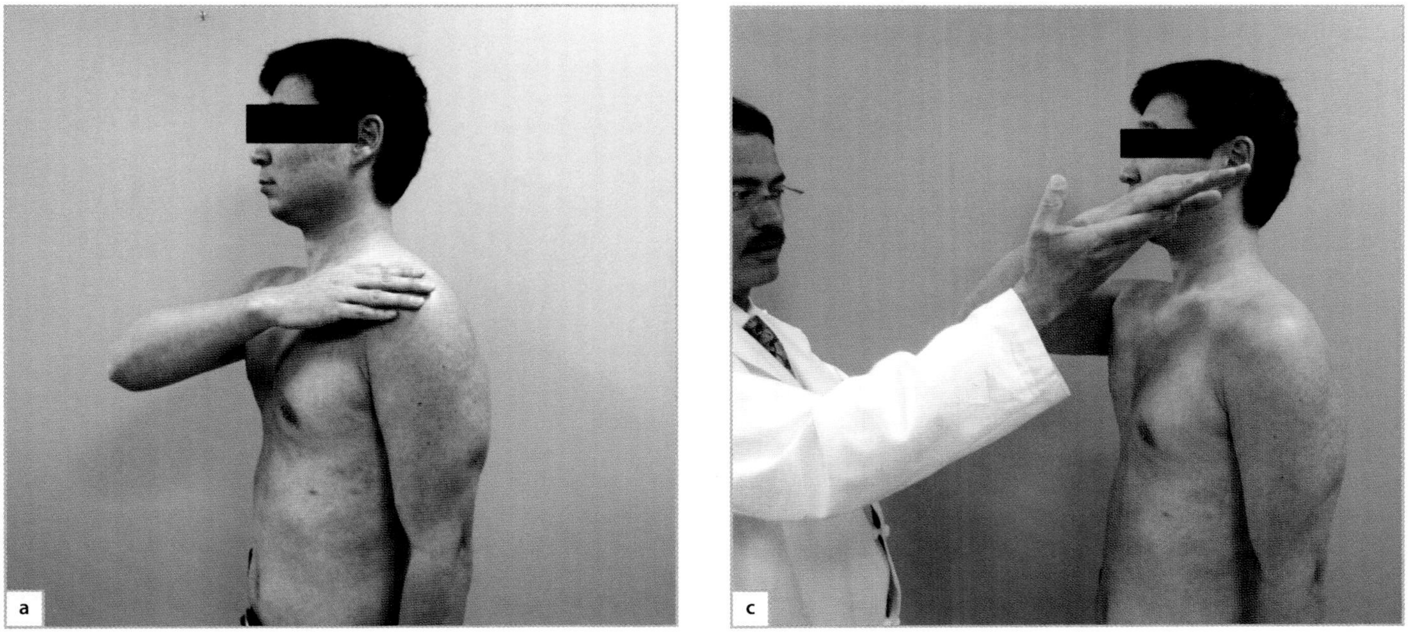

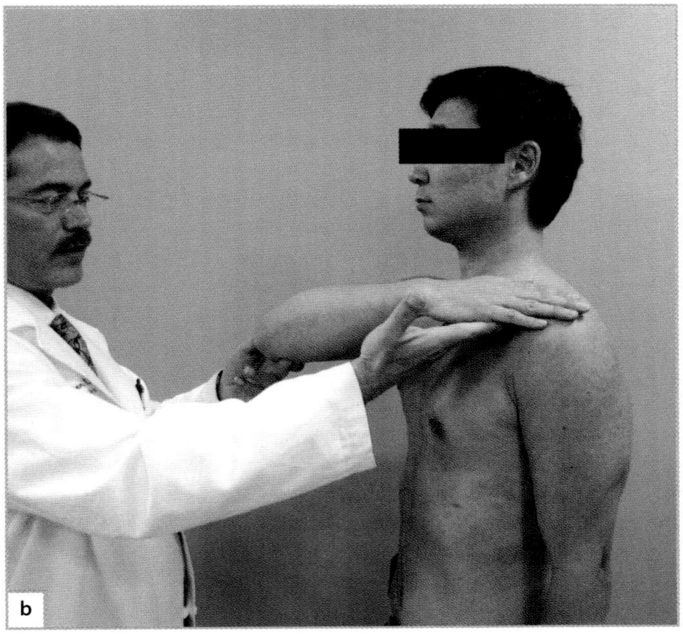

Figure 12.4 The bear hug test. (a) The patient starts with the palm of the hand of the affected shoulder on the opposite shoulder. (b) The patient tries to hold the starting position as the examiner pulls the patient's hand from the shoulder. (c) In a positive test, the patient will not be able to hold the hand on the opposite shoulder.

the presence of articular-sided fraying and partial tears. Associated lesions involving the biceps tendon and rotator interval can also be dynamically evaluated. However, Wright et al. (2001) determined that the arthroscopically visualized region represents only 26% ± 11% of the entire subscapularis. The middle and inferior glenohumeral ligaments obscure much of the remaining portion of the tendon.

Assessment of the subscapularis tendon during open surgery also has inherent limitations. Significant scar can form around the torn tendon, often in contiguity with the tendon itself and overlying fascia. The scar tissue can be mistaken for an intact tendon and adhesions to neighboring structures, including the brachial plexus, can make surgical dissection difficult (Gerber and Krushell 1991; Deutsch et al. 1997). The classification of subscapularis tears on the basis of intraoperative evaluation and CT has been proposed by Lafosse et al. (2007) and is reviewed in **Table 12.5**.

MANAGEMENT

The etiology of the subscapularis tear, whether degenerative or traumatic in nature, influences the management strategy. In addition, associated pathology including involvement of the supraspinatus tendon directs intervention and surgical approach. Degenerative tears can be initially approached conservatively; surgical intervention can proceed when these measures fail. Chronic degenerative tears involving the superior cuff can be approached in a similar manner. Acute traumatic tears, however, warrant a more aggressive approach, as surgical delay is associated with worse outcomes (Gerber et al. 1996; Warner et al. 2001). Fatty infiltration of the muscle belly correlates with a worse prognosis, with chronic tears more likely exhibiting higher grades of fatty replacement (Goutallier et al. 1994; Warner et

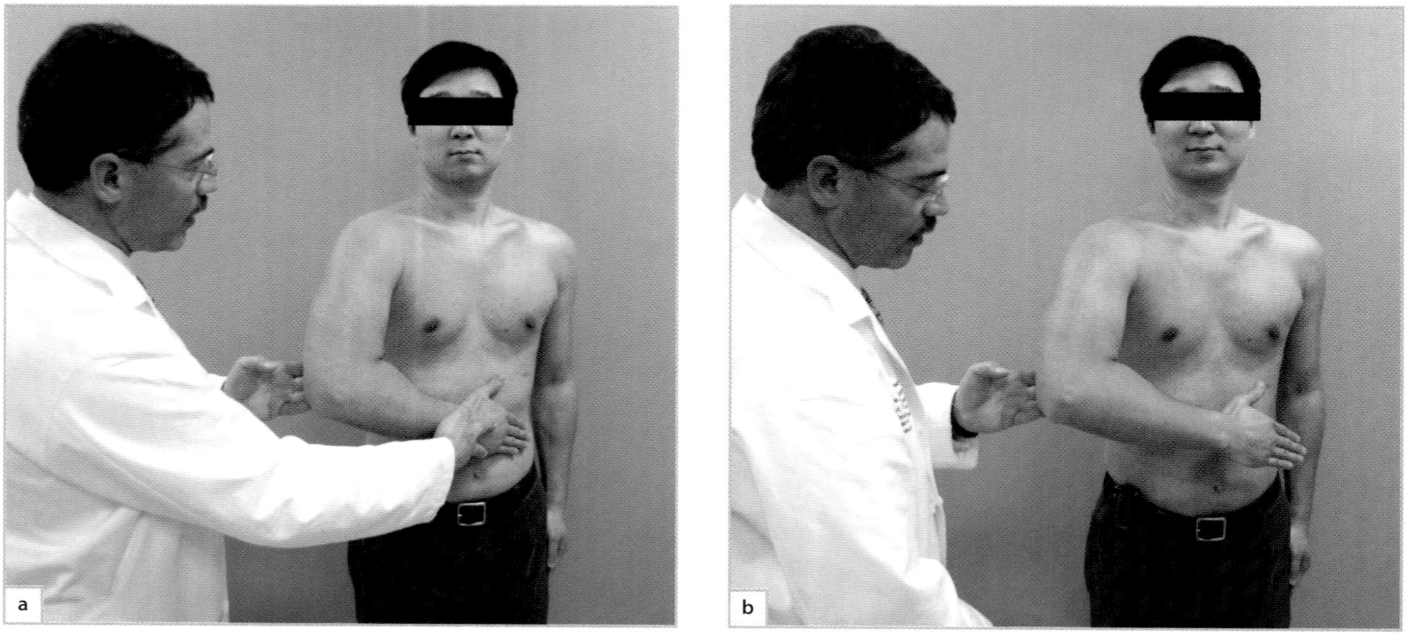

Figure 12.5 The belly-off test. (a) The arm is brought into flexion and maximum internal rotation with the elbow flexed at 90°. The elbow is supported by one of the examiner's hands; with the other hand, the examiner places the patient's hand on the patient's abdomen. (b) The test is positive if the hand lifts off the abdomen when the examiner lets go.

Table 12.2 Specificity, sensitivity, and accuracy of clinical tests

Test	Specificity (%)	Sensitivity (%)	Accuracy (%)
Napoleon's sign	98 (Barth et al. 2006) 88 (Bartsch et al. 2010)	68 (Scheibel et al. 2005) 25 (Barth et al. 2006) 80 (Bartsch et al. 2010)	77 (Barth et al. 2006) 86 (Bartsch et al. 2010)
Lift-off test	100 (Barth et al. 2006) 79 (Bartsch et al. 2010)	57 (Scheibel et al. 2005) 18 (Barth et al. 2006) 40 (Bartsch et al. 2010)	78 (Barth et al. 2006) 66 (Bartsch et al. 2010)
Belly-off test	91 (Bartsch et al. 2010)	84 (Scheibel et al. 2005) 86 (Bartsch et al. 2010)	90 (Bartsch et al. 2010)
Bear hug test	92 (Barth et al. 2006)	60 (Barth et al. 2006)	82 (Barth et al. 2006)

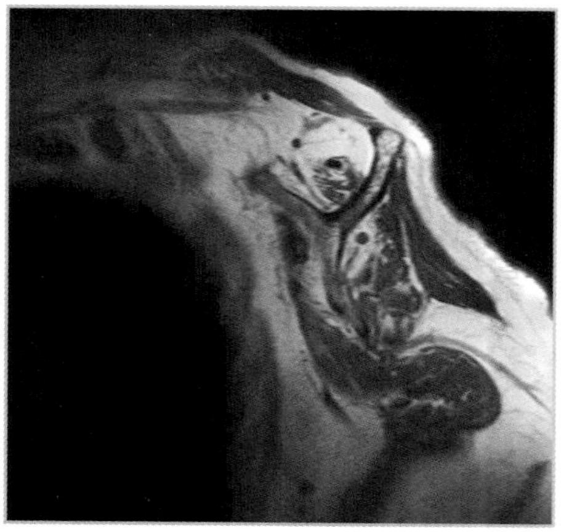

Figure 12.6 Oblique sagittal T1-weighted MR image demonstrating significant fatty infiltration and muscular atrophy of subscapularis, supraspinatus, and infraspinatus muscles.

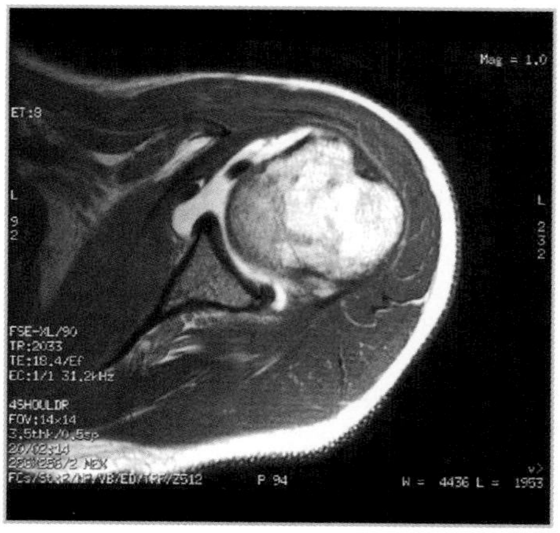

Figure 12.7 Axial T1-weighted MR image of a full-thickness subscapularis tear with biceps subluxation.

al. 2001). Muscle atrophy, similar to fatty infiltration, has also been found to correlate with poor tendon quality at the time of surgery. Decreased strength of abduction and external rotation postoperatively correlate with this preoperative atrophy (Warner et al. 2001).

Conservative management

A conservative approach to the management of subscapularis tears includes activity modification, pain management, and physical therapy. A therapy program should focus on restoring range of

Table 12.3 Pfirrmann classification scheme of subscapularis tears

Grade	
0	Normal tendon
1	Degeneration or tear less than a quarter of tendon diameter (craniocaudal)
2	Large tear greater than a quarter of tendon diameter (craniocaudal); not detached
3	Complete tendon detachment

Table 12.4 Goutallier fatty infiltration classification

Goutallier grade	
0	Normal muscle
1	Fatty streaking
2	More normal muscle than fatty infiltration
3	Equivalent muscle and fat
4	More fatty infiltration than normal muscle

Table 12.5 Lafosse classification scheme of subscapularis tears

Type	Lesion
I	Partial lesion of superior third ≤ grade 3
II	Complete lesion of superior third
III	Complete lesion of the superior two-thirds
IV	Complete lesion of tendon but head centered and fatty degeneration classified as ≤ grade 3
V	Complete lesion of tendon but eccentric head with coracoid impingement and fatty degeneration classified as ≥ grade 3

motion, strengthening the remaining rotator cuff and scapular stabilizers, and modalities as needed for pain control.

Surgical management

Open surgical technique

Regional anesthesia is administered in the form of an interscalene block before positioning in the operating room. The patient is then carefully placed into the beach-chair position after induction of general anesthesia and prepped in the standard fashion. A surgical approach is selected based on the characteristics of the tear, its chronicity, and associated involvement of the superior or posterosuperior cuff.

The deltopectoral approach and the superior deltoid-splitting approach have both been used to manage tears of the subscapularis. The advantages of the deltopectoral approach include preserving the deltoid muscle and excellent visualization of the torn subscapularis tendon. Significant scar and tendon retraction can make surgical dissection challenging. A deltopectoral approach allows for circumferential access to the subscapularis, permitting careful isolation of the tendon and muscle from neurovascular structures (Gerber and Krushell 1991; Gerber et al. 1996; Warner et al. 2001).

The superior deltoid-splitting approach allows the surgeon to address combined anterosuperior cuff tears, particularly if the subscapularis tear is small or limited to its cranial portion. This approach also allows for an acromioplasty to be performed. In large tears involving both the posterosuperior and the anterosuperior cuffs, a combined deltopectoral and superior deltoid-splitting approach may be necessary to adequately address all pathology (Warner et al. 2001).

Mobilization of the subscapularis proceeds with release of the coracohumeral ligament and capsular attachments. Freeing the subscapularis requires identification of the neurovascular structures, particularly the axillary nerve, and protecting them throughout the case. Fixation of the tendon back to the lesser tuberosity is performed with three to four transosseous holes and number 2 or number 3 non-absorbable, braided sutures (Gerber et al. 1996; Warner et al. 2001). Superior cuff lesions should be addressed before final fixation of the subscapularis tendon.

Lesions of the biceps tendon, including dislocation, fraying, or rupture, can be managed with relocation, tenotomy, or tenodesis. The authors prefer tenodesis because it definitively addresses biceps pathology and avoids postoperative spasm and cosmesis concerns. Edwards et al. (2005) reported an association between biceps tenodesis and tenotomy during open isolated subscapularis repair with improved subjective and objective outcomes.

The results of open repair of the subscapularis tendon tears exhibit a wide range of outcomes, primarily dependent on involvement of the superior or posterosuperior cuff, time to surgical intervention, and mechanism of injury. Initial reports of subscapularis repair noted good function postoperatively, but these studies only evaluated results subjectively and were limited to one or two patients (Biondi and Bear 1988; Collier and Wynn-Jones 1990).

In a series of 16 consecutive patients with isolated traumatic subscapularis tears, Gerber et al. (1996) reported a postoperative Constant score of 82%, adjusted for age and gender, at an average follow-up of 43 months (Constant and Murley 1987). Of 16 patients 12 had normal flexion and 3 had only a minor limitation characterized by a decrease of 15° or less (Gerber et al. 1996). With respect to the timing of surgery, the average Constant score was 88% for patients having surgery within 20 months of the injury, and only 59% for those having surgery after 36 months (Gerber et al. 1996).

Kreuz et al. (2005) compared total with partial isolated traumatic tears of subscapularis treated with an open approach. The nine patients with a total tear had a mean improvement in their Constant score from 38.7 to 89.3, compared with seven patients with a partial tear who had an improvement from 50.7 to 87.9. Furthermore, the final Constant score was found to be inversely proportional to the time between injury and surgery (Kreuz et al. 2005).

Edwards et al. (2005) reported on a large series of 84 isolated subscapularis repairs from either traumatic (57) or degenerative (27) causes. This group noted an increase in the mean Constant score from 55 to 79.5 with open surgical repair.

Isolated subscapularis tears are rare when compared with anterosuperior lesions. Timing is also important in this group of patients as demonstrated by Warner et al. (2001). In a series of 19 patients with anterosuperior cuff tears, patients treated within 6 months had a postoperative Constant score of 99%, compared with 44% in patients treated after 1 year. Overall, a 31% increase in age- and gender-adjusted Constant scores was noted after surgical fixation (Warner et al. 2001). Kreuz et al. (2005) compared isolated traumatic subscapularis tears with those also involving the supraspinatus in a series of 34 patients. Average Constant scores increased from 43.9 to 88.7 for patients with isolated tears and from 40.6 to 74.7 in patients with combined tears. The 14-point greater improvement in the Constant score for the isolated tear group was statistically significant.

Cases involving chronic tears with treatment delay may not be amenable to surgical repair due to significant retraction and scarring. In these patients, pectoralis major tendon transfer has been described to help restore function and relieve pain (Resch et al. 2000; Galatz et al. 2003). The surgical technique transfers a half to two-thirds of pectoralis major either anterior or posterior to the coracoid process. In a series of 12 patients with an average age of 65 and an average follow-up of 28 months, Resch et al. (2000) reported significant improvements in pain and an increase in the Constant score from 26.9% to 67.1% of normal. Of 12 patients 9 rated their outcome as excellent or good, whereas the other 3 noted a fair result (Resch et al. 2000).

Despite some variation in outcomes, patients with subscapularis tears, whether in isolation or combined with supraspinatus tears, can expect moderate improvement and satisfaction with surgical repair, especially if performed acutely. In addition, surgical fixation has been shown to help patients return to work and has demonstrated substantial cost savings (Gerber et al. 1996).

Arthroscopic technique

Although an open surgical approach was initially described for fixation of subscapularis tears, more recent studies have started to report on the outcomes of arthroscopic subscapularis fixation. We place the patient in a beach-chair position, which allows for visualization of the superior two-thirds of the subscapularis tendon compared with only 44% of the superior portion of the subscapularis tendon in the lateral decubitus position (Wright et al. 2001). Access to the anterior portion of the shoulder and the ability to manipulate the arm into varying degrees of rotation and flexion are also advantages of the beach-chair position (Lafosse et al. 2007).

Routine glenohumeral diagnostic arthroscopy is performed through a standard posterior portal. The subscapularis tendon can be visualized anteriorly. A 70° arthroscope is often useful at improving visualization over the top of the subscapularis. Another useful maneuver is for the surgical assistant to apply the "posterior lever push," in which the assistant pushes the proximal humerus posteriorly while pulling the distal humerus anteriorly, which opens the subcoracoid space and provides enough working area for the surgeon to diagnose and fix a subscapularis tendon tear (Adams et al. 2008).

Establishing proper portal placement is essential. First, the anterosuperior portal is established off the anterolateral tip of the acromion directed toward the lesser tuberosity. This portal is used for subscapularis mobilization and preparation of the bone bed (Burkhart and Brady 2006). The anterior portal is established next, just lateral to the coracoid and directed toward the joint. This portal is used for anchor placement and suture management.

The Lafosse classification helps guide treatment (Lafosse et al. 2007). Type I–III lesions can often be managed within the joint via arthroscopy. Type IV lesions require an extra-articular approach to successfully mobilize the subscapularis. Those with type V lesions are not candidates for subscapularis repair and should be managed with tendon transfer or arthroplasty (see **Table 12.5**).

Edwards et al. (2006a) reported on arthroscopic debridement of the subscapularis without repair in 11 patients with a mean age 64 years. Four tears involved the superior third, two the superior two-thirds, and five were complete tears. At a mean follow-up of 34 months, mean Constant score increased from 49 points preoperatively to 80 points postoperatively ($p < 0.00001$). Nine patients were satisfied or very satisfied.

Bennett (2003) reported results in eight patients with isolated subscapularis tears treated with arthroscopic repair with a 2-year minimum follow-up. The average postoperative Constant score was 74 patients.

Kim et al. (2005) reported on 29 patients with isolated partial articular surface tears of subscapularis. At a mean follow-up of 2.3 years, 18 reported excellent, 10 good, and 1 a fair result.

At a mean follow-up of 5 years, 80% (32 of 40) of patients had good or excellent results after an arthroscopic subscapularis repair in a study by Adams et al. (2008). In their study, they described the subscapularis tears by length from cephalad to caudad, resulting in a median of 50% of the total tendon length (range 20–100%) (Adams et al. 2008).

Ide et al. (2007) reported on 20 patients with a mean age of 62 years who underwent arthroscopic repair of anterosuperior rotator cuff tears. Five tears involved the superior third (grade 1) of the subscapularis tendon with three having moderate retraction; fifteen tears involved the superior two-thirds (grade 2) of the subscapularis tendon, with ten having severe retraction and five moderate retraction. There were no complete tears of the entire subscapularis insertion. The mean follow-up in this study was 3 years with 13 excellent, 5 good, 1 fair, and 1 poor result. The fair and poor results were in a grade 1 tear with moderate retraction and a grade 2 tear with severe retraction, respectively.

Lafosse et al. (2007) followed 17 patients for an average of 29 months who underwent arthroscopic subscapularis repair. Intraoperative classification included two type I, four type II, seven type III, four type IV, and no type V tears (see **Table 12.1**). Structural integrity of the repairs was intact in 15 of 17 patients, and partially re-ruptured in 2 based on CT arthrography. Subjectively, 12 patients were very satisfied with the result, 4 were satisfied, and 1 was not satisfied (Lafosse et al. 2007).

Postoperative care

Postoperative care is similar for open and arthroscopic approaches to subscapularis repair. Immediately postoperatively, the shoulder is immobilized in a brace or sling with the arm held in internal rotation. An individualized approach to physical therapy is needed based on the quality of the tendon, the extent and chronicity of the injury, associated rotator cuff tears, and the quality of the surgical repair. In general terms, however, pendulums are allowed during the first 1–2 weeks after surgery. Passive range of motion begins at 2 weeks with limits set based on post-repair tendon tension with intraoperative passive range of motion testing. Active-assisted and active range of motion begins at 6 weeks, usually with clinical evaluation at this time. Sling wear is also weaned at 6 weeks. Strengthening begins 3–4 months after surgery; lifting weights heavier than 20 pounds is not allowed until 6 months after surgery (Warner et al. 2001).

ADDITIONAL READING

Morag Y, Jamadar DA, Miller B, Dong Q, Jacobson JA. The subscapularis: Anatomy, injury, and imaging. Skeletal Radiol 2011;40:255–269.

Edwards TB, Walch G, Sirveaux F, et al. Repair of tears of the subscapularis. surgical technique. J Bone Joint Surg Am 2006;88(suppl 1 Pt 1):1–10.

Burkhart SS, Tehrany AM, Parten PM. Arthroscopic subscapularis repair. In: Imhoff AB, Ticker JB, Fu FH (eds), An Atlas of Shoulder Arthroscopy. London: Martin Dunitz, 2003: 327–334.

REFERENCES

Adams CR, Schoolfield JD, Burkhart SS. The results of arthroscopic subscapularis tendon repairs. Arthroscopy 2008;24:1381–1389.

Arai R, Sugaya H, Mochizuki T, Nimura A, Moriishi J, Akita K Subscapularis tendon tear: An anatomic and clinical investigation. Arthroscopy 2008;24:997–1004.

Barth JRH, Burkhart SS, De Beer JF. The bear-hug test: A new and sensitive test for diagnosing a subscapularis tear. Arthroscopy: J Arthroscop Rel Surg 2006;22:1076–1084.

Bartsch M, Greiner S, Haas NP, Scheibel M. Diagnostic values of clinical tests for subscapularis lesions. Knee Surg Sports Traumatol Arthrosc 2010;18:1712–1717.

Bennett WF. Subscapularis, medial, and lateral head coracohumeral ligament insertion anatomy: Arthroscopic appearance and the incidence of. Arthroscopy: J Arthroscop Rel Surg 2001;17:173–80.

Bennett WF. Arthroscopic repair of isolated subscapularis tears: A prospective cohort with 2- to 4-year follow-up. Arthroscopy 2003;19:131–143.

Biondi J, Bear TF. Isolated rupture of the subscapularis tendon in an arm wrestler. Orthopedics 1988;11:647–649.

Burkhart SS, Brady PC. Arthroscopic subscapularis repair: Surgical tips and pearls A to Z. Arthroscopy: J Arthroscop Rel Surg 2006;22:1014–1027.

Burkhart SS, Tehrany AM. Arthroscopic subscapularis tendon repair: Technique and preliminary results. Arthroscopy 2002;18:454–63.

Chao S, Thomas S, Yucha D, et al. An electromyographic assessment of the "bear hug": An examination for the evaluation of the subscapularis muscle. Arthroscopy 2008;24:1265–1270.

Charousset C, Bellaiche L, Duranthon LD, Grimberg J. Accuracy of CT arthrography in the assessment of tears of the rotator cuff. J Bone Joint Surg Br 2005;87:824–828.

Codman EA. The Shoulder. Boston, MA: Thomas Todd, 1934: 184.

Collier SG, Wynn-Jones CH. Displacement of the biceps with subscapularis avulsion. J Bone Joint Surg Br 1990;72:145.

Constant CR, Murley AH. A clinical method of functional assessment of the shoulder. Clin Orthop Relat Res 1987;214:160–164.

D'Addesi LL, Anbari A, Reish MW, Brahmabhatt S, Kelly JD. The subscapularis footprint: An anatomic study of the subscapularis tendon insertion. Arthroscopy: J Arthrosc Relat Surg 2006;22:937–940.

Deutsch A, Altchek DW, Veltri DM, Potter HG, Warren RF. Traumatic tears of the subscapularis tendon. clinical diagnosis, magnetic resonance imaging findings, and operative treatment. Am J Sports Med 1997;25:13–22.

Edwards TB, Walch G, Sirveaux F, et al. Repair of tears of the subscapularis. J Bone Joint Surg Am 2005;87:725–730.

Edwards TB, Walch G, Nove-Josserand L, et al. Arthroscopic debridement in the treatment of patients with isolated tears of the subscapularis. Arthroscopy 2006a;22:941–946.

Edwards TB, Walch G, Sirveaux F, et al. Repair of tears of the subscapularis. surgical technique. J Bone Joint Surg Am 2006b;88(suppl 1 Pt 1):1–10.

Ferrick MR. Coracoid impingement. A case report and review of the literature. Am J Sports Med 2000;28:117–119.

Flury MP, John M, Goldhahn J, Schwyzer HK, Simmen BR. Rupture of the subscapularis tendon (isolated or in combination with supraspinatus tear): When is a repair indicated? J Shoulder Elbow Surg 2006;15:659–664.

Galatz LM, Connor PM, Calfee RP, Hsu JC, Yamaguchi K. Pectoralis major transfer for anterior-superior subluxation in massive rotator cuff insufficiency. J Shoulder Elbow Surg 2003;12:1–5.

Gerber C, Krushell RJ. Isolated rupture of the tendon of the subscapularis muscle. clinical features in 16 cases. J Bone Joint Surg Br 1991;73:389–394.

Gerber C, Sebesta A. Impingement of the deep surface of the subscapularis tendon and the reflection pulley on the anterosuperior glenoid rim: A preliminary report. J Shoulder Elbow Surg 2000;9:483–490.

Gerber C, Hersche O, Farron A. Isolated rupture of the subscapularis tendon. J Bone Joint Surg Am 1996;78:1015–1023.

Goutallier D, Postel JM, Bernageau J, Lavau L, Voisin MC. Fatty muscle degeneration in cuff ruptures. pre- and postoperative evaluation by CT scan. Clin Orthop Relat Res 1994;304:78–83.

Haas SL. Fracture of the lesser tuberosity of the humerus. Am J Surg 1944;63:253–256.

Hauser ED. Avulsion of the tendon of the subscapularis muscle. J Bone Joint Surg Am 1954;36:139–141.

Iannotti JP, Ciccone J, Buss DD, et al. Accuracy of office-based ultrasonography of the shoulder for the diagnosis of rotator cuff tears. J Bone Joint Surg Am 2005;87:1305–1311.

Ide J, Tokiyoshi A, Hirose J, Mizuta H. Arthroscopic repair of traumatic combined rotator cuff tears involving the subscapularis tendon. J Bone Joint Surg Am 2007;89:2378–2388.

Kadaba MP, Cole A, Wootten ME, et al. Intramuscular wire electromyography of the subscapularis. J Orthop Res 1992;10:394–397.

Kasper JC, Itamura JM, Tibone JE, Levin SL, Stevanovic MV. Human cadaveric study of subscapularis muscle innervation and guidelines to prevent denervation. J Shoulder Elbow Surg 2008;17:659–662.

Kim SH, Oh I, Park JS, Shin SK, Jeong WK. Intra-articular repair of an isolated partial articular-surface tear of the subscapularis tendon. Am J Sports Med 2005;33:1825–1830.

Kim TK, Rauh PB, McFarland EG. Partial tears of the subscapularis tendon found during arthroscopic procedures on the shoulder: A statistical analysis of sixty cases. Am J Sports Med 2003;31:744–750.

Kreuz PC, Remiger A, Erggelet C, et al. Isolated and combined tears of the subscapularis tendon. Am J Sports Med 2005;33:1831–1837.

Lafosse L, Jost B, Reiland Y, et al. Structural integrity and clinical outcomes after arthroscopic repair of isolated subscapularis tears. J Bone Joint Surg Am 2007;89:1184.

Li XX, Schweitzer ME, Bifano JA, et al. MR evaluation of subscapularis tears. J Comput Assist Tomogr 1999;23:713–717.

Lo IK, Burkhart SS. The etiology and assessment of subscapularis tendon tears: A case for subcoracoid impingement, the roller-wringer effect, and TUFF lesions of the subscapularis. Arthroscopy 2003;19:1142–1150.

Morag Y, Jamadar DA, Miller B, Dong Q, Jacobson JA. The subscapularis: Anatomy, injury, and imaging. Skeletal Radiol 2011;40:255–269.

Neviaser RJ, Neviaser TJ. Recurrent instability of the shoulder after age 40. J Shoulder Elbow Surg 1995;4:416–418.

Nove-Josserand L, Boulahia A, Levigne C, Noel E, Walch G. Coraco-humeral space and rotator cuff tears. Rev Chir Orthop Reparatr Appar Mot 1999;85:677–683.

Patten RM. Tears of the anterior portion of the rotator cuff (the subscapularis tendon): MR imaging findings. AJR Am J Roentgenol 1994;162:351–354.

Pfirrmann CW, Zanetti M, Weishaupt D, Gerber C, Hodler J. Subscapularis tendon tears: Detection and grading at MR arthrography. Radiology 1999;213:709–714.

Resch H, Povacz P, Ritter E, Matschi W. Transfer of the pectoralis major muscle for the treatment of irreparable rupture of the subscapularis tendon. J Bone Joint Surg Am 2000;82:372.

Sakurai G, Ozaki J, Tomita Y, Kondo T, Tamai S. Incomplete tears of the subscapularis tendon associated with tears of the supraspinatus tendon: Cadaveric and clinical studies. J Shoulder Elbow Surg 1998;7:510–515.

Scheibel M, Magosch P, Pritsch M, Lichtenberg S, Habermeyer P. The belly-off sign: A new clinical diagnostic sign for subscapularis lesions. Arthroscopy 2005;21:1229–1235.

Studler U, Pfirrmann CW, Jost B, et al. Abnormalities of the lesser tuberosity on radiography and MRI: Association with subscapularis tendon lesions. AJR Am J Roentgenol 2008;191:100–106.

Symeonides PP. The significance of the subscapularis muscle in the pathogenesis of recurrent anterior dislocation of the shoulder. J Bone Joint Surg Br 1972;54:476–483.

Teefey SA, Rubin DA, Middleton WD, et al. Detection and quantification of rotator cuff tears. comparison of ultrasonographic, magnetic resonance imaging, and arthroscopic findings in seventy-one consecutive cases. J Bone Joint Surg Am 2004;86:708.

Tokish JM, Decker MJ, Ellis HB, Torry MR, Hawkins RJ. The belly-press test for the physical examination of the subscapularis muscle: Electromyographic validation and comparison to the lift-off test. J Shoulder Elbow Surg 2003;12:427–430.

Uno A, Bain GI, Mehta JA. Arthroscopic relationship of the axillary nerve to the shoulder joint capsule: An anatomic study. J Shoulder Elbow Surg 1999;8:226–230.

Walch G, Nove-Josserand L, Boileau P, Levigne C. Subluxations and dislocations of the tendon of the long head of the biceps. J Shoulder Elbow Surg 1998;7:100–108.

Ward SR, Hentzen ER, Smallwood LH, et al. Rotator cuff muscle architecture: Implications for glenohumeral stability. Clin Orthop Relat Res 2006;448:157–163.

Warner JJ, Higgins L, Parsons IM, 4th, Dowdy P. Diagnosis and treatment of anterosuperior rotator cuff tears. J Shoulder Elbow Surg 2001;10:37–46.

Weishaupt D, Zanetti M, Tanner A, Gerber C, Hodler J. Lesions of the reflection pulley of the long biceps tendon. MR arthrographic findings. Invest Radiol 1999;34:463–469.

Wright JM, Heavrin B, Hawkins RJ, Noonan T. Arthroscopic visualization of the subscapularis tendon. Arthroscopy 2001;17:677–684.

Yoo JC, Ahn JH, Lee SH, Kim JH. Arthroscopic full-layer repair of bursal-side partial-thickness rotator cuff tears: A small-window technique. Arthroscopy 2007;23:903.e1, 903.e4.

Yung SW, Lazarus MD, Harryman DT, 2nd. Practical guidelines to safe surgery about the subscapularis. J Shoulder Elbow Surg 1996;5:467–470.

Chapter 13 Rotator cuff arthropathy and glenohumeral arthritis: prevention and treatment

Andrea Grasso, Matteo Salvatore, Gianluca Falcone

KEY FEATURES

- Rotator cuff arthropathy is a painful, degenerative condition characterized by degeneration of articular cartilage and a massive rotator cuff tear.
- The association between massive tears of rotator cuff tendons and severe glenohumeral degenerative arthritis is complex and still poorly understood.
- In massive rotator cuff tears, unbalanced muscle forces can lead to anteroposterior instability of the humeral head, tearing of the long head of biceps, and gradual degeneration of the glenohumeral joint.
- Non-surgical measures are the first line in management, and are often a good option in low-demand and less symptomatic patients.
- Arthroscopic joint debridement, although not curative, remains a surgical option and may improve pain and motion in patients with longstanding symptoms.
- Newer shoulder joint resurfacing and replacement procedures can result in improved clinical results.

INTRODUCTION

Shoulder arthropathy is a painful condition characterized by damage and degeneration of the articular cartilage and is usually associated with a massive irreparable rotator cuff tear. The condition is most commonly detected in elderly people. With the increases in life expectancy, rotator cuff arthropathy has become more prevalent in the general population.

Adams (1857) provided the earliest description of the anatomical and pathological features of rotator cuff tear arthropathy. Adams described two types of chronic rheumatoid arthritis: a generalized form resembling rheumatoid arthritis and a localized form involving the shoulder, which had the morphological characteristics of what is now known as rotator cuff tear arthropathy.

In 1934 Codman reported on a 51-year-old woman who had what he named a subacromial space hygroma. He described recurrent swelling of the shoulder, absence of the rotator cuff, cartilaginous bodies attached to the synovial tissue, and severe destructive glenohumeral arthritis. These descriptions of what is now known as rotator cuff tear arthropathy were made without the benefit of modern diagnostic tests, such as serological analysis or synovial crystal analysis.

"L'epaule senile hemorragique" (the hemorrhagic shoulder of elderly people) was described by De Seze et al. in 1968. This condition was seen in three elderly women who did not have a history of trauma, and consisted of recurrent blood swelling of the shoulder, and radiographic findings of severe degenerative glenohumeral arthritis and a chronic tear of the rotator cuff.

The term "Milwaukee shoulder" was introduced in 1981 by Halverson et al. to describe the condition in four elderly women who had recurrent bilateral shoulder effusions, severe radiographic destructive changes of the glenohumeral joints, and massive tears of the rotator cuff.

In 1982, spontaneous large glenohumeral effusions, mild pain, and tears of the rotator cuff were reported by Massias et al. (1982) in six elderly women, and the condition was described as "l'arthropathie destructrice rapide de l'epaule" (rapid destructive arthritis of the shoulder).

Neer et al., in 1983, introduced for the first time the term "rotator cuff arthropathy," describing severe disorganization of the glenohumeral joint with collapse of the humeral head occurring after massive tears of the rotator cuff. Neer hypothesized that the massive tear allows superior displacement of the humerus into the subacromial space with "femoralization" of the humeral head (erosion of the greater tuberosity) and "acetabularization" of the coracoacromial arch, a deformity that allows the humeral head to be stable in a socket (Parsons et al. 2004).

PHYSIOLOGY

Normal function of the shoulder is guaranteed by four characteristics: motion, stability, muscular strength, and articular cartilage integrity (smoothness). If for any reason one of the components fails, arthritis can develop.

Motion

The shoulder is the most mobile joint of the human body. Its anatomy confers this peculiarity. In this, capsular laxity is the major factor influencing motion. The capsule remains lax for most of the range of motion, becoming tight during the extreme degrees of motion. If, for a pathological process or trauma, the capsule stiffens up, movement will be restricted.

As an example, posterior translation occurs during end extension and external rotation. If there is a capsular contracture, this movement can start prematurely causing forced humeral head translation with eccentric loading and loss of concentric rotation, producing articular cartilage shear that, with time, can produce arthritis (Harryman et al. 1992).

Stability

The shoulder joint is an intrinsically unstable articulation. Different factors act to contrast this instability. First is the orientation of the articular surfaces. The humeral head is oriented with 30° retroversion and 130° head-shaft angle. If these angles are modified, instability can ensue.

On the other hand, the glenoid is retroverted. In arthritis, posterior glenoid wear is predominant, increasing retroversion and posterior instability. The articular surface of the humeral head is larger than the glenoid, allowing a wide range of motion (ROM). In the arthritic glenohumeral joint, stability can be compromised by a reduced amount of available humeral articular surface. The other important factors include glenoid concavity and the possible effective arcs. The arc is defined by the maximal angle of motion possible before dislocation occurs. With asymmetric glenoid rim wear, less effective arcs are possible.

The arc of the glenoid determines the maximum angles that the net humeral joint reaction force can make with the glenoid centerline before dislocation occurs. In an arthritic joint, the effective glenoid arc can be diminished by wear or inflammation, e.g., posterior wear is typical of glenohumeral osteoarthritis and capsulorrhaphy arthropathy, whereas central erosion of the glenoid is typical of rheumatoid arthritis. Finally, the joint reaction force is the sum of the multiple forces produced by muscle groups that condition the direction of the resulting force. If there is a rupture or weakness of one muscle group, this produces eccentric loading and accelerates wear (Matsen et al. 2006).

Strength

Strength is related to stability. Deltoid and rotator cuff integrity and strength are important for normal movement. If the muscles are contracted, they will reduce arm excursion.

The requisites of strength include:

- a functional deltoid
- a functional rotator cuff
- normal length relationships of muscle origin and insertions.

If the rotator cuff is deficient, progressive degeneration of the articular cartilage occurs (Brems 1994).

Articular cartilage integrity (smoothness)

Normal articular glide is required for the shoulder to reach the entire effective arc of motion. Synovial fluid provides a thin layer of lubrication between the articular surfaces. The relatively smooth articular surface, combined with the synovial fluid, allows smooth, fluid motion with very little resistance. However, if the surfaces become rough, as with loss of articular cartilage, the coefficient of friction and relative resistance between two gliding objects greatly increase. In addition, with increased resistance, the amount of wear increases tremendously.

The anatomical requisites of smooth motion are as follows.

Smooth joint surfaces

In the normal shoulder, the intact articular cartilage covering the humeral head and the glenoid lubricated with normal joint fluid provide the lowest possible resistance to motion at the joint surface. In arthritis, these factors are compromised.

Smoothness of the humeroscapular motion interface

In a physiological situation, the subacromial bursa guarantees a gliding interface between the humeral head and the acromion. This allows the proximal humerus and rotator cuff to slide smoothly beneath deltoid, the acromion, coracoacromial ligament, the coracoid, and coracoid muscles. Smoothness of the humeroscapular motion interface is often compromised in rotator cuff arthropathy. The result is wear and accelerated articular cartilage damage (Matsen 2009).

PATHOGENESIS

The glenohumeral joint has more motion than any other joints, made possible by the unusual arrangement of the shallow glenoid and rotator cuff. The rotator cuff provides a closed joint space, moves the glenohumeral joint, and stabilizes the humeral head against proximal displacement, and anterior and posterior subluxations and dislocations.

The association between massive tears of rotator cuff tendons and severe glenohumeral degenerative arthritis is complex and still poorly understood. Its exact etiology is unknown, and several hypotheses have been put forward. A major source of confusion is the fact that different authors have described its clinical characteristics in general terms, and have given it various names.

Crystal-mediated theory

The association between rotator cuff tear arthropathy and the intra-articular presence of basic calcium phosphate crystals has been identified (Visotsky et al. 2004; Ecklund et al. 2007). These reports on the Milwaukee shoulder included clinical aspects and studies of synovial fluid as well as morphological and biochemical studies of excised synovial tissue from four patients, three of whom had bilateral disease. McCarty et al. (1981) identified collagenolytic and neutral protease activity in the synovial fluid, measuring the release of soluble enzymatic products. Electron microscopic analysis of synovial tissue from the glenohumeral joints of patients with rotator cuff tear arthropathy showed microspheroids of basic calcium phosphate crystals, suggesting phagocytosis of these crystals by synovial cells. Histology showed foci of calcific deposits in the synovial microvilli and the subsynovial layers.

The hypothesis proposed that an explanation of the Milwaukee shoulder starts with the concept that a hydroxyapatite mineral phase develops in the altered capsule, synovial tissue, or degenerative articular cartilage and releases basic calcium phosphate crystals into the synovial fluid. These crystals are then phagocytosed by synovial cells, forming calcium phosphate crystal microspheroids, which induce the release of activated enzymes from these cells, causing destruction of the periarticular tissues and articular surfaces.

Basic calcium phosphate crystal is a generic term used to identify a crystal composed of carbonate-substituted hydroxyapatite, octacalcium phosphate, or, more rarely, tricalcium phosphate. These crystals are not birefringent, so polarized light microscopy is not useful for their identification. Furthermore, the resolution power of light microscopy is inadequate to detect the individual crystals, which are needle shaped and <0.1 nm long. Both scanning and transmission electron microscopy with energy-dispersive X-ray microanalysis have been used to identify basic calcium phosphate crystals in synovial fluid pellets.

Unfortunately, there is no simple, cost-effective, readily available method to detect basic calcium phosphate crystals that is comparable with the use of polarized light microscopy for the detection of calcium pyrophosphate dihydrate and monosodium urate monohydrate crystals. Aggregates of basic calcium phosphate crystals have been found in the synovial fluid of joints undergoing acute attacks of mixed crystal deposition disease, calcific periarthritis, or acute arthritis. These aggregates have also been identified in the synovial fluid of patients who have erosive polyarticular disease, osteoarthritis of the knee, and rotator cuff tear arthropathy. The response of synovial tissue to calcium-containing crystals, such as basic calcium phosphate and calcium pyrophosphate dihydrate crystals is low-grade inflammation with cellular proliferation.

The cellular hyperplasia observed in the synovial tissue of patients who have rotator cuff tear arthropathy may be explained by the mitogenic properties of basic calcium phosphate crystals, which stimulate proliferation of human foreskin fibroblasts. Synovial fibroblasts and chondrocytes, in response to certain growth factors, cytokines, and other chemical agents, synthesize the enzymes collagenase and stromelysin (Dieppe et al. 1988). Collagenase is a proteolytic enzyme that degrades interstitial collagen and stromelysin, a metalloprotease, degrades connective tissue components and activates procollagenase. As already noted, McCarty et al. (1981) initially identified collagenase activity in the synovial fluid from patients with rotator cuff tear arthropathy. However, this finding was not confirmed in subsequent reports.

Halverson et al. (1981) suggested that this inconsistency may arise from the presence of a low-molecular-weight inhibitor of collagenase, the avid binding of collagenase to collagen, or an artifact resulting from poor handling of specimens in preparation for the enzyme assays. Recent investigations have focused on identifying the induction of collagenase or stromelysin gene transcription by basic calcium phosphate crystals to elucidate the loss of collagenous structures in patients who have rotator cuff tear arthropathy. Basic calcium phosphate crystals stimulate the proliferation of cultured adult porcine articular chondrocytes and increase collagenase messenger RNA (mRNA) in a dose-responsive manner. Human fibroblasts have been induced by basic calcium phosphate crystals to accumulate collagenase as well as stromelysin mRNA and to secrete collagenase, stromelysin, and 92-kDa gelatinase. Basic calcium phosphate crystals induce the synthesis of proteolytic enzymes responsible for the degradation of cartilage–matrix components.

The aggregates of hydroxyapatite crystals observed throughout articular cartilage, but most commonly in the midzone, may also directly cause mechanical wear of cartilage. Using cadaveric knee joints, Clift et al. (1989) found that a higher deposition of basic calcium phosphate crystals and an increase in the mean friction coefficient occurred together with severe fibrillation of articular cartilage.

An in vitro investigation also suggested that crystals in the synovial fluid may cause wear of the articular cartilage (Hayes et al. 1992). As the presence of crystals increased, the concentration of wear debris and the size and shape of the crystals influenced the type of articular damage observed.

The large crystal aggregates, frequently found in the midzone of the articular cartilage, were studied using a linear elastic finite element model under short-term loading conditions. These aggregates increase the shear stress and strain concentrations in the surrounding cartilage. The exact origin of basic calcium phosphate crystals remains unclear, and whether these crystals are the cause or the result of arthritis remains unanswered. It has been suggested that basic calcium phosphate crystals are an epiphenomenon resulting from biochemical changes in the matrix of the damaged cartilage, and that the crystals are then shed into the synovial fluid.

Peach et al. (2007) explored the possibility that some people may have a genetic predisposition to developing arthritis if experiencing a chronic rotator cuff tear. They studied variation in the genes *ANKH* and *TNAP* which are involved in pyrophosphate metabolism and can influence the levels of extracellular calcium crystal formation. Comparing the levels of genetic variation in *ANKH* and *TNAP* in individuals with and without cuff tear arthropathy, they found significantly higher levels of variant genotypes for *ANKH* and *TNAP* in affected individuals compared with healthy controls. Transfection of variants of *ANKH* into human chondrocytes resulted in altered pyrophosphate metabolism. These results support the hypothesis that genetic variation in *ANKH* and *TNAP* may lead to calcium crystal formation, which could predispose a patient to developing arthritis after a chronic rotator cuff tear.

In periarthropathies such as calcific rotator tendinopathy or degenerative tears of the rotator tendon, basic calcium phosphate crystals are known to form. Additional investigations are required to elucidate the origin of the basic calcium phosphate crystals and the effect that they elicit in individuals who have degenerative disease of the shoulder (Brett 2008).

Rotator cuff arthropathy theory

In addition to the pathological changes seen in the tendon and muscle after a rotator cuff tear, the glenohumeral joint can also undergo degenerative changes after chronic massive rotator cuff tear. It is uncertain why some patients with chronic rotator cuff tears develop severe, debilitating osteoarthritis, whereas others show few degenerative changes in the glenohumeral joint.

A massive tear of the rotator cuff exposes a large portion of the articular cartilage of the humeral head, impairs normal movement of the glenohumeral joint, and makes the humeral head unstable.

Nutritional factors imposed by the massive tear induce loss of a closed joint space and impaired movement of the glenohumeral joint. The loss of a closed joint space, with leaking synovial fluid under reduced pressure, would be expected to alter the perfusion of nutrients into the articular cartilage.

Joint inactivity leads to structural alterations of the articular cartilage and changes in water and glycosaminoglycan content of the cartilage and capsule. Both the loss of a closed joint space and inactivity contribute to the atrophy of the articular cartilage of the humeral head. Inactivity also causes disuse osteoporosis of the subchondral bone, with its eventual collapse.

Only after collapse of the subchondral bone of the head should the term "rotator cuff tear arthropathy" be used (Neer et al. 1983).

The mechanical factors contributing to rotator cuff tear arthropathy include gross instability of the humeral head on the glenoid and upward migration of the head against the acromion and acromioclavicular joint. Loss of the stabilizing functions of the long head of biceps after its tear, or subluxation and tear of the rotator cuff, contribute to these two types of instability. Anterior and posterior subluxations and dislocations produce abnormal trauma and injury to the articular surfaces of the humeral head and glenoid. Eventually, the incongruous head may erode through the glenoid into the coracoid process. The upward instability and upward migration of the head escalate the previously described process of subacromial impingement. Impingement wear erodes the anterior part of the acromion, acromioclavicular joint, and outer aspect of the clavicle.

Instability of the head seems to be essential for the development of its collapse. Although frozen shoulders and immobilized joints also have been described as showing biochemical changes and alterations in the articular cartilage, which is also possible with disuse osteoporosis of the subchondral bone, collapse of the humeral head in frozen shoulder is at best rare. Presumably, this is because the rotator cuff is intact and the instability that produces the abnormal trauma necessary for the collapse of the head is absent.

It is impossible to estimate accurately the number of shoulders with a rotator cuff tear that proceed to rotator cuff tear arthropathy, because several cadaveric studies have documented age-related prevalence of rotator cuff tears. Those studies did not show a relationship between the presence or size of the rotator cuff tear and symptoms or prevalence of associated glenohumeral arthritis. Neer et al. (1983) estimated, on the basis of his observation of approximately 52 cases of cuff tear arthropathy over 8 years, that cuff tear arthropathy would develop in only 4% of patients who have a complete tear of the rotator cuff and suggested that, because of their small size, most tears of the cuff do not lead to arthropathy.

Several authors have performed longitudinal follow-up studies of patients who had a massive rotator cuff tear, with different results. Hamada et al. (1990) reported the long-term radiographic results of non-surgical management of 22 patients with arthrographically proved massive rotator cuff tears. In five of the seven shoulders followed for more than 8 years, degenerative changes had progressed radiographically. Those authors concluded that a massive tear of the cuff would progress to cuff tear arthropathy with progressive radiographic changes.

In 1993, Bokor et al. reported that the functional results of non-surgical treatment of arthrographically documented rotator cuff tears did not deteriorate after an average follow-up period of 7–8 years. However, objective data, such as the size of the tear and the radiographic appearance of the shoulder, were not included, and only one patient developed symptoms of rotator cuff tear arthropathy.

Arthroscopic subacromial decompression without debridement of the tendon has also been performed to manage full-thickness rotator cuff tears; however, reports on that procedure described only short-term results, and lacked radiographic follow-up. In a retrospective study of 25 patients who had had arthroscopic acromioplasty and debridement of a tear of the rotator cuff with 6–9 years of follow-up, 7 exhibited clinical and radiographic features of rotator cuff tear arthropathy. The tears in that series were classified according to size, and the integrity of the subscapularis tendon was not specifically reported.

Open and arthroscopic debridement of massive tears of the rotator cuff combined with acromioplasty has been reported in patients who did not have glenohumeral arthritis. Those studies provided more objective data about the size of the tear and the clinical outcome. Augereau and Apoil (1988) reported that rotator cuff tear arthropathy developed in more than 25% of 56 patients 10 years after open debridement of a degenerative lesion of the rotator cuff. Matsen (2009) reported that none of 53 shoulders with a chronic, massive, irreparable tear of the supraspinatus and infraspinatus tendons had progressive deterioration of the glenohumeral joint after open acromioplasty and debridement of the rotator cuff. These patients were followed for an average of 6.5 years, and shoulders followed for less than 5 years were compared with those followed for at least 5 years. Neither deterioration in the functional results nor the appearance of radiographic degenerative changes could be associated with time.

Force couple theory

The effect of a tear of the rotator cuff on the biomechanics of the shoulder has been investigated in radiographic and biomechanical studies. Inman et al. (1996) used the concept of force couples to develop a theoretical model that determined the force requirements necessary for function of the shoulder joint. The force couple in the coronal plane consisted of the superiorly directed force vector of deltoid and the inferiorly directed force vector of the short external rotators of the rotator cuff. Rotation or abduction of the shoulder joint occurred as the two oppositely directed forces acted on opposite sides of the center of rotation. A weak or detached supraspinatus tendon would be unable to maintain centering of the humeral head on the glenoid, and a superiorly directed force vector would result from the unbalanced force couple.

This force couplet concept was supported by a radiographic study comparing patients who had an arthrographically proven tear of supraspinatus with those who had a normal shoulder. Inman et al. (1996) concluded that some patients with a rotator cuff tear have superior translation of the humeral head on the glenoid as a result of the loss of the normal depressing effect of supraspinatus.

Free body analysis of the glenohumeral joint has shown that the resultant force vector is directed superiorly during the first 60° of shoulder elevation, and it also has been used to explain superior migration of the humeral head in association with a tear of the rotator cuff. Although these investigators provided insight into glenohumeral biomechanics, they disregarded the contributions of the other rotator cuff muscles in maintaining joint stability.

The presence and importance of the transverse-plane force couple, in which the anterior aspect of the cuff (subscapularis) is balanced against the posterior aspect (infraspinatus and teres minor), were first shown in an electromyographic study. In a subsequent study, fluoroscopic examination of patients who had a massive tear of the rotator cuff revealed varying degrees of glenohumeral instability which corresponded directly to the degree of involvement of the posterior portion of the rotator cuff and the subscapularis tendon.

A suspension bridge model of the shoulder, in which the leading edge of the detached rotator cuff tendon behaves biomechanically like the cable of a suspension bridge, was used to explain the non-progressive nature of some rotator cuff tears. The tension that develops on the edge of the supraspinatus tendon during the contraction of the torn rotator cuff muscle was theorized to propagate along the cable of the bridge to its point of attachment on the greater tuberosity. This allows some patients who have a large or massive tear to maintain the transverse force couple and thus to retain the ability to actively elevate the shoulder. The location of the cable (tendon) attachments on the tuberosities results in either stable or unstable glenohumeral kinematics, depending on the presence of an intact transverse force couple. This principle has been supported clinically.

Biomechanical studies to investigate the effect of a rotator cuff tear on the performance of the glenohumeral joint have been performed in cadavers. A dynamic shoulder-testing apparatus with preserved transverse force couples was used to investigate the effect of a torn supraspinatus tendon. Full abduction was possible, and the glenohumeral kinematics were not markedly altered. In another study with use of this testing apparatus, it was found that, if the transverse force couple remained functionally intact, there was sufficient compressive force to maintain concentric reduction of the humeral head and the ball-and-socket kinematics. No association was found between the size of the rotator cuff tear and the geometry of the humeral head, disproving the concept that there is a critical ratio between the two. The information from these cadaveric studies is limited, however, as assessment of scapulothoracic motion was not included, and the artificial environment does not take into account the attritional, degenerative changes that occur in the rotator cuff tendons.

Rotator cuff tear arthropathy is a clinical manifestation of instability of the glenohumeral joint and loss of articular cartilage. On the basis of the existing clinical and biomechanical data, it is apparent that, if the remaining balance of the rotator cuff in the coronal and transverse planes is sufficient to maintain glenohumeral stability, the presence of a rotator cuff tear or degenerative defect may not alter the biomechanics of the glenohumeral joint. If stability cannot be maintained and repetitive abnormal excursions of the humeral head occur on the glenoid, in both the transverse and the coronal planes, then wear and loss of the glenohumeral cartilage will result. The combination of glenohumeral instability resulting from loss of the primary and secondary stabilizers and loss of normal articular cartilage results in the production of basic calcium phosphate crystals. These crystal aggregates, which may originate from damage to the articular cartilage or from degenerative changes in the rotator cuff tendons, accelerate additional degenerative changes through the induction of enzymatic activity.

CLINICAL FINDINGS AND EVALUATION

History

Rotator cuff tear arthropathy is a clinical manifestation of instability of the glenohumeral joint and loss of articular cartilage resulting from insufficiency of the rotator cuff. It represents only one of the forms of arthritis that can involve the shoulder: any other type of shoulder arthritis should be analyzed and excluded in the decision-making.

On the basis of the existing clinical and biomechanical data, it is apparent that, if the remaining balance of the rotator cuff in the coronal and transverse planes is sufficient to maintain glenohumeral stability, the presence of a rotator cuff tear or degenerative defect may not alter the biomechanics of the glenohumeral joint. If, however, stability cannot be maintained, and repetitive abnormal excursions of the humeral head occur on the glenoid, in both the transverse and the coronal planes, then wear and loss of the glenohumeral cartilage will result. This pathology is more common in women than in men. Patients typically are elderly women with shoulder symptoms of long duration. The dominant side is most commonly affected. However, bilateral involvement is seen in approximately 60% of patients.

Pain and loss of function are the main symptoms for patients with symptomatic glenohumeral arthritis secondary to rotator cuff disease. It is helpful to describe the onset of the problem, if started with an injury and the amount of discomfort in the activity of daily living (ADL). Systemic or polyarticular manifestations of sepsis, degenerative joint disease, or rheumatoid arthritis can provide helpful clues. A past history of steroid medication, fracture, or working at depths might suggest the diagnosis of avascular necrosis. Past injury or surgery suggests the possibility of secondary arthritis or capsulorrhaphy arthropathy. Usually, the patient does not recognize a major trauma as the onset of the problem but, more often, the pain is the main symptom, increasing over time. Finally, a loss of shoulder function, not compatible with the normal ADL, is the reason why the patient consults a physician.

Physical examination

Early clinical findings in the patient with rotator cuff arthropathy include decreased ROM, crepitus, and muscle wasting about the shoulder. The active and passive ROMs can be severely limited and should be assessed. The amount of capsular contracture determines the limitation in passive ROM. Specific motion planes correspond to areas of the capsule. Internal rotation with the arm at 90° abduction tightens the posteroinferior capsule, whereas external rotation with the arm at the side tightens the anterosuperior capsule.

Limitation in active ROM arises from insufficiency of the rotator cuff. Often there is coexistent atrophy of supraspinatus and infraspinatus (**Figs 13.1a and b**). The isometric strength in every direction of movement should be tested knowing that, in patients with advanced rotator cuff arthropathy, it is not always possible. The loss of strength in external

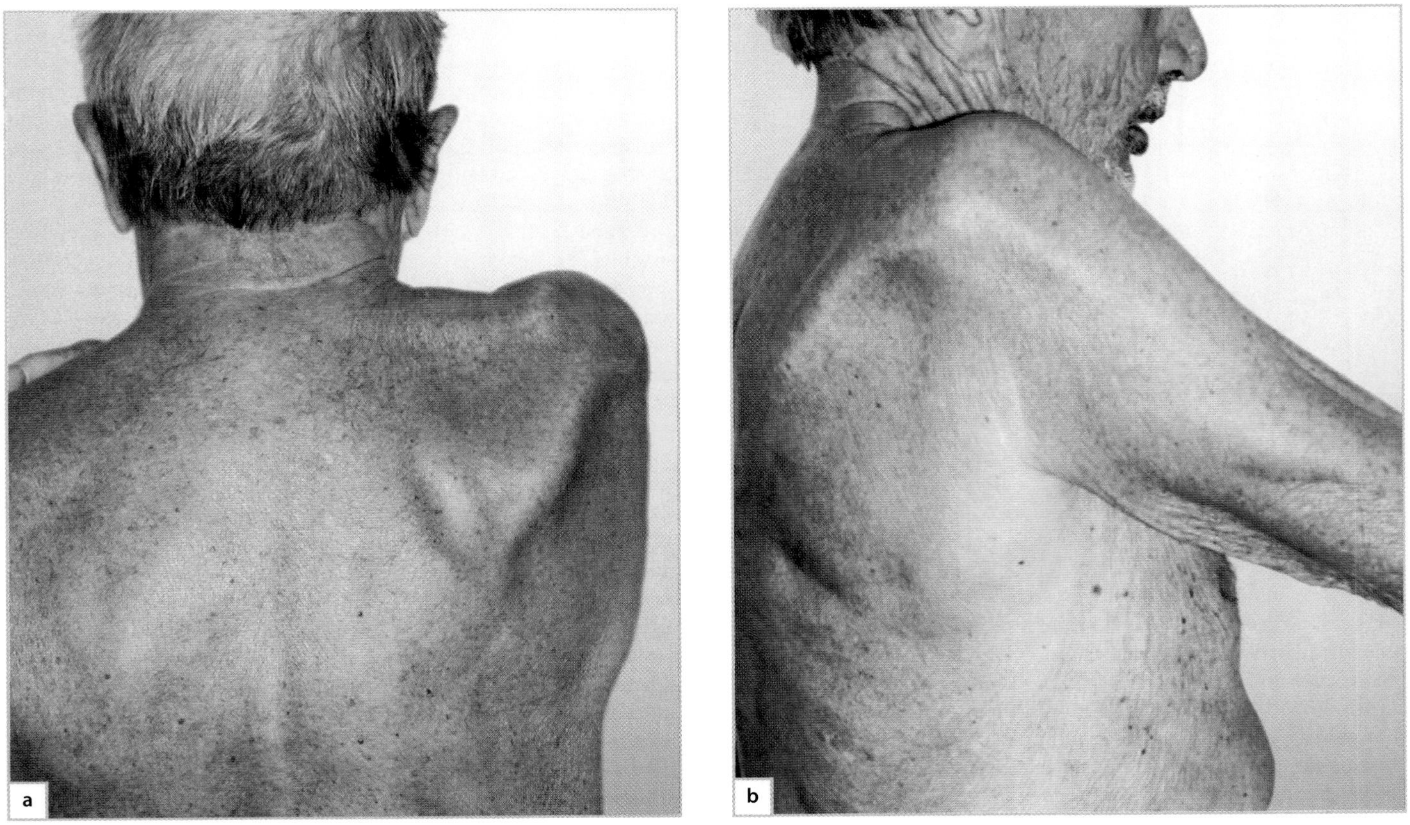

Figure 13.1 Rotator cuff arthropathy. (a) Atrophy of supraspinatus and (b) infraspinatus with severe limitation in active forward flexion.

rotation with the arm at the side and at 90° abduction (both with elbow flexed at 90°) indicates the deficiency of the superior and posterosuperior part of the cuff, and is usually indicative of the pathology.

Physical examination should assess the ability of the arch to contain the humerus during shoulder elevation. Posterior or anterosuperior migration, depending on the integrity of subscapularis, should be assessed by observation. Crepitation during passive ROM should suggest the presence of severe degenerative changes including cartilage disruption, exposure of subchondral bone, and loose bodies. Hygroma, ecchymosis, and recurrent blood-tinged effusions are the main symptoms present in the very late phase (**Fig. 13.2**). Any other medical condition that might affect the outcome should be identified before the surgery.

Radiographic evaluation

Early radiographic changes consist of a high-riding humeral head from rotator cuff tear, with mild subchondral bone sclerosis and narrowing of the glenohumeral joint space, but with few or no osteophytes. These changes may stabilize or show minimal cartilage erosions for several years, followed by sudden deterioration in a dramatic fashion. Occasionally, in severely affected shoulders, erosive changes are seen in both the glenohumeral joint and adjacent structures such as the base of the coracoid process, lateral end of the clavicle, and anterior aspect of the acromion.

These radiographs demonstrate narrowing of the space between the glenoid and the humerus, the position of the humerus with respect to the acromion, the presence of inferior osteophytes, the bone stock quality, and the shape and thickness of the humeral cortex.

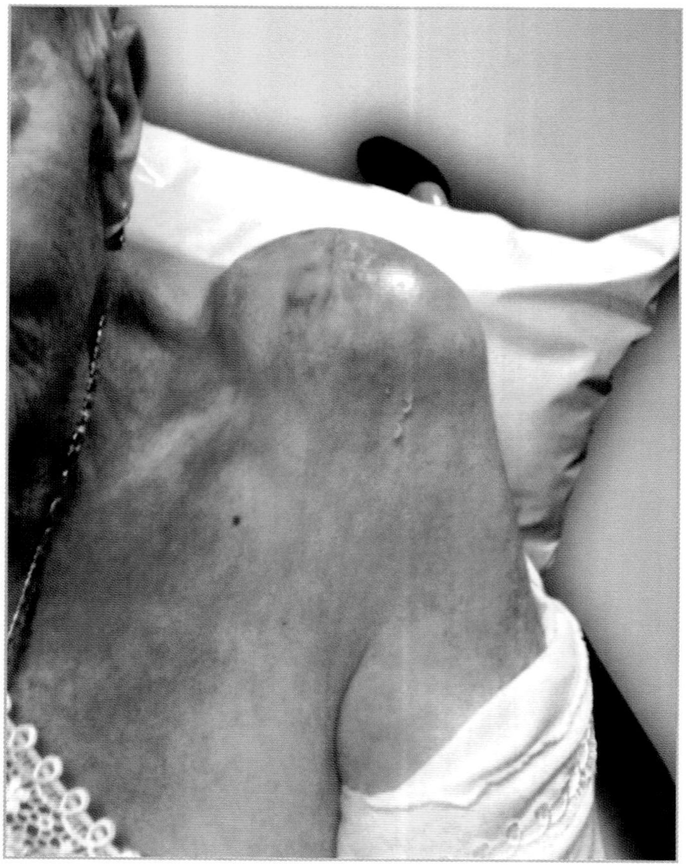

Figure 13.2 Hygroma of a shoulder with rotator cuff arthropathy.

A true anteroposterior (AP) view and an axillary view are standard studies (**Figs 13.3a** to **c**). The AP view places the humeral neck in maximal profile and centers the humerus in the glenoid fossa. This view shows the thickness of the cartilage space, the degree of deformity of the humeral articular surface, and superior humeral migration. The axillary lateral view is crucial for assessing glenoid erosion, abnormal glenoid version, and humeral subluxation. Other features that should be noted include the presence and location of osteophytes, the degree of osteopenia, the degree of medial glenoid erosion, and the presence of cyst-like changes around the tuberosities, which may indicate a chronic rotator cuff tear.

Additional views may be helpful. The AP view at 35° external rotation is particularly useful for those shoulders that need prosthetic replacement. Using this view, it is possible to decide the size of the humeral stem, measuring it with specific templates. The radiographs should be performed with a magnification marker to assure a realistic comparison between the anatomy of that region and the templates.

Three radiographic classifications have been developed to define the bone changes that occur in these shoulder conditions; each focuses on a different set of findings associated with these disorders. The Seebauer classification targets superior migration of the humeral head and its containment within the coracoacromial (CA) arch (Visotsky et al. 2004). The Hamada classification system characterizes the structural changes associated within the CA arch (Hamada et al. 1990). The Favard classification focuses on bone loss of the glenoid (Sirveaux et al. 2004). Iannotti et al. (2010) concluded that, of these three, the Seebauer classification of cuff tear arthropathy best defines the role of the CA arch in the stability of the humeral head in the setting of a massive rotator cuff tear (**Table 13.1**). These radiographic findings, when combined with the clinical examination for active elevation and superior instability of the humeral head, were the most important factors in recommending hemiarthroplasty or reverse total shoulder arthroplasty for rotator cuff tear arthropathy (Iannotti et al. 2010).

Figure 13.3 shows the method used to measure the distance, on AP views, between the center of the glenoid, humerus, and CA arch. Some authors studied the diameter of the humeral stem in a cadaveric computed tomography (CT) model, and concluded that the lateral view seems more predictable than AP views for sizing the humeral stems. On the AP view, the canal seems bigger than in the lateral one (Lee et al. 2008). To perform an AP view correctly, the arm should be placed at 45° abduction. In this position, the central part of the glenoid fossa is in contact with the same part of the articular surface of the humeral head, revealing earlier cartilage narrowing and degenerative condition of the peripheral part of the humeral head than in any other position. Glenoid wear may also occur medially, as evidenced by destruction of the coracoid process, which is best seen on axillary radiographs.

When surgical reconstruction is needed, CT may be a valuable imaging adjunct, especially in cases with poor bone stock quality. CT may be particularly useful to assess cavitary bone defects or to measure glenoid version (Hernigou et al. 2002).

Many authors have studied groups of patients to define the standard range of glenoid version, and concluded that the glenoid is oriented through a range of 30°. They also try to identify the best method to analyze the version. Studies that assess the CT scan seem to be the only reproducible method of assessing the glenoid orientation. The

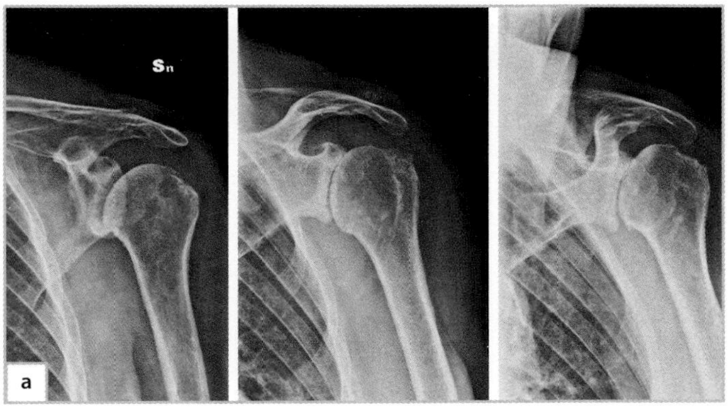

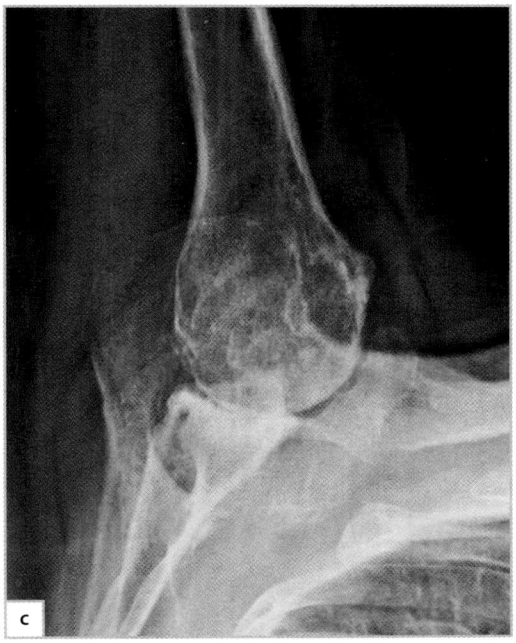

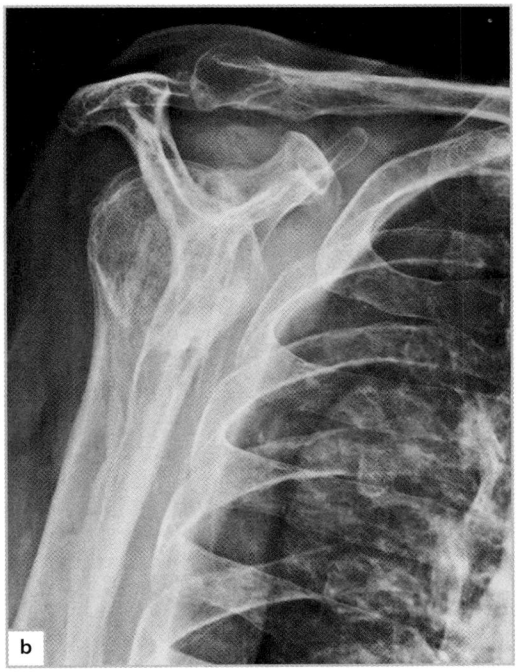

Figure 13.3 Radiographic evaluation of a rotator cuff arthropathy. (a,b) Anteroposterior views; (c) axillary view. (a) Line drawing shows the radiographic parameters used in the anteroposterior radiographs to evaluate the relationship between the glenoid and the humerus: x, linear distance in millimeters between the center of the humeral head and the center of the glenoid; y, linear distance from a line tangent to the top of the humeral head and a line parallel to the undersurface of the acromion; z, linear distance from a vertical line from the most lateral aspect of the greater tuberosity and the most lateral aspect of the acromion.

standard axillary radiographs cannot accurately determine the glenoid version (Nyffeler et al. 2003). The easiest method to calculate the glenoid version consists in connecting a line drawn form the scapular body with a line in contact with the anterior and posterior glenoid rims. The normal range varies from 0 to –7°.

It is important to know the correct version of the scapula. This knowledge not only helps the surgeon in positioning the screws during glenoid fixation, but also allows the surgeon to modify the glenoid version in patients with severe degenerative changes.

Comparing shoulders with and without arthritis, Badet et al. (1998) evaluated the CT findings of 113 patients; they showed that glenoid retroversion is increased and humeral version decreased with respect to the shoulder without arthritis. Other authors reported a significant variability in the measurement of glenoid version. As reported by Bokor et al. (1993), version might vary depending on the angle between the scapular position and plane of the CT scanner. In fact, on high-resolution, three-dimensional CT reconstructions, the location of maximum wear was most commonly posterior and was missed on the clinical two-dimensional CT slices in 52% of cases (Hoenecke et al. 2010).

Although arthrography, ultrasonography, and magnetic resonance imaging (MRI) are not necessary for diagnosis, each reveals characteristic findings of a chronic rupture of the rotator cuff. Arthrography often reveals an abnormal communication (the so-called geyser sign; Craig 1984) between the glenohumeral and acromioclavicular joints that is associated with pathological distension or formation of a pseudoganglion of the acromioclavicular joint (see **Fig. 3.2**). Ultrasonography is less invasive than MRI (especially when performed with the use of contrastografic solution) and can reveal the integrity of the rotator cuff. Ultrasonography is less helpful, however, for evaluating any extension of a tear. For this reason, unless the medical conditions of the patient do not allow it (as in a patient with a cardiac pacemaker or who undergoes cardiac valve replacement), we prefer MRI to ultrasonography.

Further, MRI can be helpful in identifying the number of tendons involved, classifying the retraction of the tendons (cuff, humerus, or glenoid) (Patte 1990), and evaluating the degree of fatty infiltration of the rotator cuff muscle. This information is helpful clinically for the surgeon when choosing a shoulder prosthesis.

Table 13.1 The Seebauer classification system

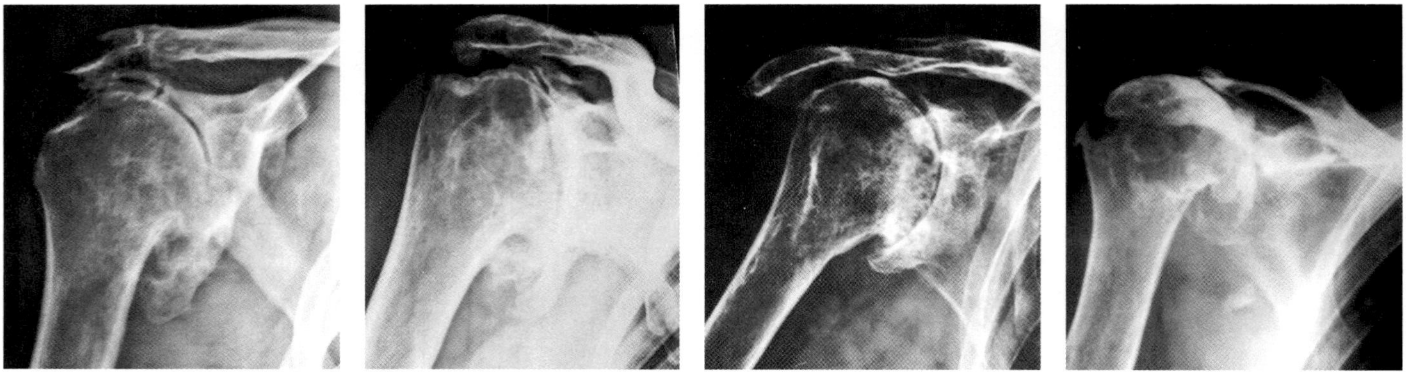

Type IA	Type IB	Type IIA	Type IIB
Centered stable	Centered medialized	Decentered limited stable	Decentered unstable
Intact anterior restraints	Intact anterior restraints (force couple intact – compensated)	Compromised anterior restraints – compromised force couple	Incompetent anterior structures
Minimal superior migration	Minimal superior migration	Superior translation	Anterior superior escape
Dynamic joint stabilization	Compromised dynamic joint stabilization	Insufficient dynamic joint stabilization	Absent dynamic joint stabilization
	Medial erosion of the glenoid	Minimum stabilization by coracoacromial arch Superior medial erosion of the glenoid	No stabilization by coracoacromial arch – deficient anterior structure
Acetabularization of coracoacromial arch	Acetabularization of coracoacromial arch	Acetabularization of coracoacromial arch	
Femoralization of humeral head	Femoralization of humeral head	Femoralization of humeral head	

CONSERVATIVE AND SURGICAL TREATMENT

Indications

The decision about the management of cuff tear arthropathy depends on the type of pathological changes, severity, and symptoms. Not all patients with rotator cuff arthropathy present the same signs and symptoms. Some may have few or no symptoms and others severe symptoms, including recurrent hemarthrosis, loss of function, and persistent pain.

Symptomatic cuff-tear arthropathy is extremely disabling and painful. The extent of the disability is consistently based on the degree of superior migration and loss of centralization of the humeral head. In some cases, anterosuperior instability becomes so great that the head "escapes," leading to the clinical picture of pseudoparalysis of the shoulder, in which deltoid is functional but the patient has a significantly limited ability to forward flex and abduct the arm. This is a devastating clinical syndrome that can often be treated only by shoulder arthroplasty.

The mechanical factors associated with massive rotator cuff tears lead to unbalanced muscle forces. These factors are anteroposterior instability of the humeral head, resulting from a massive tear of the rotator cuff, and rupture or dislocation of the long head of biceps, leading to proximal migration of the humeral head and acromial impingement. The wear on the glenoid is often eccentric, involving the anterosuperior part. This leads to an accelerated process of further cuff destruction and arthropathy. In some cases, the anterosuperior instability is so great that the head lies under the skin. In these patients, the clinical picture is a pseudoparalysis of the shoulder, making it almost impossible to elevate the arm for forward flexion and abduction.

The principles of management are based on pain relief and restoration of the function of the arm. Starting with non-surgical management, these patients can be treated with non-steroidal anti-inflammatory drugs (NSAIDs), cortisone injections, and physical therapy.

Intra-articular injections

Patients may benefit from fluid aspiration and corticosteroid injection. Repeated intra-articular injections of corticosteroids are discouraged, because they are largely ineffective (Williams and Rockwood 1996; Koester et al. 2007).

Thus, aspiration and corticosteroid administration may be a useful adjunct to physical therapy for patients who are unable or unwilling to undergo surgery (Feeley et al. 2009). Many surgeons are hesitant to give repeated cortisone injections into the shoulder with cuff tear arthropathy because of the risk of infection in a joint with a persistently large and often hemorrhagic effusion; however, it remains an excellent tool at the surgeon's discretion (Dines et al. 2009).

Hyaluronan injections are safer, and may be repeated as necessary, and, although of benefit for early and late osteoarthritis of the shoulder, have not been investigated for cuff arthropathy yet (Funk 2004; Valiveti et al. 2006). Hyaluronans act by blocking pain receptors, stimulating endogenous hyaluronan production, and have a direct anti-inflammatory effect by inhibiting leukocyte action (Funk et al. 2007).

Deltoid rehabilitation program

In the presence of pain, it is almost impossible to undertake an efficient rehabilitation program. Rehabilitation is mainly effective when pain can be adequately controlled.

The rationale for re-education of deltoid is validated by recent biomechanical research that challenges the traditional description of the deltoid as being a humeral head elevator (Levy et al. 2008). Gagey and Hue (2000) reported that one of deltoid's functions is to prevent upward migration of the humeral head and to compress it against the glenoid, even in the presence of a large cuff tear. Burkhart (1992) described three kinematic patterns in massive rotator cuff tears based on a fluoroscopic study. Stable fulcrum kinematics were seen in patients with normal shoulder motion with a stable glenohumeral fulcrum. Unstable fulcrum kinematics were seen in patients who have an unstable fulcrum of glenohumeral motion. This situation allowed anterior and superior translation of the humeral head with attempted active elevation.

Captured fulcrum kinematics was seen in a third group. This means that, although the coronal plane force couple could not adequately keep the humeral head centered in the glenoid, there was enough deltoid strength to allow elevation of the shoulder about the fulcrum that the humeral head developed on the undersurface of the acromion or at the anterior acromiodeltoid origin. The patients who improved substantially with deltoid rehabilitation changed from unstable to captured fulcrum kinematics. This deltoid muscle rehabilitation regimen, associated with pain medication, was effective in improving the function and pain in elderly patients with massive cuff tears (Levy et al. 2008).

Surgical options

Arthroscopy

Arthroscopic debridement is not a substitute for joint replacement arthroplasty, but it may provide an alternative for some patients, delaying prosthetic replacement. Epis et al. (2007) reported the efficacy of tidal irrigation in patients with Milwaukee shoulder syndrome. The authors concluded that this is a minimally invasive procedure, and led to a significant improvement in both pain and active motion in patients with longstanding symptoms.

Klinger et al. (2005) suggested that arthroscopic debridement is an excellent treatment for elderly patients with modest functional demands. However, its long-term consequences still need to be evaluated by studies with lengthy follow-up. Patients with recent-onset disease, as opposed to chronic disease, do best with this form of treatment.

Prognostic factors that may lead to a negative outcome are preoperative superior migration of the humeral head, presence of a subscapularis tear, presence of glenohumeral arthritis, and decreased ROM.

Arthroscopic acromioplasty and tendon debridement are commonly used for cuff arthropathy. In many cases, this has led to resection of the CA ligament, which increases the risk of anterosuperior escape as cuff tear arthropathy progresses (Hockman et al. 2004), and should be avoided. In patients with massive or irreparable rotator cuff tears, arthroscopic debridement and acromioplasty can result in short-term pain relief and improvement in shoulder function.

Boileau et al. (2007) retrospectively reviewed 68 patients with massive rotator cuff tears treated with an isolated biceps tenotomy or tenodesis. In patients with a massive rotator cuff tear and a biceps lesion, tenotomy or tenodesis could be effective in managing pain and poor shoulder function. Leim et al. (2008) retrospectively reviewed 31 patients with a massive irreparable rotator cuff tear. Patients were treated with arthroscopy, debridement, biceps tenotomy, and maintenance of the CA arch. The mean American Shoulder and Elbow Surgeon (ASES) score was significantly improved from 24.0 to 69.8 points at follow-up. Pain scores decreased from 7.8 to 2.0 on a 10-point visual analog scale. Therefore, arthroscopic debridement of shoulders with massive irreparable rotator cuff tears is indicated in elderly patients with low functional demands.

During the procedure, a thorough debridement of bursal tissue should be performed, and tenotomy of the biceps tendon should be considered in those with evidence of a biceps lesion during arthroscopy. Maintenance of the CA arch is important to avoid anterosuperior escape. Patients with an absent or atrophic teres minor, complete subscapularis tear, or advanced glenohumeral arthritis are at risk for poorer outcomes.

Arthrodesis

Although rarely indicated, some patients may still benefit from a glenohumeral arthrodesis. In cases in which there is a deficient anterior deltoid, or in patients in whom multiple previous operations have failed, prosthetic replacement would have a poor result. These patients may be considered for arthrodesis.

Shoulder arthroplasty

Hemiarthroplasty

Total shoulder replacements have been abandoned because the excessive shearing forces produced what is known as the "rocking horse" phenomenon, leading to superior eccentric loading on the glenoid and glenoid loosening. Hemiarthroplasty has consequently become a recommended option for cuff tear arthropathy, and has yielded satisfactory results for rotator cuff-deficient shoulders.

The implant for cuff tear arthropathy is a hemiarthroplasty with extended coverage of the humeral head (**Fig. 13.4**). The extended humeral head may allow improved results in cuff tear arthropathy patients, although at this time it is unclear whether this is better than a conventional hemiarthroplasty. The extended coverage provides a larger, low-friction surface area for articulation against the acromion in abduction and external rotation without increasing the size of the head.

These implants provide an arc of surface area greater than 180° that allow articulation with the lateral aspect of the humeral head against the acromion. Visotsky et al. (2004) reported the 2-year follow-up of 60 patients with cuff tear arthropathy in whom a large humeral head prosthesis was used. The average external rotation improved from 8% to 30%, and the average forward flexion improved from 56% to 116%. The average ASES score improved from 29 preoperatively to 79 at the time of follow-up, and no complications were reported.

The correct size of the humeral head is one of the most important goals of a hemiarthroplasty (**Fig. 13.5**). The risk of overstuffing arises from a too large humeral head, but a too small one can determine a loss of power by shortening the lever arm of the deltoid. To determine the correct size, it is important to obtain radiographs of the healthy contralateral shoulder, and to adequately remove the osteophytes intraoperatively. This latter step is also important to achieve correct version of the humeral head and take the tension off the anterior capsule and subscapularis.

Appropriate soft-tissue balancing is fundamental to the success of surgery. The CA arch provides significant stability to the glenohumeral joint, and has been demonstrated in both the laboratory and the clinic. Sectioning of cadaveric CA ligaments with a massive rotator cuff tear resulted in anterosuperior migration of an average of 3.44 mm

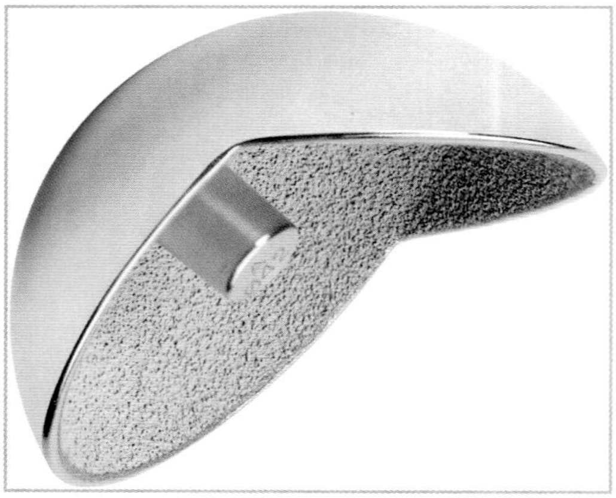

Figure 13.4 Extended coverage arthroplasty.

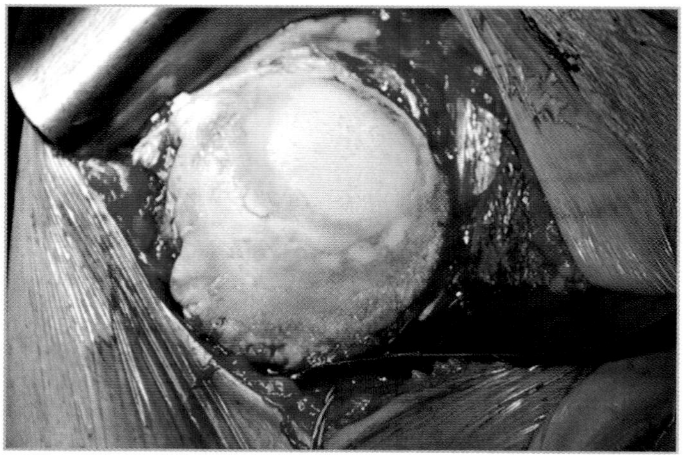

Figure 13.5 Humeral head in rotator cuff arthropathy: the importance of the correct size for arthroplasty.

(Hockman et al. 2004). Unfortunately, in many cases the CA arch has already been compromised in patients with prior attempts at rotator cuff repair. When the arch has not been maintained, the patient may present with instability or progression of superior migration of the humeral head with anterior escape. If the arch has been disrupted in this manner and escape is present, these patients are best treated with a reverse shoulder prosthesis.

Before the advent of the reverse prosthesis, the Field and Dines study found 81% pain relief in 16 patients who underwent a hemiarthroplasty for cuff-tear arthropathy, with the worst results from those patients who had undergone a prior acromioplasty (Field et al. 1997). These results demonstrated the importance of maintaining the acromial arch. We now often apply this principle when treating chronic rotator cuff tears. For those tears that we deem irreparable, it is imperative that the CA arch remains intact in the event that cuff tear arthropathy ensues. Recently, Goldberg et al. (2008) reported the results of hemiarthroplasty of 34 shoulders in 31 patients with cuff tear arthropathy. All patients were evaluated by physical examination at a mean of 3.7 years postoperatively, and 25 shoulders were measured with an ASES score at a mean of 10 years. Only two complications were noted. Thus, hemiarthroplasty appears to provide satisfactory long-term outcomes for selected patients with cuff tear arthropathy.

Sanchez-Sotelo et al. (2001) reported 30 patients (33 shoulders) with cuff tear arthropathy treated with humeral hemiarthroplasty. At the time of follow-up (5 years), 67% were rated as successful and 33% as unsuccessful. The authors noted that 8 shoulders had progressive superior erosion of the glenoid and 14 had progressive erosion of the acromion. This is another challenge that has not been fully answered, and is increased after previous acromioplasty and CA ligament resection.

Reverse total shoulder prosthesis

The semi-constrained reverse ball-and-socket design was introduced by Grammont in 1985 (Boileau et al. 2005). The semi-constrained design of the prosthesis ensures stability (**Fig. 13.6**), even in the presence of anterosuperior escape. Until Grammont's device, all reverse designs had a lateral offset of the glenoid component relative to the glenoid surface. This attachment site proved to be the site of failure, because the lateral offset increased the moment arm of the resultant joint reactive force, which further stressed the glenoid–prosthetic bone attachment.

Unlike previous designs, Grammont's device shifted the center of rotation medially to the glenoid fossa to reduce the effective lever arm and distally to tension deltoid and improve its mechanics (Boileau et al. 2005). In this inverted design, the resultant force applied to the neck of the scapula limits the shear forces that are responsible for loosening of the glenoid. This design alleviates pain and improves function in patients with cuff tear arthropathy.

There are three biomechanical advantages of using the reverse prosthesis design: (1) the large glenosphere allows greater stability and range of motion; (2) the glenosphere makes contact with the glenoid surface, placing the center of rotation of the shoulder within the glenoid, thereby reducing the torque on the baseplate bone interface; and (3) the medialized center of rotation increases the number of deltoid muscle fibers recruited for abduction, and lowering of the humerus places increased tension on deltoid (Boileau et al. 2005).

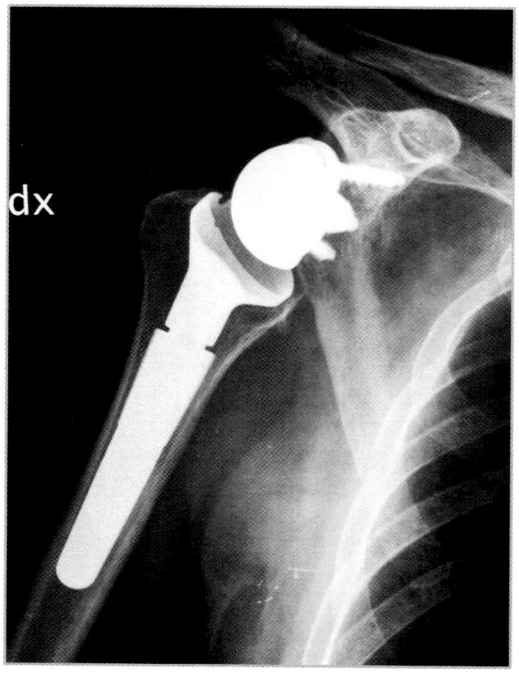

Figure 13.6 Radiograph of reverse shoulder prosthesis (36-mm glenosphere).

In a study on the in vivo dynamics of normal, rotator cuff-deficient, total shoulder arthroplasty, and reverse shoulder arthroplasty shoulders, the reverse shoulder replacement shoulder exhibited kinematic and kinetic patterns similar to normal shoulders. The semi-constrained design kept the intersection of the differing planes of motion axis relatively constant (Mahfouz et al. 2005).

The basic reverse shoulder design consists of the proximal humerus and the glenoid attachments. The proximal humerus is a modular prosthesis in which the humeral stem (diaphysis) is attached to the epiphyseal stem, with the attachment of a polyethylene cup spacer on the proximal portion. The concave shape of the spacer is a third of a sphere to accommodate articulation with the glenosphere. The glenoid prosthesis consists of a glenoid base plate (or metaglene), which is placed with screw fixation, and the ball or glenosphere, which represents the humeral head that is fixed to the base plate (Dines et al. 2009).

In the reverse total shoulder, the center of rotation is in the center of the spherical glenoid component fixed to the scapula, whereas, before surgery, the center of rotation is in the center of the humeral head. Changes in the center of rotation affect the resting tension in the deltoid and residual cuff muscles, as well as their respective moment arms. The position of the center of rotation after a reverse total shoulder arthroplasty is determined by the design of the glenoid prosthesis and the position in which it is placed (Saltzman et al. 2010). This implant should be used only in patients with an intact deltoid muscle. There must be adequate glenoid bone stock available to implant the glenoid component securely.

Contraindications include deltoid dysfunction (neurological or structural), glenoid wear or destruction that does not allow secure implantation of the glenoid component, and active infection. Relative contraindications include younger age, rheumatoid arthritis, and surgeon inexperience with shoulder arthroplasty.

Rheumatoid arthritis would at first evaluation seem to be an indication for the reverse shoulder. There is almost always rotator cuff dysfunction and deficiency, and there is joint injury. The nature of the disease and the treatment regimens can, however, result in poor bone stock on the glenoid side.

The prosthesis can be implanted through a superior or deltopectoral approach. The superior approach can be utilized in primary cases. In revision and primary surgery, the deltopectoral approach may allow improved exposure of the inferior glenoid, with better inferior placement and inferior tilt to the glenoid component. In revision cases with an existing implant in place, the deltopectoral approach is more extensile and recommended (Nicholson 2006). The humeral neck cut is made at 155° (**Fig. 13.7**), to place a small cup that covers less than half of the glenosphere. This has the advantage of lowering the humerus, resulting in overtensioning of deltoid. It allows a greater ROM to occur before component bone impingement.

Sufficient exposure of the glenoid is necessary for placement of the metaglene (**Fig. 13.8**). The glenoid component is a third of a sphere with a large diameter of 36 or 42 mm and no neck. The posterior aspect of the glenosphere is in direct contact with the prepared glenoid surface. This design has the advantage of placing the center of rotation of the joint in contact with the center of the humeral head, and provides a fixed center of rotation. Furthermore, the large diameter allows greater range of movement before impingement of the components occurs and provides more stability.

The frequency of scapular notching, likely related to mechanical impingement by the medial rim of the humeral cup against the scapular neck in adduction, is of concern, and has been suggested as a cause of glenoid loosening. Glenoid erosion by impingement of the humeral component on the inferior glenoid is often seen. It usually is not progressive, but needs to be observed and revised if severe. The low positioning of the glenosphere (Werner et al. 2005) is probably the most important factor, and should avoid most of the notches.

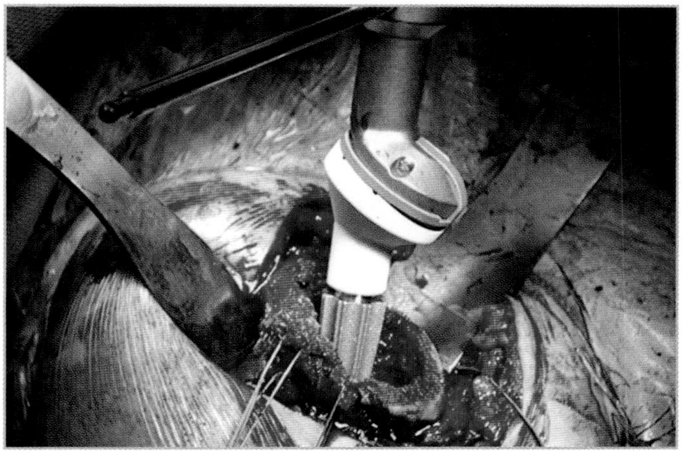

Figure 13.7 Intraoperative picture of humeral prosthesis implant. The humeral neck cut is made at 155°.

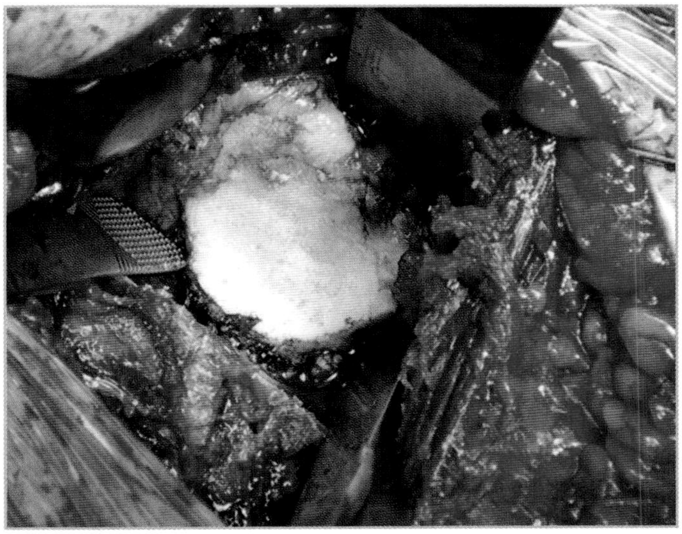

Figure 13.8 Intraoperative picture of exposure of the glenoid necessary for placement of the metaglene, to reduce the risk of scapular notching.

As a practical point, the authors recommend positioning the baseplate flush with the inferior glenoid rim so that the glenosphere extends 4 mm beyond the glenoid inferiorly (Levigne et al. 2008). In addition, tilting the glenoid of 15° should reduce the risk of impingements and increase the adduction of the arm. Newer designs of glenospheres (e.g., the SMR [Systema Multiplana Randelli], LIMA, Udine, Italy) have become available: eccentric glenospheres and larger diameter glenospheres (36 and 44 mm) (**Figs 13.9a** and **b**). (Chou et al. 2009) These newer glenospheres are designed to offer greater ROMs, and theoretically may reduce the risk of mechanical impingement and hence scapular notching. The 36-mm eccentric glenosphere has an eccentric attachment of 4 mm, and the 44-mm eccentric glenosphere (made of polyethylene material) has an eccentric attachment of 2 mm. The eccentric and larger diameter glenospheres of the SMR reverse prosthesis allow greater ROMs. The eccentric designs have a greater effect on increasing adduction. Improved adduction may reduce mechanical impingement and the risk of scapular notching (**Fig. 13.10**).

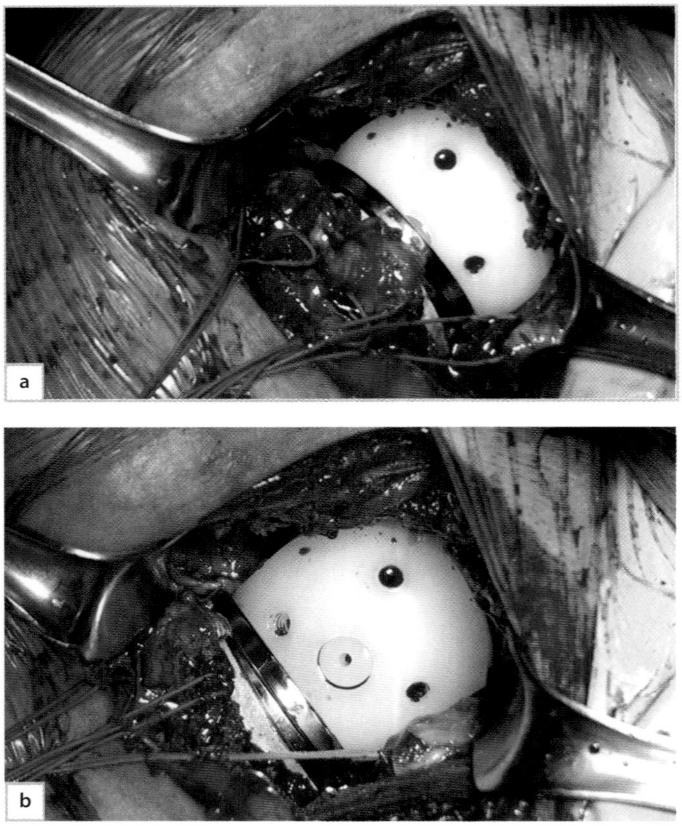

Figure 13.9 Intraoperative picture of eccentric glenospheres and larger diameter glenospheres (36 and 44 mm).

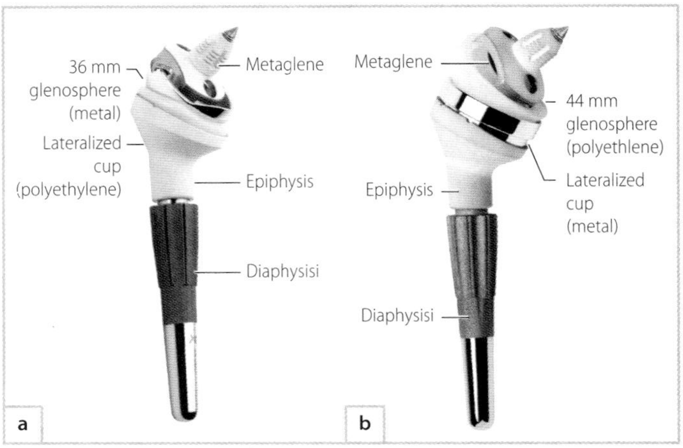

Figure 13.10 Reverse shoulder arthroplasty and its components: (a) 36-mm glenosphere (metallic) and (b) 44-mm glenosphere (polyethylene)

Despite the clinical success of the reverse total shoulder implant in alleviating pain and restoring function, its widespread use is limited by a high reported complication rate. Werner et al. (2005) reported an overall complication rate of 50%, which occurred in 29 of the 58 patients, and a reoperation rate of 33% with the use of a reverse prosthesis: 19 patients underwent a total of 31 (range 1–3 per patient) reoperations after implantation of the Delta III prosthesis.

Dislocation is also relatively common, especially after the revision of a previous arthroplasty, when the osseous and soft-tissue anatomy has been distorted by prior trauma, when components are malpositioned, or when the humeral component levers against glenoid bone. Fractures of the acromion occur commonly as a result of a pre-existing acromial lesion, overtensioning of deltoid, or osseous fatigue from loading of an osteopenic acromion. Contraindications for patients under consideration for receiving the reverse prosthesis include a non-functional deltoid, active infection, excessive glenoid bone loss, severe neurological deficiencies, refusal to modify postoperative physical activities, and metal allergy (Frankle et al. 2005).

CONCLUSION

Rotator cuff arthropathy involves a complex series of pathological, biochemical, and biomechanical changes that appear to develop in response to tendon rupture. This lesion is peculiar to the glenohumeral joint because of the unique anatomy of the rotator cuff.

Cuff tear arthropathy is especially difficult to treat and, although many tears of the rotator cuff do not enlarge sufficiently to allow this condition to develop, it is a factor to consider when deciding whether or not a documented tear of the rotator cuff should be surgically repaired.

Conservative treatment is still a good option in low-demand and less symptomatic patients due to a palliation of pain and disability.

The surgical treatment of rotator cuff arthropathy has changed over time. Since Grammont introduced reversed shoulder arthroplasty in 1985 (Boileau et al. 2005), the design, materials, and surgical techniques have changed significantly. Nowadays this procedure can be considered a real option for patients with this peculiar pathology who can achieve functionally satisfactory and long-lasting results.

REFERENCES

Adams R. Illustrations of the Effects of Rheumatic Gout or Chronic Rheumatic Arthritis on All the Articulations: With descriptive and explanatory statements. London: J Churchill, 1857: 1–31.
Augereau B, Apoil A. Repair using a deltoid flap of an extensive loss of substance of the rotary cuff of the shoulder. Rev Chir Orthop Reparatrice Appar Mot 1988;74:298–301.
Badet R, Walch G, Boulahia A. Computed tomography in primary glenohumeral osteoarthritis without humeral head elevation. Rev Rheum Engl Ed 1998;65:187–194.
Boileau P, Watkinson DJ, Hatzidakis AM, Balg F. Grammont reverse prosthesis: design, rationale, and biomechanics. J Shoulder Elbow Surg 2005;14:147–161.
Boileau P, Baqué F, Valerio L, et al. Isolated arthroscopic biceps tenotomy or tenodesis improves symptoms in patients with massive irreparable rotator cuff tears. J Bone Joint Surg Am 2007;89:747–757.
Bokor DJ, Hawkins RJ, Huckell GH, et al. Results of nonoperative management of full-thickness tears of the rotator cuff. Clin Orthop Relat Res 1993;294:103–110.
Brems JJ. Rehabilitation following total shoulder arthroplasty. Clin Orthop Relat Res 1994;307:70–85.
Brett MA, Murrell GAC. Shoulder – The biology of rotator cuff tears. Curr Orthop Pract 2008;19:516–523.
Burkhart SS. Fluoroscopic comparison of kinematic patterns in massive rotator cuff tears. A suspension bridge model. Clin Orthop 1992;284:144–152.
Codman EA. Rupture of the supraspinatus tendon and other lesions in or about the subacromial bursa. In: The Shoulder. Boston, MA: Thomas Todd, 1934.
Chou J, Malak SF, Anderson IA, Astley T, Poon PC. Biomechanical evaluation of different designs of glenospheres in the SMR reverse total shoulder prosthesis: Range of motion and risk of scapular notching. J Shoulder Elbow Surg 2009;18:354–359.

Clift SE, Harris B, Dieppe PA, Hayes A. Frictional response of articular cartilage containing crystals. Biomaterials 1989;10:329-334.
Craig EV. The geyser sign and torn rotator cuff: clinical significance and pathomechanics. Clin. Orthop 1984;191:213–215.
De Seze S, Robault A, Rampon S. L'epaule senile hemorragique. In: L'actualite Rhumatologique. Paris: Expansion Scientifique Française, 1968: 107–114.
Dieppe PA, Cawston T, Mercer E, et al. Synovial fluid collagenase in patients with destructive arthritis of the shoulder joint. Arthritis Rheum 1988;31:882–890.
Dines DM, et al. Arthritis and arthroplasty. The Shoulder, vol 11. Philadelphia, PA: Saunders, 2009: 116–122.
Ecklund KJ, Lee TQ, Tibone J, Gupta R. Rotator cuff tear arthropathy. J Am Acad Orthop Surg 2007;15:340–349.
Epis O, Caporali R, Scirè CA, et al. Efficacy of tidal irrigation in Milwaukee shoulder syndrome. J Rheumatol 2007;34:1545–1550.
Feeley BT, Gallo RA, Craig EV. Cuff tear arthropaty: Current trends in diagnosis and surgical management J Shoulder Elbow Surg 2009;18:484–494.
Field L, Dines D, Zabinski S et al. Hemiarthroplasty of the shoulder for rotator cuff arthropathy. J Shoulder Elbow Surg 1997;6:18–23.
Frankle M, Levy JC, Pupello D, et al. The reverse shoulder prosthesis for glenohumeral arthritis associated with severe rotator cuff deficiency. A minimum two-year follow-up study of sixty patients. J Bone Joint Surg Am 2005;87:1697–1705.
Funk L. Ostenil hyaluronan for inoperable osteoarthritis of the shoulder. Osteoarthr Cartilage 2004;12(suppl B).
Funk L, Haines J, Trail I. Rotator cuff arthropathy. Curr Orthop 2007;21:415–421.
Gagey O, Hue E. Mechanics of the deltoid muscle. A new approach. Clin Orthop 2000;375:250–257.
Goldberg SS, Bell JE, Kim HJ, et al. Hemiarthroplasty for the rotator cuff-deficient shoulder. J Bone Joint Surg Am 2008;90:554–559.
Goutallier D, Postel JM, Bernageau J, et al. Fatty muscle degeneration in cuff rupture. Pre and postoperative evaluation by CT scan. Clin Orthop Relat Res 1994;304:78–83.
Halverson PB, Cheung HS, McCarty DJ, et al. "Milwaukee shoulder" association of microspheroids containing hydroxyapatite crystals, active collagenase, and neutral protease with rotator cuff defects. II. Synovial fluid studies. Arthr Rheum 1981;24:474–483.
Hamada K, Fukuda H, Mikasa M, Kobayashi Y. Roentgenographic findings in massive rotator cuff tears. Clin Orthop Relat Res 1990;254:92–96.
Harryman DT, Sidles JA, Harris SL, Matsen FA. The role of the rotator interval capsule in passive motion and stability of the shoulder. J Bone Joint Surg Am 1992;74:53–66.
Hayes AI, Turner G, Powell KA, Dieppe PA. Crystal aggregates in articular cartilage as observed in the SEM. J Mater Sci: Mater Med 1992;3:75–378.
Hernigou P, Duparc F, Hernigou A. Determining humeral retroversion with computed tomography. J Bone Joint Surg Am 2002;84:1753–1762.
Hockman DE, Lucas GL, Roth CA. Role of the coracoacromial ligament as restraint after shoulder hemiarthroplasty. Clin Orthop Relat Res 2004;419:80–82.
Hoenecke HR Jr, Hermida JC, Flores-Hernandez C, D'Lima DD. Accuracy of CT-based measurements of glenoid version for total shoulder arthroplasty. J Shoulder Elbow Surg 2010;19:166–171.
Iannotti JP, McCarron J, Raymond CJ, et al. Agreement study of radiographic classification of rotator cuff tear arthropathy. J Shoulder Elbow Surg 2010;19:1–7.
Inman VT, Saunders JB, Abbott LC. Observations of the function of the shoulder joint. Clin Orthop Relat Res 1996;330:3–12.
Klinger HM, Steckel H, Ernstberger T, Baums MH. Arthroscopic debridement of massive rotator cuff tears: negative prognostic factors. Arch Orthop Trauma Surg 2005;125:261–266.
Koester MC, Dunn WR, Khun JE, Spindler KP. The efficacy of subacromial corticosteroid injection in the treatment of rotator cuff disease: a systematic review. J Am Acad Orthop Surg 2007;15:3–11.
Leim D, Lengers N, Dedy N, et al. Arthroscopic debridement of massive irreparable rotator cuff tears. Arthroscopy 2008;24:743–738.
Lee M, Chebli C, Mounce D, et al. Intramedullary reaming for press-fit fixation of a humeral component removes cortical bone asymmetrically. J Shoulder Elbow Surg 2008;17:150–155.
Levigne C, Boileau P, Favard L, et al. Scapular notching in reverse shoulder arthroplasty. J Shoulder Elbow Surg 2008;17:925–935.
Levy O, Mullett H, Roberts S, Copeland S. The role of anterior deltoid reeducation in patients with massive irreparable degenerative rotator cuff tears. J Shoulder Elbow Surg 2008;17:863–870.
McCarty DJ, Halverson PB, Carrera GF, Brewer BJ, Kozin F. "Milwaukee shoulder" – association of microspheroids containing hydroxyapatite crystals, active collagenase, and neutral protease with rotator cuff defects. I. Clinical aspects. Arthr Rheum 1981;24:464–473.
Mahfouz M, Nicholson GP, Komistek R, et al. In vivo determination of the dynamics of normal, rotator cuff deficient, total and reverse replacement shoulder. J Bone Joint Surg Am 2005;87(suppl 2):107–113.
Massias P, Sallierre D, Clerc D, Languille D. L'arthropathie destructrice rapide de l'epaule. Rev Rhum Mal Osteoartic 1982;49:547–548.
Matsen FA, Rockwood CA. The Shoulder, 4th edn. Philadelphia, PA: WB Saunders, 2009.
Matsen FA, Chebli C, Lippitt S. Principles for the evaluation and management of shoulder instability. J Bone Joint Surg Am 2006;88:648–659.
Neer CS, Craig EV, Fukuda H. Cuff-tear arthropathy. J Bone Joint Surg Am 1983;65:1232–1244.
Nicholson GP. Current concepts in reverse shoulder replacement. Curr Opin Orthop 2006;17:306–309.
Nyffeler RW, Jost B, Pfirrmann CW, Gerber C. Measurement of glenoid version: conventional radiographs versus computed tomography scans. J Shoulder Elbow Surg 2003;12:493–496.
Patte D. Classification of rotator cuff lesions. Clin Orthop Relat Res 1990;254:81–86.
Parsons IM, Weldon EJ, III, Titelman RM, Smith KL. Glenohumeral arthritis and its management. Phys Med Rehabil Clin North Am 2004;15:447–474.
Peach CA, Zhang Y, Dunford JE, et al. Cuff tear arthropathy: evidence of functional variation in pyrophosphate metabolism genes. Clin Orthop Relat Res 2007;462:67–72.
Saltzman MD, Mercer DM, Warme WJ, et al. A method for documenting the change in center of rotation with reverse total shoulder arthroplasty and its application to a consecutive series of 68 shoulders having reconstruction with one of two different reverse prostheses. J Shoulder Elbow Surg 2010;19:1–6.
Sanchez-Sotelo J, Cofield RH, Rowland CM. Shoulder hemi-arthroplasty for glenohumeral arthritis associated with severe rotator cuff deficiency. J Bone Joint Surg Am 2001;83:1814–1822.
Sirveaux F, Favard L, Oudet D, et al. Grammont inverted total shoulder arthroplasty in the treatment of glenohumeral osteoarthritis with massive rupture of the cuff. Results of a multicentre study of 80 shoulders. J Bone Joint Surg Br 2004;86:388–395.
Valiveti M, Reginato AJ, Falasca GF. Viscosupplementation for degenerative joint disease of shoulder and ankle. J Clin Rheumatol 2006;12:162–263.
Visotsky JL, Basamania C, Seebauer L, et al. Cuff tear arthropathy: pathogenesis, classification, and algorithm for treatment. J Bone Joint Surg Am 2004;86:35–40.
Werner CM, Steinmann PA, Gilbart M, Gerber C. Treatment of painful pseudoparesis due to irreparable rotator cuff dysfunction with the Delta III reverse ball and socket total shoulder prosthesis. J Bone Joint Surg Am 2005;87:1476–1486.
Williams GR, Rockwood CA. Hemiarthroplasty in rotator cuff-deficient shoulders. J Shoulder Elbow Surg 1996;5:362–367.

Chapter 14 Single-row versus double-row rotator cuff repair

Robert B. Kohen, Asheesh Bedi, Joshua S. Dines

KEY FEATURES

- The clinical outcomes after arthroscopic rotator cuff repair are equivalent to those reported for both mini-open and open techniques.
- A major target of arthroscopic rotator cuff repair is to reproduce the anatomical tendon footprint.
- The double-row repair technique involves placement of a linear row of anchors at the articular margin of the humeral head, and a second row of anchors along the lateral aspect of the rotator cuff footprint on the tuberosity.
- Cadaveric studies suggest a biomechanical superiority of double-row configurations for increased load-to-failure, better-restored footprint anatomy, and more favorable load sharing.
- Although there is strong evidence of biomechanical effectiveness after a double-row repair, multiple level I clinical trials have demonstrated no superiority of double-row repairs over the single-row ones.

INTRODUCTION

Recent literature suggests that the clinical outcomes after arthroscopic rotator cuff repair are now equivalent to those reported for both mini-open and open techniques. Clinical outcomes are generally favorable, but reliable structural integrity of the repairs remains undefined. Despite improvements in surgical technique, implants, and biological augmentation, failure rates for large (>3 cm) tears range from 13% to 94% at 2-year follow-up. Especially with larger tears, structural integrity is associated with a superior clinical outcome (Dines et al. 2010).

One of the major targets in improving the structural and healing properties of arthroscopic rotator cuff repairs is to reproduce the anatomical tendon footprint with a double-row technique. This technique involves a linear row of anchors placed at the articular margin of the humeral head and a second row placed along the lateral aspect of the rotator cuff footprint on the tuberosity. The impetus for this technique was a desire to create a construct equivalent to a transosseous repair and prevent simple point fixation of the rotator cuff to bone. Indeed, biomechanical studies demonstrate increased load to failure, improved contact area, and decreased gap formation at the enthesis with double-row constructs (Dines et al. 2010).

ROTATOR CUFF ANATOMY AND TENDON-TO-BONE HEALING

The tendons of the rotator cuff muscles insert into a fibrocartilaginous tissue known as the enthesis. This tissue maximizes stress concentration at the tendon–bone interface. The transition from tendon to bone proceeds through four continuous zones: the tendon proper, fibrocartilage, mineralized fibrocartilage, and bone. This organization is not recapitulated in rotator cuff repair. The repaired insertion is inferior biomechanically and histologically, with healing primarily by interposed fibrovascular scar tissue. Although the biological factors that affect healing are complex, the anatomy of the footprint is well described (Mochizuki et al. 2008).

Several recent studies have elucidated the anatomy of the rotator cuff footprint. Initially thought to measure 25 mm from anterior to posterior and 14.7 mm in transverse diameter, the supraspinatus footprint is in reality smaller (Dugas et al. 2002; Mochizuki et al. 2008), with a sagittal insertion of 12.6 mm medially and 1.3 mm at its lateral margin. The larger trapezoidal insertion for the infraspinatus ranges from 20.2 mm to 32.7 mm in the sagittal plane and covers a greater percentage of the greater tuberosity due, in part, to the lateral sweep of the tendon as it inserts anteriorly (**Fig. 14.1**). The medial-to-lateral length of the rotator cuff insertion ranges from 6.9 mm to 10.2 mm at supraspinatus and infraspinatus insertions respectively.

Restoration of this footprint should be one focus of rotator cuff repair because the potential for tendon-to-bone healing increases as the available contact area between the cuff and its insertion increases (Oguma et al. 2001). Other aspects of rotator cuff repair that are targets for optimization include suture materials, anchor fixation, biological augmentation, inflammatory modulation, and modified rehabilitation.

BIOMECHANICS OF SINGLE- VERSUS DOUBLE-ROW REPAIRS

Footprint restoration

The theoretical advantage of footprint restoration has been extensively biomechanically tested (Apreleva et al. 2002). A notable difference in early arthroscopic repairs relative to historical open repairs was a transition from transosseous suture fixation to point fixation with anchors. Apreleva et al. (2002) noted that the repair site contact area is 20% larger with transosseous simple suture repairs when compared with point fixation with suture anchors. To further optimize insertion site reconstruction, Toheti et al. (2005) demonstrated that double-row repairs increased the footprint contact area by 42% and 60% relative to transosseous and single-row techniques in a cadaveric model. This work was validated by Mazzocca et al. (2010) who described consistently larger footprint coverage in double-row constructs relative to single-row repairs. Meier et al. (2006) furthered these findings by comparing the footprints of transosseous, single-row, and double-row repairs using three-dimensional mapping. They found that double-row repairs restored 100% of the anatomical footprint, whereas the transosseous and single-row techniques restored 71% and 46% of the footprint, respectively.

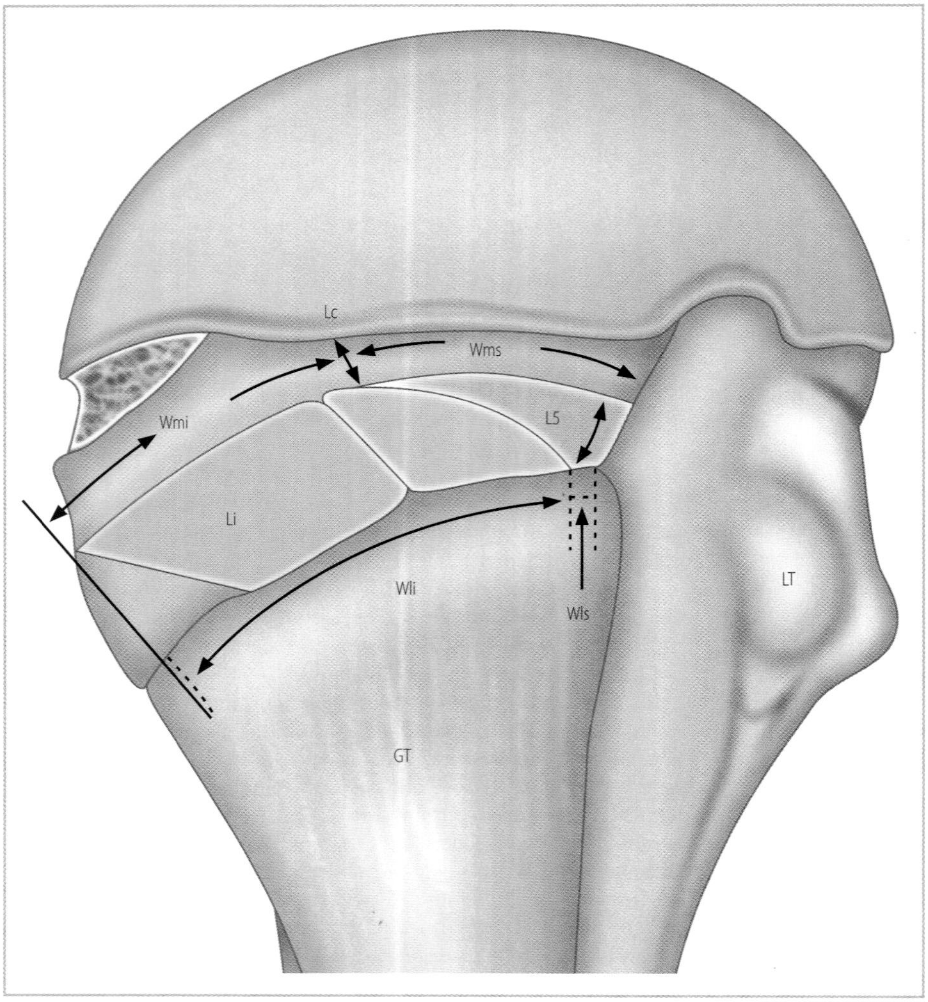

	Average and standard deviation (mm)
Supraspinatus	
Maximum medial-to-lateral length	6.9 ± 1.4
Anteroposterior width of medial margin	12.6 ± 2.0
Anteroposterior width of lateral margin	1.3 ± 1.4
Infraspinatus	
Maximum medial-to-lateral length	10.2 ± 1.6
Anteroposterior width of medial margin	20.2 ± 6.2
Anteroposterior width of lateral margin	32.7 ± 3.4
Articular capsule	
Medial-to-lateral length at posterior edge of supraspinatus footprint	4.5 ± 0.5

Figure 14.1 Insertional anatomy of the rotator cuff. The average dimensions are listed. GT, greater tuberosity; Lc, length of attachment of the capsule; Li, maximum length of infraspinatus insertion; Ls, maximum length of supraspinatus insertion; LT, lesser tuberosity; Wli, width of lateral infraspinatus footprint; Wls, width of lateral supraspinatus footprint; Wmi, width of medial infraspinauts footprint; Wms, width of medial supraspinatus footprint. (Reproduced with permission from Mochizuki T, Sugaya H, Uomizu M, et al. Humeral insertion of the supraspinatus and infraspinatus: New anatomical findings regarding the footprint of the rotator cuff. J Bone Joint Surg Am 2008;90:962–969.)

In a novel analysis of footprint reconstruction, Ahmad et al. (2009) evaluated fluid extravasation in single- and double-row constructs in eight cadaveric shoulders. The single-row repairs resulted in significantly greater fluid extravasation, which may have hindered rotator cuff repair healing. Therefore, there is consistent validation in the literature that the anatomical footprint contact area is better recreated with double-row repairs.

Mechanical strength

After confirming the superiority of double-row repairs in reproducing the anatomical rotator cuff footprint, multiple studies evaluated the mechanical properties of these constructs. Baums et al. (2010) utilized a sheep model to study the impact of suture material and the addition of medial mattress sutures to a lateral Mason–Allen single-row construct. They showed a significant increase in tensile strength in the double-row repairs. Gerber et al. (1994) found that the addition of a second row to six simple sutures increased the load to failure of repairs from 273 N to 336 N. Similarly, Kim et al. (2006) reported that a second row of anchors increased ultimate load to failure by 48%. Milano et al. (2008) likewise showed significant mechanical superiority in double-row repairs relative to single-row repairs, particularly when fixed under tension. Gap formation is reduced in double-row repairs, regardless of rotational position (Dines et al. 2010).

In contrast, two studies have shown no apparent mechanical strength advantage of double-row repairs. Nelson et al. (2008) compared the time-zero mechanical strength of double-row repairs with single-row modified Mason–Allen rotator cuff repairs in a sheep model. They found a significant increase in footprint restoration with the double-row technique, but no significant differences in displacement, elongation, or mean load to failure. In addition, Mazzoca et al. (2010) reported no difference between single- and double-row repairs, but specimens were cycled 3000 times before load-to-failure testing, possibly influencing the results. Mahar et al. (2007) reported a similar conclusion in a bovine model, but the single-row group did have the greatest elongation in cyclical loading.

With the literature tending to support improved mechanical strength in double-row repairs, some authors have begun to compare specific double-row configurations and clarify functions of the medial and lateral rows. For example, Burkhart et al. (2009) evaluated the biomechanical strength of a knotless double-row construct in matched human cadaveric shoulders. The study demonstrated no difference between a knotless double-row construct and a standard double-row construct in ultimate load or cyclic displacement. Kulwicki et al. (2010) subsequently evaluated the suture tension in single-row, double-row, and transosseous equivalent cadaveric repairs. Significantly greater suture tension was seen in the single-row repairs. There was no difference in the load borne by the medial and lateral anchors in double-row repairs, suggesting load sharing between the rows. Hepp et al. (2009) evaluated three double-row repair techniques in sheep shoulders. This study compared a double-row technique with a double-layer, double-row technique using either simple or mattress sutures. They concluded that there was no difference between the double-layer and standard double-row techniques in elongation and load to failure. There was, however, a significant increase in ultimate load, ultimate elongation, and energy absorbed in the double-layer mattress repairs relative to the double-layer simple suture repairs.

Footprint contact pressure

The basic science literature suggests that controlling the mechanical forces at a tendon–bone interface can significantly impact healing. Footprint contact pressure may be even more important than simply recreating the footprint contact area (Park MC et al. 2007). Park and colleagues (Park MC et al. 2009) compared single-row, double-row, and transosseous equivalent rotator cuff repairs in human cadaveric shoulders at variable abduction and rotation positions. A Tekscan pressure sensor demonstrated significantly increased contact pressure in the transosseus equivalent repairs at all abduction angles greater than zero and all rotations tested (**Figs 14.2a** and **b**). Likewise, Baums et al. (2009) studied the rotator cuff contact pressure in 5 types of repairs in 40 sheep cadaveric shoulders. They showed that double-row constructs with a Mason–Allen suture configuration resulted in the greatest footprint contact pressure. Grimberg et al. (2010; Mazzocca et al. 2010) also assessed bone–tendon contact surface and pressure in single-row, double-row bridge, and double-row cross-suture constructs. There was a significant increase in contact surface and pressure in the double-row cross suture configuration relative to the other tested constructs. Finally, Mazzocca et al. (2010) evaluated 4 different rotator cuff repair techniques in 16 cadaveric shoulders. Transosseous equivalent repairs had the highest contact pressure and force compared with single-row, triangular double-row, and suture-chain transosseous repair. Notably, the contact pressure and force decreased in all constructs 160 minutes after the repair.

An important distinction must be made between two simple rows of suture and newer "transosseous equivalent" repairs. These "transosseous" or "suture bridge" repairs were developed to optimize the tendon–bone interface pressure. With these techniques, the medial row suture limbs are drawn across the bursal-side cuff insertion and incorporated into the lateral row of anchors, providing compression between the tendon and bone (**Figs 14.3a** and **b**). Key points are to place the medial row at the articular margin and the medial sutures as medially as possible, and to maintain an adequate bone bridge between the medial and lateral rows. New implants from nearly every arthroscopic instrument company have been helpful in simplifying the execution of these repairs. Studies of these new repairs have shown improved load to failure and pressurized contact area relative to traditional double-row constructs. Further, there may be an advantage to interconnecting the sutures from each anchor to allow load sharing during rotation.

Despite improved biomechanical stability in load-to-failure testing, the "transosseous equivalent" repairs may present other concerns. These issues include a compromise of vascular supply by excessive compression, increased operating room time, tuberosity crowding, implant cost, and difficulty in revision. Other have described a new mode of failure after "transosseous equivalent repair" in which intramuscular tear occurs while the footprint remains intact. Clearly, good clinical studies are warranted to better clarify these issues.

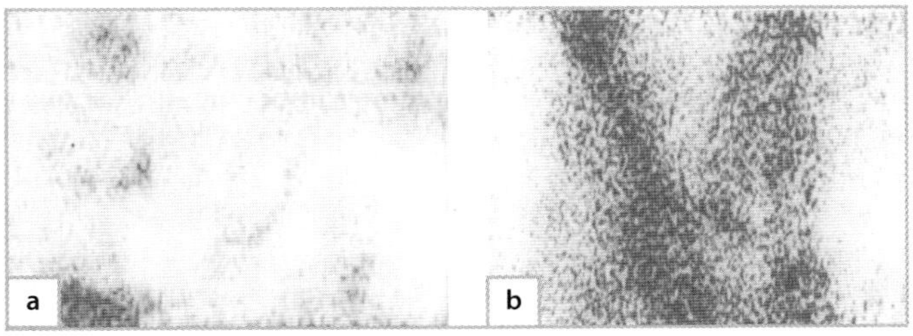

Figure 14.2 Qualitative pressure imprints for different double-row rotator cuff repair techniques. (a) Double-row technique and (b) double-row suture bridge technique. The top of each film represents the medial rotator cuff footprint. (Reproduced with permission from Park MC, ElAttrache NS, Tibone JE, et al. Part I: Footprint contact characteristics for a transosseous-equivalent rotator cuff tear technique compared with a double row repair technique. J Shoulder Elbow Surg 2007;16:461–468).

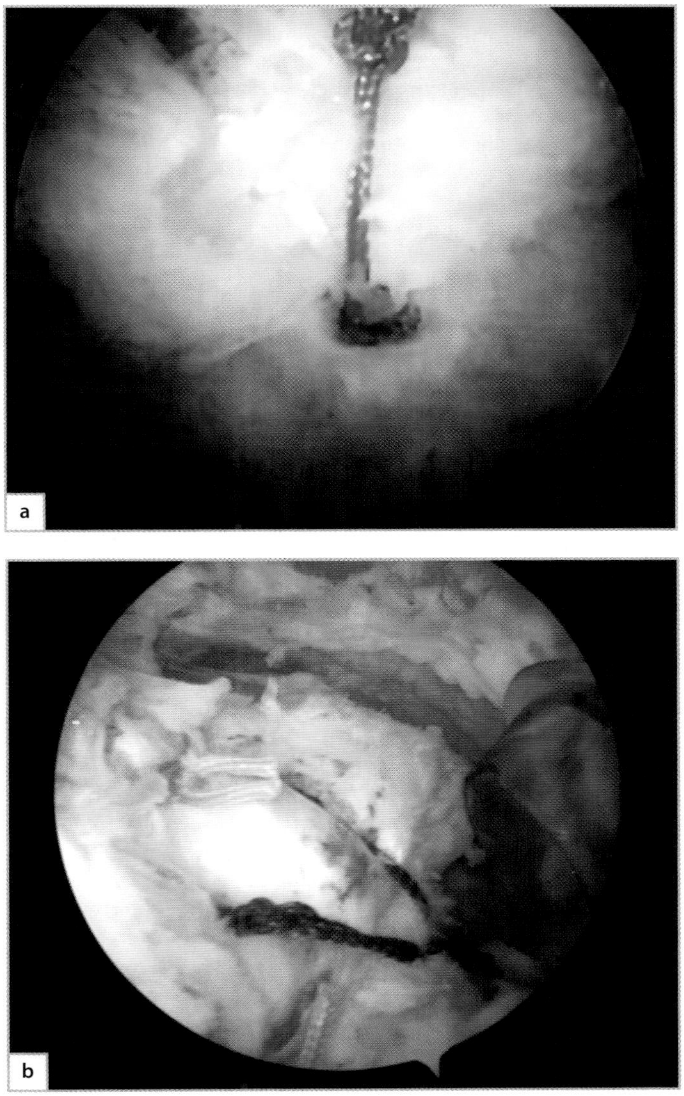

Figure 14.3 Intraoperative arthroscopic photos of (a) single-row and (b) double-row suture bridge rotator cuff repairs.

CLINICAL OUTCOMES OF SINGLE-VERSUS DOUBLE-ROW REPAIRS

In response to the evidence suggesting improved biomechanical properties of double-row repairs, multiple clinical studies have evaluated the clinical and structural outcomes of these repairs compared with traditional single-row and transosseous repairs. Although several studies have documented favorable clinical case series of double-row repairs, multiple level I studies have demonstrated no superiority of double-row repairs relative to single-row repairs.

Level 1 studies

The first of these studies was a randomized controlled trial of 60 patients with similar demographics and tear sizes, who underwent either single-row or double-row (medial mattress, lateral simple suture) rotator cuff repair. No significant differences were found at 2-year follow-up with magnetic resonance (MR) arthrography or UCLA shoulder assessment scores (Franceschi et al. 2007). Likewise, Burks et al. (2009) randomized 40 patients to single-row and double-row repairs. Clinical evaluation and three postoperative MRI studies showed no difference in footprint coverage or tendon thickness. At 1-year follow-up the authors concluded that there were no clinical differences between the repairs. Several other level I randomized studies demonstrated no significant differences between single-row and double-row rotator cuff repairs (Grasso et al. 2009) and between transosseous-equivalent repairs and single-row repairs at 2-year follow-up (Aydin et al. 2010).

Case series/retrospective comparisons

Despite no definite clinical advantage of double-row repairs in randomized controlled trials, multiple case series and retrospective comparisons in the literature provide evidence for excellent clinical outcomes. Grasso et al. (2009) compared 40 patients who underwent single-row repair with 40 patients treated with double-row repairs. At 2-year follow-up no significant differences were seen in DASH scores, Constant scores, or strength testing. Only age, gender, and baseline strength influenced the outcome. Similarly, Buess et al. (2009) retrospectively studied 32 single-row and 33 double-row repairs with the simple shoulder test and visual analog scale. A subset was also evaluated by Constant score. This study found significantly more "yes" answers on the simple shoulder test and slightly better pain reduction in the double-row group. Patient satisfaction was greater than 97% in both groups. Aydin et al. (2010) followed two groups of 34 patients with small or medium rotator cuff tears treated with single- or double-row rotator repairs for at least 2 years. Both groups had improved functional outcomes and Constant scores between the two groups did not reveal any significant difference.

STRUCTURAL INTEGRITY

In addition to studying clinical outcomes, several groups have evaluated the structural integrity of single-row and double-row repairs. Charousset et al. (2007) reported no differences in structural integrity or clinical outcomes using computed tomography (CT) arthrography and multiple outcome measures. This study did demonstrate better restoration of the anatomical footprint radiographically in double-row repairs. Bosse and colleagues (Voigt et al. 2010) studied 51 patients treated with a double-row suture bridge technique and compared them with historical controls. The clinical outcome was measured by the simple shoulder test, Constant score, and MRI. The radiographic structural failure rate was 28.9%. The structural status of the repair did not affect Constant scores. The authors concluded that they could not confirm an advantage of double-row repairs in the study group relative to published results.

CLINICAL STUDIES SUGGESTING SUPERIOR OUTCOMES IN DOUBLE-ROW REPAIRS

There does appear to be some evidence that double-row repairs may be advantageous specifically in larger rotator cuff tears. Duquin et al. (2010) performed a systematic review of the literature and identified 23 studies that evaluated repair structural integrity and stratified the results according to tear size. Re-tear rates were compared among transosseous, single-row, double-row, and suture bridge techniques. Analysis of open or arthroscopic technique was also performed. Significantly lower re-tear rates were seen for all tears >1 cm (**Table 14.1**). There was no difference between transosseous and single-row repairs, and structural outcomes were independent of arthroscopic or open technique (Duquin et al. 2010).

Another recent systematic review of the literature concluded that double-row repairs may result in improved structural healing at the site of repair, but that there is no evidence of any functional outcome advantage (Saridakis and Jones 2010) Additional evidence for an advantage of double-row repairs was provided by Park et al. who demonstrated significantly better functional outcome scores (Constant, ASES, and shoulder severity index [SSI]) in their double-row repairs at 2 years postoperatively in tears >3 cm (Park JY et al. 2008). This study is limited by lack of randomization and no evaluation of structural integrity. Similarly favorable, but limited, data were provided by Lafosse et al. (2007) who described decreased structural failure in double-row repairs compared with historical controls. Further support for a structural advantage of double-row repairs was reported by Sugaya et al. (2005) who utilized postoperative MRI to document a decreased prevalence of rotator cuff defects after repair. Again, no clinical difference was detected at final follow-up.

Ji et al. (2010) retrospectively compared the clinical outcomes of 22 patients after single-row repair and 25 patients who underwent double-row repair. There was no significant difference in UCLA rating scale and ASES shoulder index scores between the two groups. Subscores of the UCLA score did demonstrate better strength and patient satisfaction in the double-row group. Pennington et al. (2010) prospectively evaluated a non-randomized group of 78 single-row, Mason–Allen, rotator cuff repairs and 54 double-row, transosseous-equivalent rotator cuff repairs. There was no significant difference seen between the single- and double-row repairs in visual analog, UCLA, or ASES score. Likewise, active range of motion and dynamometric strength were similar between the groups. A subset of patients underwent MRI evaluation of repair integrity at a minimum of 12 months and demonstrated improved radiographic healing in the double-row group when matched for tear size.

Table 14.1 Summary of healing and re-tear rate in rotator cuff tears >3 cm with various repair techniques

Repair	n	Complete healing	Incomplete healing	Re-torn	% Re-torn
Transosseous	98	44	7	47	48
Single-row, suture anchor	138	61	17	60	44
Double-row, suture anchor	230	129	39	62	27
Suture bridge	10	9	0	1	10
Transosseous + suture anchor	236	105	24	107	45
Double-row, suture anchors + suture bridge	240	138	39	63	26*

*p <0.01 compared to transosseous and single-row suture anchor.

Reproduced with permission from Duquin TR, Buyea C, Bisson LJ. Which method of rotator cuff repair leads to the highest rate of structural healing? A systematic review. Am J Sports Med. 2010;38:835–841.)

CONCLUSION

The goal of rotator cuff surgery is to achieve superior clinical outcomes and durable structural integrity of the repair. Improved understanding of soft-tissue healing and the rotator cuff insertion led to the development of double-row repair techniques. Recent cadaveric literature suggests a biomechanical advantage of double-row repairs with superior load to failure, footprint anatomy restoration, footprint pressure, and load sharing. Although multiple level 1 studies have not shown a significant clinical advantage in double-row repairs, there is evidence suggesting superior structural outcomes when using a double-row repair in tears larger than 1 cm. However, this tendency needs to be confirmed by appropriately powered, well-executed, level I investigations.

REFERENCES

Ahmad CS, Vorys GC, Covey A, et al. Rotator cuff repair fluid extravasation characteristics are influenced by repair technique. J Shoulder Elbow Surg 2009;18:976–981.

Apreleva M, Ozbaydar M, Fitzgibbons PG, Warner JJ. Rotator cuff tears: the effect of the reconstruction method on three-dimensional repair site area. Arthroscopy 2002;18:519–526.

Aydin N, Kocaoglu B, Guven O. Single-row versus double-row arthroscopic rotator cuff repair in small- to medium-sized tears. J Shoulder Elbow Surg 2010;19:722–725.

Baums MH, Spahn G, Steckel H, et al. Comparative evaluation of the tendon-bone interface contact pressure in different single- versus double-row suture anchor repair techniques. Knee Surg Sports Traumatol Arthrosc 2009;17:1466–1472.

Baums MH, Geyer M, Buschken M, et al. Tendon-bone contact pressure and biomechanical evaluation of a modified suture-bridge technique for rotator cuff repair. Knee Surg Sports Traumatol Arthrosc 2010;18:992–998.

Buess E, Waibl B, Vogel R, Seidner R. A comparative clinical evaluation of arthroscopic single-row versus double-row supraspinatus tendon repair. Acta Orthop Belg 2009;75:588–594.

Burkhart SS, Adams CR, Schoolfield JD. A biomechanical comparison of 2 techniques of footprint reconstruction for rotator cuff repair: the SwiveLock-FiberChain construct versus standard double-row repair. Arthroscopy 2009;25:274–281.

Burks RT, Crim J, Brown N, et al. A prospective randomized clinical trial comparing arthroscopic single- and double-row rotator cuff repair: magnetic resonance imaging and early clinical evaluation. Am J Sports Med 2009;37:674–682.

Charousset C, Grimberg J, Duranthon LD, et al. Can a double-row anchorage technique improve tendon healing in arthroscopic rotator cuff repair?: A prospective, nonrandomized, comparative study of double-row and single-row anchorage techniques with computed tomographic arthrography tendon healing assessment. Am J Sports Med 2007;35:1247–1253.

Dines JS, Bedi A, ElAttrache NS, Dines DM. Single-row versus double-row rotator cuff repair: techniques and outcomes. J Am Acad Orthop Surg 2010;18:83–93.

Dugas JR, Campbell DA, Warren RF, et al. Anatomy and dimensions of rotator cuff insertions. J Shoulder Elbow Surg 2002;11:498–503.

Duquin TR, Buyea C, Bisson LJ. Which method of rotator cuff repair leads to the highest rate of structural healing? A systematic review. Am J Sports Med 2010;38:835–841.

Franceschi F, Ruzzini L, Longo UG, et al. Equivalent clinical results of arthroscopic single-row and double-row suture anchor repair for rotator cuff tears: a randomized controlled trial. Am J Sports Med 2007;35:1254–1260.

Gerber C, Schneeberger AG, Beck M, Schlegel U. Mechanical strength of repairs of the rotator cuff. J Bone Joint Surg Br 1994;76:371–380.

Grasso A, Milano G, Salvatore M, et al. Single-row versus double-row arthroscopic rotator cuff repair: a prospective randomized clinical study. Arthroscopy 2009;25:4–12.

Grimberg J, Diop A, Kalra K, et al. In vitro biomechanical comparison of three different types of single- and double-row arthroscopic rotator cuff repairs: analysis of continuous bone-tendon contact pressure and surface during different simulated joint positions. J Shoulder Elbow Surg 2010;19:236–243.

Hepp P, Osterhoff G, Engel T, et al. Biomechanical evaluation of knotless anatomical double-layer double-row rotator cuff repair: a comparative ex vivo study. Am J Sports Med 2009;37:1363–1369.

Ji JH, Shafi M, Kim WY, Kim YY. Clinical outcomes of arthroscopic single and double row repair in full thickness rotator cuff tears. Indian J Orthop 2010;44:308–313.

Kim DH, Elattrache NS, Tibone JE, et al. Biomechanical comparison of a single-row versus double-row suture anchor technique for rotator cuff repair. Am J Sports Med 2006;34:407–414.

Kulwicki KJ, Kwon YW, Kummer FJ. Suture anchor loading after rotator cuff repair: effects of an additional lateral row. J Shoulder Elbow Surg 2010;19:81–85.

Lafosse L, Brozska R, Toussaint B, Gobezie R. The outcome and structural integrity of arthroscopic rotator cuff repair with use of the double-row suture anchor technique. J Bone Joint Surg Am 2007;89:1533–1541.
Mahar A, Tamborlane J, Oka R, et al. Single-row suture anchor repair of the rotator cuff is biomechanically equivalent to double-row repair in a bovine model. Arthroscopy 2007;23:1265–1270.
Mazzocca AD, Bollier MJ, Ciminiello AM, et al. Biomechanical evaluation of arthroscopic rotator cuff repairs over time. Arthroscopy 2010;26:592–599.
Meier SW, Meier JD. Rotator cuff repair: the effect of double-row fixation on three-dimensional repair site. J Shoulder Elbow Surg 2006;15:691–696.
Milano G, Grasso A, Zarelli D, et al. Comparison between single-row and double-row rotator cuff repair: a biomechanical study. Knee Surg Sports Traumatol Arthrosc 2008;16:75–80.
Mochizuki T, Sugaya H, Uomizu M, et al. Humeral insertion of the supraspinatus and infraspinatus. New anatomical findings regarding the footprint of the rotator cuff. J Bone Joint Surg Am 2008;90:962–969.
Nelson CO, Sileo MJ, Grossman MG, Serra-Hsu F. Single-row modified mason-allen versus double-row arthroscopic rotator cuff repair: a biomechanical and surface area comparison. Arthroscopy 2008;24:941–948.
Oguma H, Murakami G, Takahashi-Iwanaga H, et al. Early anchoring collagen fibers at the bone-tendon interface are conducted by woven bone formation: light microscope and scanning electron microscope observation using a canine model. J Orthop Res 2001;19:873–880.
Park JY, Lhee SH, Choi JH, et al. Comparison of the clinical outcomes of single- and double-row repairs in rotator cuff tears. Am J Sports Med 2008;36:1310–1316.
Park MC, ElAttrache NS, Tibone JE, et al. Part I: Footprint contact characteristics for a transosseous-equivalent rotator cuff repair technique compared with a double-row repair technique. J Shoulder Elbow Surg 2007;16:461–468.
Park MC, Pirolo JM, Park CJ, et al. The effect of abduction and rotation on footprint contact for single-row, double-row, and modified double-row rotator cuff repair techniques. Am J Sports Med 2009;37:1599–1608.
Pennington WT, Gibbons DJ, Bartz BA, et al. Comparative analysis of single-row versus double-row repair of rotator cuff tears. Arthroscopy 2010;26:1419–1426.
Saridakis P, Jones G. Outcomes of single-row and double-row arthroscopic rotator cuff repair: a systematic review. J Bone Joint Surg Am 2010;92:732–742.
Sugaya H, Maeda K, Matsuki K, Moriishi J. Functional and structural outcome after arthroscopic full-thickness rotator cuff repair: single-row versus dual-row fixation. Arthroscopy 2005;21:1307–1316.
Tuoheti Y, Itoi E, Yamamoto N, et al. Contact area, contact pressure, and pressure patterns of the tendon-bone interface after rotator cuff repair. Am J Sports Med 2005;33:1869–1874.
Voigt C, Bosse C, Vosshenrich R, et al. Arthroscopic supraspinatus tendon repair with suture-bridging technique: functional outcome and magnetic resonance imaging. Am J Sports Med 2010;38:983–991.

Chapter 15 Growth factors and tendon healing

Francesco Oliva, Nicola Maffulli

KEY FEATURES

- Growth factors directly affect cellular mitogenesis and chemotaxis. They are able to influence the healing cascade, but the exact process by which this happens remains to be clarified.
- The release of growth factors significantly increases the in vitro proliferation of human tendon cells and stimulates them to produce angiogenic factors such as vascular endothelial growth factor and hepatocyte growth factor.
- Few studies have been conducted that elucidate the timing of the expression of the various growth factors during the different phases of the tendon healing process.

INTRODUCTION

Tendons connect muscle to bone. They modulate the transmission of muscle-derived forces to bone. The basic cell biology of tendons is still not fully understood, and the management of tendon injury still constitutes a considerable challenge for clinicians.

Tendon injuries can be acute or chronic, and are caused by intrinsic or extrinsic factors, either alone or in combination. In acute trauma, extrinsic factors predominate. Overuse injuries and chronic tendon disorders generally have a multifactorial origin (Benjamin and Ralphs 1995).

The pathological label "tendinosis" has been in use for more than three decades to describe the typical lesion of tendinopathy, and is only one of the features of tendinopathy (Maffulli et al. 1998). Many clinicians still use the term "tendonitis" or "tendinitis," thus implying that the fundamental problem is inflammatory. As the essential lesion of tendinopathy is a failed healing response, we advocate the use of the term "tendinopathy" as a generic descriptor of the clinical conditions in and around tendons arising from overuse, and suggest that the terms "tendinosis," "tendonitis," and "tendinitis" be used after only histopathological examination (Maffulli et al. 1998).

Growth factors are synthesized and secreted by a wide variety of inflammatory cells, platelets, fibroblasts, epithelial cells, and vascular endothelial cells. Growth factors bind to external receptors on the cell membrane, which leads to intracellular changes in DNA synthesis and expression.

Growth factors directly affect cellular mitogenesis and chemotaxis, and are able to influence the healing cascade. The exact process by which this happens remains to be clarified (Mehta and Mass 2005).

Historical studies

Researchers have been studying the growth factor requirements of tendon cells for over three decades. Initial experiments focused on the actions of epidermal growth factor (EGF), insulin, and platelet-derived growth factor (PDGF) in the in vitro setting (Gauger et al. 1985; Stein et al. 1985). These experiments showed that EGF and insulin could reduce the reliance of the cultured tendon cell on serum. The positive impact of insulin and insulin-like growth factor (IGF-1) was again demonstrated in an in vitro rabbit flexor tendon model in which matrix synthesis stimulation and increased cell proliferation were observed (Abrahamsson et al. 1991).

In an alternative approach to growth factor supplementation, protein extracts were prepared from both normal and injured canine flexor tendons (Duffy et al. 1995). Through this methodology, it became apparent that normal tendons contained basic fibroblastic growth factor (bFGF) whereas in healing tendons there where notable levels of PDGF and EGF. Subsequent to this study, PDGF was demonstrated to promote repair of the medial collateral ligament of rats (Batten et al. 1996). Bone morphogenetic protein 7 (BMP 7) was excluded as a reparative growth factor in the rat's Achilles tendon repair model, with bone formation observed (Forslund and Aspenberg 1998). Reinforcing the findings of previous in vivo studies, it was noted that low levels of bFGF were present in uninjured rabbit flexor tendons, and bFGF was then upregulated following on from injury (Chang et al. 1998). The technique of deriving platelet-rich plasma (PRP), developed in the late 1990s (Marx et al. 1998), and an effective means to concentrate endogenous growth factors, is now commonly used in North America (Mishra and Pavelko 2006) and continental Europe (Anitua et al. 2006 ;Sanchez et al. 2007).

TENDON INJURIES

Tendon injuries can be acute or chronic, and are caused by intrinsic or extrinsic factors, either alone or in combination. Intrinsic factors such as alignment and biomechanical faults play a causative role in many tendon injuries including in two-thirds of Achilles tendon disorders in athletes (Kvist 1991, 1994). Excessive loading of tendons during vigorous physical training is regarded as the main pathological stimulus for tendinopathy, but tendon damage may also occur from stresses within the physiological limits, because frequent cumulative microtrauma may not allow enough time for repair (Selvanetti et al. 1997; Tallon et al. 2001).

Tendon repair

Tendon repair can occur either intrinsically via the resident tenocytes (Gelberman et al. 1984) or via extrinsic mechanisms, whereby cells from the surrounding sheath or synovium invade the tissue (Potenza 1962). Three biologically and temporally overlapping phases are described during tendon repair (Sharma and Maffulli 2006). Various attempts to improve the healing process can have different effects on different phases (**Fig. 15.1**):

1. The inflammatory phase is characterized by: hematoma, platelet activation, and invasion of cells that form a granuloma. Usually, this phase occurs 3–7 days after the injury; cells migrate from the extrinsic peritendinous tissue such as the tendon sheath, periosteum, subcutaneous tissue, and fascicles, as well as from the epitenon and endotenon (Reddy et al. 1999).
2. In the formative phase, cells proliferate and differentiate. The migrated fibroblasts in the granuloma produce collagen (mostly collagen type III), which gradually increases its mechanical strength, so that loading can lead to elastic deformation; this allows mechanical signaling to start to influence the process. Production of collagen type I gradually takes over, and the repair callus reaches its largest size. Tenocytes become the main cell type, and over the next 5 weeks collagen is continuously synthesized. This phase of repair continues for 8 weeks after the initial injury (Maffulli and Benazzo 2000).
3. Finally, in the remodeling phase, collagen type III is reabsorbed and replaced to produce better organization, and cross-linking increases. The callus transverse area gradually decreases as the mechanical tissue properties improve. Despite intensive remodeling over the following months, complete regeneration of the tendon is never achieved. The tissue replacing the defect remains hypercellular. The diameter of the collagen fibrils is altered, favoring thinner fibrils with reduction in the biomechanical strength of the tendon (Maffulli et al. 2002).

The timing of growth factor release in the healing process is poorly understood. In a rabbit model, during healing of acute midsubstance rotator cuff tears, Kobayashi et al. (2006) assessed semiquantitatively the time expression of bFGF, IGF-1, PDGF, and transforming growth factor (TGF-β) for 28 days. IGF-1 and TGF-β appear first in the blood cells in the inflammation phase; bFGF and PDGF appear later during the formative phase.

Würgler-Hauri et al. (2007) studied bFGF, bone morphogenic proteins BMP-12, BMP-13, and BMP-14, cartilage oligomeric matrix protein (COMP), connective tissue growth factor (CTGF), PDGF-B, and TGF-β1 in tendon-to-bone healing in a rat supraspinatus model for 16 weeks. Immunoassays showed an increase in the expression of all growth factors at 1 week, followed by a return to control or undetectable levels by 16 weeks in both the insertion and midsubstance.

The release of growth factors significantly increases the in vitro proliferation of human tendon cells and stimulates them to produce angiogenic factors such as vascular endothelial growth factor (VEGF) and hepatocyte growth factor (HGF). This might be particularly relevant in the tendon repair process, assuming that the reduced blood supply to the tendon is associated with its low healing capability. Moreover, HGF is a potent anti-fibrotic agent with potential to reduce the formation of scarring around tendon tissue. Scarring itself is correlated with inferior repair quality (Awad et al. 2003).

Growth factors in tendon healing

Numerous growth factors are involved in tendon repair. These include BMPs, EGF, FGF1, FGF2, IGF-I, IGF-II, PDGF-AA, PDGF-BB, PDGF-AB, and TGF-β. These may be produced locally by cells in areas of injury, growth, and repair, or may be delivered by blood. In the rat supraspinatus tendon model, numerous growth factors increased markedly 1 week after injury in both the insertion and midsubstance zones. These growth factors included BMP-12, BMP13, BMP-14, bFGF, COMP, CTGF, PDGF-B, and TGF-β1. All increases had returned to pre-injury levels by 16 weeks, establishing a clear connection between in vivo upregulation and repair (Würgler-Hauri et al. 2007). Exogenous supplementation of these factors in failed healing responses, such as in resistant tendinopathies, may lead to a definitive healing response.

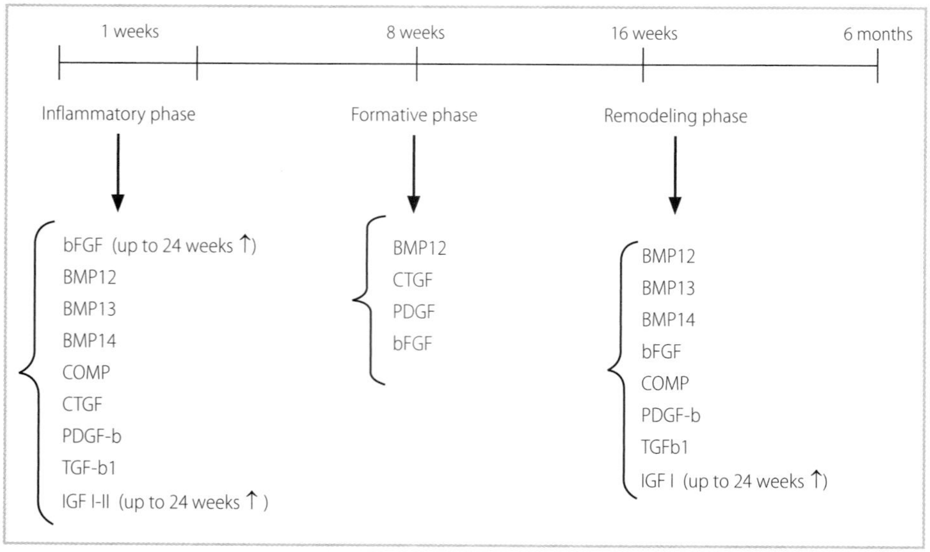

Figure 15.1 The healing process of all tendons pass through three well-known stages. Growth factors are expressed during all these phases, promoting cell proliferation, extracellular matrix production, and also participating in the final remodeling of the tendon. This figure shows how the timing of some growth factors, possibly studied in the near future, will be modified after new research but must be kept in mind, because the addition of growth factors too early or late in the tendon healing process can decrease their effectiveness. AFA, autologous fibrin adhesive; bFGF, basic fibroblast growth factor; BMP, bone morphogenic protein; CDMP, cartilage-derived morphogenetic proteins; COMP, cartilage oligomeric matrix protein; CTGF, connective tissue growth factor; EGF, epidermal growth factor; ESWT, extracorporeal shock wave therapy; FGF, fibroblast growth factor; GDF, growth differentiation factor; GF, growth factors; HGF, hepatocyte growth factor; hsp47, heat shock protein 47; IGF-1, insulin-like growth factor-1; IGFBPs, insulin-like growth factor-binding proteins; iNOS, inducible nitric oxide synthase; MMP, matrix metalloproteinase; mRNA, messenger ribonucleic acid; PDGF, platelet-derived growth factor; PDGF-BB, platelet-derived growth factor isoform B; PIGF, placenta growth factor; PRP, platelet-rich plasma; RC, rotator cuff; Smad, small mothers against decapentaplegic; TGF-β, transforming growth factor β; TIEG, TGF-β-inducible early gene; VEGF, vascular endothelial growth factor.

Basic fibroblastic growth factor

Basic FGF is a single-chain polypeptide of 146 amino acids, and is a member of the part of heparin-binding growth factor family. In humans, 22 members have been identified, all of which are structurally related signaling molecules. Basic FGF is angiogenic (Gabra et al. 1994) and has mitogenic effects on many mesenchymal cells such as ligament fibroblasts (Lee et al. 1995).

This growth factor has been shown to be involved in wound healing. Chan BP et al. (1997) showed that, in vitro, supplementation of bFGF increases the proliferation of rat patellar tendon fibroblasts. Chang et al. in 1998 showed that bFGF mRNA is upregulated in the tendon wound environment, and upregulated in tenocytes as well as in tendon sheath fibroblasts and inflammatory cells in vivo (Chang et al. 1998).

Basic FGF has also a stimulatory effect on human rotator cuff tendon cells in vitro, but suppresses collagen synthesis (Takahasih et al. 2002). Kobayashi et al. (2006) show an immunohistochemical peak expression of bFGF in the first week in a midsubstance injury of supraspinatus tendon in the rabbit, and it was suggested that bFGF could be used to promote the healing process of a torn rotator cuff tendon (Gullotta and Rodeo 2009). In a rabbit supraspinatus tendon bone injury, Würgler-Hauri et al. (2007) supported this finding and, in addition, they detected another increase of bFGF at 8 weeks.

Bone morphogenetic proteins

BMPs are a group of factors of the TGF-β superfamily that stimulate bone formation but also stimulate tendon cell mitogenesis and tendon healing. Although it is clear that BMPs stimulate tendon healing, the exact mechanism remains unclear (Chhabra et al. 2003; Yu et al. 2007). A combination of BMP signaling and influences of mechanical loading is likely crucial for tendon healing. This is reinforced by the BMP-14 knockout mice studies in which a delayed tendon healing response and irregular type I collagen fibrils were observed (Chhabra et al. 2003). However, in rat Achilles tendon injury models, BMP-13, not BMP-14, appeared to be involved in early tendon healing, whereas BMP-14 was primarily required for the maintenance of homeostasis of mature tendons, and BMP-12 was required for both (Eliasson et al. 2008). BMP-12, BMP-13, and BMP-14 have all been detected in intact human tendons by immunohistochemistry (Fu et al. 2003; Chuen et al. 2004).

Ovoid tendon cells (tenoblasts) in patellar tendons display elevated levels of both BMP-12 and BMP-13 when compared with the elongated tendon cells (tenocytes) (Chuen et al. 2004). This suggests that tenoblasts are more active in matrix remodeling and healing than tenocytes. In addition, BMP-2, BMP-7, and BMP-12 all participate in tendon–bone healing and improve formation of new bone and fibrocartilage at the healing tendon attachment site, resulting in an improved load to failure (Rodeo 2007).

Recently, gene therapy with the BMP-12 cDNA muscle graft showed histologically better organized and homogeneous pattern of collagen fibers at all time points than the control groups (Majewski et al. 2008). Recombinant BMP-12 on a sponge carrier also stimulated rotator cuff repair in the sheep model (Seeherman et al. 2008). Although BMP-14 did not appear to be involved directly in healing in the Achilles tendon model, BMP-14 gene therapy did increase tendon tensile strength in a rat model of Achilles tendon injury (Bolt et al. 2007).

Insulin-like growth factor

Insulin-like growth factor is named after its hypoglycemic effect following intravenous administration. The stimulatory effects of IGF-1 have been demonstrated in many cell types, including cartilage, bone, muscle, and tendon cells (Trippel et al. 1993). During tendon healing, its role seems to stimulate the proliferation and migration of the tenoblasts during the inflammatory phase, whereas its increase in the remodeling phase seems to be clear (Molloy et al. 2003; Dahlgren et al. 2005). In addition to the mitogenic effect, IGF-1 can also stimulate selected components of matrix synthesis, and its expression was noted in avian tenocytes (Tsuzaki et al. 2000).

Complementary to this are the observations that IGF-1 induced tenocyte migration, division, and matrix expression, and accelerated functional recovery from Achilles tendon injury in a rat model (Banes et al. 1995; Abrahamsson and Lohmander 1996; Kurtz et al. 1999). However, IGF-1 was not observed in tenocytes on day 10 after injury in a canine flexor tendon repair model, but was instead located in the surrounding inflammatory cells (Tsubone et al. 2004). Similar observations were noted in studies concerning lesions of the flexor digitorum superficialis tendons of both forelimbs (Dahlgren et al. 2005). Similar to the canine model, IGF-1 levels had decreased by approximately 40% when compared with normal tendon at 2 weeks. Continued analysis then revealed a substantial upregulation of IGF-1, exceeding normal tendons. By 4 weeks, IGF-1 levels had increased substantially and were maintained through to 8 weeks. IGF-1 also improved aspects of healing in an equine model of collagenase-induced flexor tendinopathy (Dahlgren et al. 2002).

The expression of the IGF-1-binding proteins (IGFBPs) has been studied in equine flexor tendons after acute injury and during healing over time: mRNA and protein expression for IGFBP-2, -3, and -4 was detected in normal tendon, and showed a marked increase after injury (Dahlgren et al. 2006). IGF-1, PDGF-BB, and bFGF were used alone and in combination to optimize tenocyte proliferation in cells of the synovial sheath, epitenon, and endotenon isolated from rabbit flexor digitorum profundus tendons. For all three tendon cell populations, proliferation at 72 hours was greater in the presence of individual growth factors. In addition, a synergistic effect was observed if growth factors were used in association compared with maximal doses of individual growth factors (Costa et al. 2006). Systemic administration of IGF-1 improves healing in collagenous extracellular matrices from loaded and unloaded tissues (Provenzano et al. 2007).

Platelet-derived growth factor

PDGF was first isolated from platelets, but can be produced by many different cells, including smooth muscle cells (Bowen-Pope and Ross 1984). PDGF is a basic protein of approximately 30 kDa formed by two subunits (α and β chain) that exist in three isoforms. Most studies are focused on the homodimer PDGF-BB isoform, which has stimulatory effects on both cell division and matrix synthesis.

An investigation into the consequences of administration of PDGF-BB directly into the wound gap of rat patellar tendons showed that early supplementation (day 3 post-injury) was not beneficial to restoration of mechanical properties (Chan BP et al. 2006), probably from an increase in cell proliferation without matrix production. Later supplementation with PDGF-BB (on day 7 post-injury) did stimulate matrix production, with an accompanying higher peak load and pyridinoline content. PDGF-BB stimulated matrix and DNA synthesis in a dose-dependent manner in intrasynovial intermediate and proximal segments of deep flexor tendons, and extrasynovial peroneal tendons of rabbits during short-term cultures. PDGF-BB stimulated collagen synthesis and non-collagen protein synthesis in proximal intrasynovial tendon segments more than in extrasynovial peroneal tendon segments, and DNA synthesis less in proximal than in intermediate intrasynovial tendons (Yoshikawa and Abrahamsson 2001).

PDGF holds particular promise in combination with other growth factors. Tendon cells express the receptor for PDGF, but do not normally express PDGF itself (Tsuzaki et al. 2000). When applied with IGF-1, robust stimulation of tendon fibroblast migration and cell division are produced (Banes et al. 1995; Abrahamsson and Lohmander 1996; Bynum et al. 1997). In addition, IGF-1 and PDGF act synergistically with cyclical tension to stimulate cell division. A further examination into the response of human tendon fibroblasts to cyclical mechanical stretching demonstrated that concentrations of TGF-β, bFGF, and PDGF all increased compared with non-stretched controls (Skutek et al. 2001). Moreover, serum, which contains both PDGF and IGF-1, stimulates cells in the whole tendon both mitogenically and matrigenically, and synergistically with cyclic load (Banes et al. 1999). Taken together, these suggest that PDGF and IGF-1 may exert a positive influence on tendon and ligament healing through stimulation of cell proliferation, differentiation, and matrix formation. Additional studies have shown that it is likely that matrix formation was stimulated predominantly by PDGF (Eppley et al. 2004; de Mos et al. 2008). In a tissue engineering study, PDGF-BB-transduced cells stimulated adjacent rat tendon fibroblasts to increase collagen synthesis by 300% at 24 hours compared with a 28% increase in IGF-1-transduced cells (Uggen et al. 2005).

In a study of intrasynovial canine tendon, PDGF-BB and bFGF significantly increased flexor tendon fibroblast proliferation, collagen production, and matrix synthesis when each was applied on its own. The combined administration of PDGF-BB and bFGF led to increased proliferation (Thomopoulos et al. 2005). In a study on the expression of growth factors in normal canine flexor tendon healing, PDGF-AA, PDGF-BB, and VEGF appeared in the whole tendon section 10 days after tendon injury (Tsubone et al. 2004). Mechanical stretching of tendon fibroblasts also promoted increased concentrations of TGF-β, PDGF, and bFGF, suggesting that cyclical mechanical stretching may have a positive influence on tendon and ligament healing through stimulation of cell proliferation, differentiation, and matrix formation (Skutek et al. 2001). PDGF in association with hypoxia exerts a synergistic effect that increases the expression of VEGF in Achilles tendon fibroblasts (Petersen et al. 2003).

In a similar canine model, PDGF-BB delivery increased cell proliferation, matrix remodeling, and accelerated flexor tendon healing (Thomopoulos et al. 2007). The functional properties of repaired intrasynovial flexor tendons in an animal model study were significantly improved with the sustained administration of PDGF-BB. The range of motion of the proximal and distal interphalangeal joints was significantly higher for the PDGF-BB-treated tendons compared with the repair-alone tendons. Excursion values were also significantly higher in the PDGF-BB-treated tendons. There were no significant differences in tensile properties when comparing PDGF-BB-treated with repair-alone tendons. The failure to achieve improvements in ultimate load, stiffness, and strain in the experimental group may have resulted from suboptimal PDGF-BB dosage or suboptimal release kinetics (Gelberman et al. 2007).

Exogenous PDGF genes can be transferred effectively into intrasynovial tenocytes. The transfer increases significantly the expression of genes for PDGF and type I collagen (Wang et al. 2004). In another study, PDGF gene therapy was more beneficial to tendon healing than VEGF gene therapy in an in vitro study of rat intrasynovial tendons (Wang et al. 2005).

Transforming growth factor β

Originally, TGF-β was thought to be related to cellular transformation events before neoplastic growth. It is now clear that TGF-β has numerous physiological effects (Chan et al. 2008). The expression of TGF-β appears closely tied to the expression of a differentiated phenotype in many cell lines including the mesenchymal precursor. Tendon and ligament formation has been tied directly to factors belonging to the TGF-β superfamily (Wolfman et al. 1997). Proliferation, and matrix synthesis and differentiation have also been affected in tenoblasts, chondroblasts, and osteoblasts (Herpin et al. 2004). Whether this is an inhibitory or stimulatory effect depends on the stage of differentiation, presence of other growth factors, and assay system used (Fu et al. 2005; Anitua et al. 2007).

TGF-β is a weak stimulator of tendon cell migration and mitogenesis, but can stimulate robust expression of extracellular matrix (Banes et al. 1994). TGF-β affects gene expression primarily through the activation of the Smad signaling pathway. The first step in the Smad pathway is the expression of TGF-β-inducible early gene (TIEG). Healing of tendons in the TIEG knockout mouse suggests the possibility of tendon healing in the absence of the Smad pathway, and the existence of TIEG-independent routes (Tsubone et al. 2006). TGF-β1 significantly increased the amount of SMA (alpha-smooth muscle actin) in non-vascular cells in seven human rotator cuffs, suggesting that SMA-containing cells could contribute to the retraction of the torn ends of a ruptured rotator cuff and play an important role in healing (Premdas et al. 2001).

In a canine flexor tendon injury repair model, TGF-β was detected at and proximal to the repair site (Tsubone et al. 2004). Complementary to these findings was the observation that, in Achilles rat tendon healing models, the failure load and stiffness of the healing tendon were increased by administration of TGF-β1 at 2 and 4 weeks (Kashiwagi et al. 2004). Furthermore, the application of TGF-β1 significantly increased the tangent modulus and tensile strength of the fibrous tissue produced in the rabbit patellar tendon after resecting the central portion, suggesting a role of TGF-β1 in in vivo tendon regeneration (Anaguchi et al. 2005).

TGF-β may control the switching point in the healing process from normal to pathological (Blobe et al. 2000). All three TGF-β isoforms significantly increase collagen I and III production in cultured tendon fibroblasts (Klein et al. 2002). TGF-β1 induced a greater degree of contraction in tendon fibroblasts cultured in collagen gels compared with TGF-β3 (Campbell et al. 2004). This might explain the finding that TGF-β1 induces scar tissue formation, whereas TGF-β3 reduces it (Shah et al. 1995). Intraoperative infiltration of neutralizing antibody to TGF-β1 improves flexor tendon excursion, but simultaneous infiltration of neutralizing antibody to TGF-β2 nullifies this effect. Therefore, TGF-β isoforms may interact with each other to modulate collagen synthesis in healing tendons (Chang et al. 2000).

The temporal and spatial distribution of three TGF-βreceptor isoforms (RI, RII, and RIII) was analyzed in a rabbit zone II flexor tendon wound healing model. This demonstrated that TGF-β receptors were upregulated after injury and during repair (Ngo et al. 2001). Receptor production was concentrated in the epitenon, tendon sheath, and along the repair site. Peak levels of TGF-βreceptor expression where noted on day 14 and persisted until day 56.

The pathogenesis of tissue fibrosis during flexor tendon repair is also dependent, in part, on TGF-β signaling. In a rabbit flexor tendon model, TGF-β inhibition by neutralizing antibody was effective in reducing collagen I production in cultured flexor tendon cells which, in turn, could potentially reduce scar formation (Zhang et al. 2004). Tendon sheath fibroblasts, epitenon tenocytes, and endotenon tenocytes isolated from rabbit flexor tendons have demonstrated significant increases in the functional activity of TGF-β when exposed to lactate. Modulation of local lactate levels may therefore provide a mechanism whereby the effects of TGF-β on adhesion formation in flexor tendon wound healing can be modulated (Yalamanchi et al. 2004). Further distinction was provided with the demonstration that, although exogenous addition of TGF-β1 increased the contraction of human patellar tenocytes, TGF-β3 appeared to decrease contraction (Campbell et al. 2004). This suggests that, although TGF-β1 promotes scarring, TGF-β3 can improve the mechanical properties of healing tendons. Complementary to these findings were the observations concerning the locations of TGF-β1 and TGF-β3 and the formation of collagens in the rat supraspinatus tendon during tendon-to-bone healing after an acute injury. Collagen I protein and mRNA significantly increased at 10 days, and reached a plateau by 28 and 56 days. Collagen III showed a similar trend, with an early increase, remaining high until day 56. TGF-β1 was localized to the forming scar tissue and showed a distinct peak at 10 days. TGFβ-3 was not seen at the healing insertion site. Cell proliferation and density followed the same trend as TGF-β1 (Galatz et al. 2006).

Examination of tenoblasts from adult human patellar tendons revealed higher levels of TGF-β1 (and procollagen type I, heat shock protein hsp47, MMP1, BMP12, BMP13) than tenocytes. Higher expression of TGF-β1 might therefore be associated with the major activity of tenoblasts in tendon matrix remodeling (Chuen et al. 2004).

Extracorporeal shock wave therapy (ESWT) has recently been used in the management of Achilles tendinopathy (Rompe et al. 2007). In rats with collagenase-induced Achilles tendinopathy, 200 ESWT impulses restored biomechanical and biochemical characteristics of healing tendons 12 weeks after treatment. The proliferation of tenocytes added to hypertrophied cell aggregates and newly formed tendon tissue coincided with intensive TGF-β1 and IGF-1 expression. This suggested that TGF-1 and IGF-1 played important roles in mediating ESWT-stimulated cell proliferation and tissue regeneration of tendon (Chen et al. 2004).

Formation of nitric oxide is an important event in the course of tendon healing, and its inhibition results in chronic inflammation and fibrosis due to an imbalance in TGF-β expression in vivo (Darmani et al. 2004). Examining the expression of inducible nitric oxide synthase (iNOS) and TGF-β in macrophage infiltrates within crush-injured digital flexor tendon and synovium of rats during normal tendon healing, the levels of TGF-β are high at first, and gradually decrease after 3 weeks of injury (Darmani et al. 2004).

Vascular endothelial growth factors

They are important signaling proteins involved in both vasculogenesis and angiogenesis. The broad term "VEGF" covers a number of proteins from two families, which result from alternate splicing of mRNA from a single, eight-exon, VEGF gene. The most important member is VEGF-A, a glycosylated protein of 46–48 kDa composed of two disulfide-linked subunits. Other members are placenta growth factor (PIGF), VEGF-B, VEGF-C, and VEGF-D. The last ones were discovered later than VEGF-A, and before their discovery VEGF-A was termed "VEGF." All members of the VEGF family stimulate cellular responses by binding to tyrosine kinase receptors (the VEGFRs) on the cell surface, causing them to dimerize and become activated through transphosphorylation, although to different sites, times, and extents (Ferrara and Gerber 2002). In New Zealand white rabbits that had undergone a closed tenotomy of the flexor digitorum profundus tendon, numerous fine new vessels forming at the tip of lacerated tendons were shown. Adhesions that formed between tendons and the surrounding connective tissues were also highly vascularized (Matthews 1977).

Increased vascularity at the tendon stump after tendon division and suture was also shown in the flexor tendons of the canine forefoot (Potenza 1962). Bidder et al. (2000), using *in situ* hybridization in a canine model of tendon injury, identified cell populations within the repair site expressing message for VEGF, suggesting their potential for organizing the angiogenic response during the early postoperative phase of wound tendon healing. Pufe et al. (2001) demonstrated that VEGF concentrations are negligible in healthy human adult Achilles tendons, but high in ruptured and embryonic ones. The splice forms detected in the area of rupture of torn Achilles tendons were VEGF121 and VEGF165. The same authors also showed that in vitro rat tenocytes stimulated with EGF raised VEGF secretion two- to sixfold, whereas hypoxic conditions alone (5% O_2) raised VEGF secretion only twofold. However, the combination of EGF and hypoxia increased VEGF production 30- to 40-fold, apparently a synergistic effect (Pufe et al. 2001). Fenwick et al. (2002) denounce the lack of research on the distribution of receptors for potential angiogenic growth factors and receptors for those growth factors that may be involved in tendon repair, and advocate new studies in this field.

Growth factors and rotator cuff

Rotator cuff tendon tears account for more than 4.5 million physician visits per year, and over 250 000 rotator cuff repair surgeries performed annually in the USA (Yamaguchi et al. 2006). The pathogenesis of rotator cuff tears is debated Longo et al. 2009; Oliva et al. 2009). The rotator cuff has limited ability to heal back to its insertion on the humerus after repair (Gulotta and Rodeo 2009), possibly because of the poor vascularization of tendon tissue, and also because the histopathological changes that accompany a rupture are localized not only at the site of rupture but also in the macroscopic intact tendon portion, suggesting more generalized involvement of the tendon (Longo et al. 2007, 2008a,b; Maffulli et al. 2008). Gerber et al. (2000) reported a re-tear rate of 34% in 29 patients at an average of 37 months on MRI evaluation of the repair site. Given this limited ability for healing (Longo et al. 2008b), several strategies – including growth factors and cytokines, gene therapy, tendon augmentation graft, and tissue engineering with mesenchymal stem cells – have been proposed to enhance tendon healing (Gulotta and Rodeo 2009; Longo et al. 2010a,b). Several growth factors are upregulated during rotator cuff healing, and they may be used to augment rotator cuff repairs (Gulotta and Rodeo 2009).

Randelli et al. (2008) in a pilot non-randomized single group study of 14 patients showed that application of autologous platelet-rich plasma (PRP) for arthroscopic rotator cuff repair provided good clinical results.

Anitua and colleagues (2007) found faster recovery in athletes undergoing PRP-enhanced Achilles tendon repair. Athletes treated with surgery and PRP were compared with a retrospective control group of athletes treated with surgery alone. The PRP patients recovered range of motion earlier, had no wound complications, and returned to training activities in less time than control patients. The cross-sectional area of the PRP-treated tendons was also smaller than that in non-treated tendons when measured by ultrasonography.

DISCUSSION

In vitro cell-based studies and animal models have clarified the role of growth factor application. Studies show that administered growth factors enhance cell proliferation and chemotaxis (Popova et al. 2004), aid angiogenesis (Zhang et al. 2009), and influence cell differentiation during wound healing (McGrath 1990). Few studies have been conducted to better understand the timing of growth factor expression during the various phases of the healing process in tendons (Aspenberg 2007; Würgler-Hauri et al. 2007).

The time course of growth factor expression is an important element in wound healing, and a better understanding of how, where, when, and for how long such factors are expressed may help in the development of methods to manipulate their expression, accelerate healing, and reduce adhesions. The use of growth factors in soft tissue problems remains, for the time being, largely experimental.

CONCLUSION AND PERSPECTIVES

Despite the lack of knowledge of the physiology of growth factor expression and effects during the process of tendon healing, the therapeutic use of growth factors for a wide variety of soft-tissue ailments is empirically increasingly common. The study of the clinical effects of the growth factors in humans is intrinsic to the idea of biological solutions to clinical problems, and is emerging as a new paradigm in medicine, leading to the development of novel and more optimized biological preparations that might open new avenues in surgery and the management of a wide range of conditions. From a clinical viewpoint, despite the mounting laboratory evidence of the positive effects of growth factors in tendon healing, only well-conducted, appropriately powered, randomized controlled trials, with adequate outcome measures and length of follow-up, will clarify whether growth factors play a role in routine clinical practice.

REFERENCES

Abrahamsson SO, Lohmander S. Differential effects of insulin-like growth factor-I on matrix and DNA synthesis in various regions and types of rabbit tendons. J Orthop Res 1996;14:370–376.

Abrahamsson SO, Lundborg G, Lohmander LS. Long-term explant culture of rabbit flexor tendon: effects of recombinant human insulin-like growth factor-I and serum on matrix metabolism. J Orthop Res 1991; 9:503–515.

Anaguchi Y, Yasuda K, Majima T, et al. The effect of transforming growth factor-beta on mechanical properties of the fibrous tissue regenerated in the patellar tendon after resecting the central portion. Clin Biomech 2005;20:959–965.

Anitua E, Sánchez M, Nurden AT et al. New insights into and novel applications for platelet-rich fibrin therapies. Trends Biotechnol 2006 24:227–234.

Anitua E, Sánchez M, Nurden AT, et al. Reciprocal actions of platelet-secreted TGF-β1 on the production of VEGF and HGF by human tendon cells. Plastic Reconstr Surg 2007;119:950–959.

Aspenberg P. Stimulation of tendon repair: mechanical loading, GDFs and platelets. A mini-review. Int Orthop 2007;31:783–789.

Awad HA, Boivin GP, Dressler MR, et al. Repair of patellar tendon injuries using a cell–collagen composite. J Orthop Res 2003;21:420–431.

Banes AJ, Sanderson M, Boitano S, et al. Mechanical load ± growth factors induces [Ca^{2+}] release, cyclin D1 expression and DNA synthesis in avian tendon cells. In: Van Mow NE, Guilak F, Tran Son Tay R (eds), Proceedings of the Second World Congress of Biomechanics, 1994, Amsterdam.

Banes AJ, Tsuzaki M, Hu P, et al. PDGF-BB, IGF-I and mechanical load stimulate DNA synthesis in avian tendon fibroblasts in vitro. J Biomech 1995;28:1505–1513.

Banes AJ, Horesovsky G, Larson C, et al. Mechanical load stimulates expression of novel genes in vivo and in vitro in avian flexor tendon cells. Osteoarthr Cartilage 1999;7:141–153.

Batten ML, Hansen JC, Dahners LE Influence of dosage and timing of application of platelet-derived growth factor on early healing of the rat medial collateral ligament. J Orthop Res 1996;14:736–741.

Benjamin M, Ralphs J. Functional and developmental anatomy of tendons and ligaments. In: Gordon SL, Blair SJ, Fine LJ (eds), Repetitive Motion Disorders of the Upper Extremity. Rosemont, IL: American Academy of Orthopaedic Surgeons, 1995, 185–203.

Bidder M, Towler DA, Gelberman RH, Boyer MI. Expression of mRNA for vascular endothelial growth factor at the repair site of healing canine flexor tendon. J Orthop Res 2000;18:247–252.

Blobe GC, Schiemann WP, Lodish HF. Role of transforming growth factor beta in human disease. N Engl J Med 2000;342:1350–1358.

Bolt P, Clerk AN, Luu HH, et al. BMP-14 gene therapy increases tendon tensile strength in a rat model of Achilles tendon injury. J Bone Joint Surg Am 2007;89:1315–1320.

Bowen-Pope DF, Ross R. Platelet-derived growth factor. Clin Endocrinol Metab 1984;13: 191–205.

Bynum D, Almekinders L, Benjamin M, et al. Wounding in vivo and PDGF-BB in vitro stimulate tendon surface migration and loss of connesin-43 expression. Transact Ann Mtg Orthop Res Soc 1997;22:26.

Campbell BH, Agarwal C, Wang JH. TGF-beta1, TGF-beta3, and PGE(2) regulate contraction of human patellar tendon fibroblasts. Biomech Model Mechanobiol 2004;2:239–245.

Chan BP, Chan KM, Maffulli N, Webb S, Lee KK. Effect of basic fibroblast growth factor. An in vitro study of tendon healing. Clin Orthop Relat Res1997;342:239–247.

Chan BP, Fu SC, Qin L, Rolf C, Chan KM. Supplementation-time dependence of growth factors in promoting tendon healing. Clin Orthop Rel Res 2006;448:240–247.

Chan KM, Chan BP, Rosier R, Maffulli N. Future of cytokines in tissue healing. In: Chan KM, Fu F, Maffulli N, et al. (eds), Controversies in Orthopaedics Sports Medicine. Hong Kong: Williams & Wilkins Asia-Pacific Ltd, 1998: 564–576.

Chan KM, Fu SC, Wong YP, et al. Expression of transforming growth factor beta isoforms and their roles in tendon healing. Wound Repair Regen 2008;16:399–407.

Chang J, Most D, Thunder R, et al. Molecular studies in flexor tendon wound healing: the role of basic fibroblast growth factor gene expression. J Hand Surg [Am] 1998;23:1052–1058.

Chang J, Thunder R, Most D, Longaker MT, Lineaweaver WC. Studies in flexor tendon wound healing: neutralizing antibody to TGF-β1 increases postoperative range of motion. Plast Reconstr Surg 2000;105:148–155.

Chen YJ, Wang CJ, Yang KD, et al. Extracorporeal shock waves promote healing of collagenase-induced Achilles tendinitis and increase TGF-beta1 and IGF-I expression. J Orthop Res 2004;22:854–861.

Chhabra A, Tsou D, Clark RT et al. GDF-5 deficiency in mice delays Achilles tendon healing. J Orthop Res 2003;21:826–835.

Chuen FS, Chuk CY, Ping WY, et al. Immunohistochemical characterization of cells in adult human patellar tendons. J Histochem Cytochem 2004;52:1151–1157.

Costa MA, Wu C, Pham BV, et al. Tissue engineering of flexor tendons: optimization of tenocyte proliferation using growth factor supplementation. Tissue Eng 2006;12:1937–1943.

Darmani H, Crossan J, McLellan SD, Meek D, Adam C. Expression of nitric oxide synthase and transforming growth factor-beta in crush-injured tendon and synovium. Mediators Inflamm 2004;13:299–305.

Dahlgren LA, Van der Meulen MC, Bertram JE, Starrak GS, Nixon AJ. Insulin-like growth factor-I improves cellular and molecular aspects of healing in a collagenase-induced model of flexor tendinitis. J Orthop Res 2002;20:910–919.

Dahlgren LA, Mohammed HO, Nixon AJ. Temporal expression of growth factors and matrix molecules in healing tendon lesions. J Orthop Res 2005;23:84–92.

Dahlgren LA, Mohammed HO, Nixon AJ. Expression of insulin-like growth factor binding proteins in healing tendon lesions. J Orthop Res 2006;24:183–192.

de Mos M, van der Windt AE, Jahr H, et al. Can platelet-rich plasma enhance tendon repair? A cell culture study. Am J Sports Med 2008;36:1171–1178.

Duffy FJ Jr, Seiler JG, Gelberman RH, Hergrueter CA. Growth factors and canine flexor tendon healing: initial studies in uninjured and repair models. J Hand Surg [Am] 1995;20:645–649.

Eliasson P, Fahlgren A, Aspenberg P. Mechanical load and BMP signaling during during tendon repair. A role for follistatin? Clin Orthop Relat Res 2008;466:1592–1597.

Eppley BL, Woodell JE, Higgins J. Platelet quantification and growth factor analysis from platelet-rich plasma: implications for wound healing. Plast Reconstr Surg 2004;114:1502–1508.

Fenwick SA, Hazleman BL, Riley GP. The vasculature and its role in the damaged and healing tendon Arthritis Res 2002;4:252–260.

Ferrara N, Gerber HP. The role of vascular endothelial growth factor in angiogenesis. Acta Haematol 2002;106:148–156.
Forslund C, Aspenberg P. OP-1 has more effect than mechanical signals in the control of tissue differentiation in healing rat tendons. Acta Orthop Scand 1998;69:622–626.
Fu SC, Wong YP, Chan BP, et al. The roles of bone morphogenetic protein (BMP) 12 in stimulating the proliferation and matrix production of human patellar tendon fibroblasts. Life Sci 2003;72:2965–2974.
Fu SC, Wong YP, Cheuk YC, Lee KM, Chan KM. TGF-beta1 reverses the effects of matrix anchorage on the gene expression of decorin and procollagen type I in tendon fibroblasts. Clin Orthop Relat Res 2005;431:226–232.
Gabra N, Khiat A, Calabres P. Detection of elevated basic fibroblast growth factor during early hours of in vitro angiogenesis using a fast ELISA immunoassay. Biochem Biophys Res Commun 1994;205:1423–1430.
Galatz LM, Sandell LJ, Rothermich SY, et al. Characteristics of the rat supraspinatus tendon during tendon-to-bone healing after acute injury. J Orthop Res 2006;24:541–550.
Gauger A, Robertson C, Greenlee TK Jr, Riederer-Henderson MA. A low-serum medium for tendon cells: effects of growth factors on tendon cell growth and collagen production. In Vitro Cell Dev Biol 1985;21: 291–296.
Gelberman RH. PDGF-BB released in tendon repair using a novel delivery system promotes cell proliferation and collagen remodelling. J Orthop Res 2007;25:1358–1368.
Gelberman RH, Manske PR, Van de Berg JS, Lesker PA, Akeson WH. Flexor tendon repair in-vitro: a comparative histologic study of the rabbit, chicken, dog and monkey. J Orthop Res 1984;2:39–48.
Gelberman RH, Thomopoulos S, Sakiyama-Elbert SE, Das R, Silva MJ. The early effects of sustained platelet-derived growth factor administration on the functional and structural properties of repaired intrasynovial flexor tendons: an in vivo biomechanic study at 3 weeks in canines. J Hand Surg [Am] 2007;32:373–379.
Gerber C, Fuchs B, Hodler J. The results of repair of massive tears of the rotator cuff. J Bone Joint Surg Am 2000;82:505–515.
Gulotta LV, Rodeo SA. Growth factors for rotator cuff repair. Clin Sports Med 2009;28:13–23.
Herpin A, Lelong C, Favrel P. Transforming growth factor-beta-related proteins: an ancestral and widespread superfamily of cytokines in metazoans. Dev Comp Immunol 2004;28:461–485.
Kashiwagi K, Mochizuki Y, Yasunaga Y, et al. Effects of transforming growth factor-beta 1 on the early stages of healing of the Achilles tendon in a rat model. Scand J Plast Reconstr Surg Hand Surg 2004;38:193–197.
Klein MB, Yalamanchi N, Pham H, Longaker MT, Chang J. Flexor tendon healing in vitro: effects of TGF-β on tendon cell collagen production. J Hand Surg Am 2002;27:615–620.
Kobayashi M, Itoi E, Minagawa H, et al. Expression of growth factors in the early phase of supraspinatus tendon healing in rabbits. J Shoulder Elbow Surg 2006;15:371–377.
Kvist M. Achilles tendon injuries in athletes. Sports Med 1994;18:173–201.
Kvist M. Achilles tendon overuse injuries: a clinical and pathophysiological study in athletes. Thesis, University of Turku, Turku, Finland, 1991.
Kurtz CA, Loebig TG, Anderson DD, DeMeo PJ, Campbell PG. Insulin-like growth factor I accelerates functional recovery from Achilles tendon injury in a rat model. Am J Sports Med 1999;27:363–369.
Lee J, Green MH, Amiel D. Synergistic effect of growth factors on cell outgrowth from explants of rabbit anterior cruciate and medial collateral ligaments. J Orthop Res 1995;13:435–41.
Longo UG, Franceschi F, Ruzzini L, et al. Light microscopic histology of supraspinatus tendon ruptures. Knee Surg Sports Traumatol Arthrosc 2007;15:1390–1394.
Longo UG, Oliva F, Denaro V, Maffulli N. Oxygen species and overuse tendinopathy in athletes. Disabil Rehabil 2008a;30:1563–1571.
Longo UG, Franceschi F, Ruzzini L, et al. Histopathology of the supraspinatus tendon in rotator cuff tears. Am J Sports Med 2008b;36:533–538.
Longo UG, Franceschi F, Ruzzini L, et al. Higher fasting plasma glucose levels within the normoglycaemic range and rotator cuff tears. Br J Sports Med 2009;43: 284–287.
Longo UG, Franceschi F, Spiezia F, et al. Triglycerides and total serum cholesterol in rotator cuff tears: do they matter? Br J Sports Med 2010a;44:948–951.
Longo UG, Lamberti A, Maffulli N, Denaro V. Tendon augmentation grafts: a systematic review. Br Med Bull 2010b;94:165–188.
McGrath MH. Peptide growth factors and wound healing. Clin Plast Surg 1990;17:421–432.
Maffulli N, Benazzo F. Basic sciences of tendons. Sports Med Arthrosc Rev 2000;8:1–5.
Maffulli N, Khan KM, Puddu G. Overuse tendon conditions: time to change a confusing terminology. Arthroscopy 1998;14:840–843.
Maffulli N, Moller HD, Evans CH. Tendon healing: can it be optimised? Br J Sports Med 2002;36:315–316.
Maffulli N, Longo UG, Franceschi F, Rabitti C, Denaro V. Movin and Bonar scores assess the same characteristics of tendon histology. Clin Orthop Relat Res 2008;466:1605–1611.
Majewski M, Betz O, Ochsner PE, et al. *Ex vivo* adenoviral transfer of bone morphogenetic protein 12 (BMP-12) cDNA improves Achilles tendon healing in a rat model. Gene Ther 2008;15:1139–1146.
Matthews JP. Vascular changes in flexor tendons after injury and repair: an experimental study. Injury 1977;8:227–233.
Marx RE, Carlson ER, Eichstaedt RM et al. Platelet-rich plasma: Growth factor enhancement for bone grafts. Oral Surg Oral Med Oral Pathol Oral Radiol Endod 1998;85:638–646.
Mehta V, Mass D The use of growth factors on tendon injuries. J Hand Ther 2005;18: 87–92.
Mishra A, Pavelko T. Treatment of chronic elbow tendinosis with buffered platelet-rich plasma. Am J Sports Med 2006;34:1774–1778.
Molloy T, Wang Y, Murrell G. The roles of growth factors in tendon and ligament healing Sports Med 2003;33:381–394.
Ngo M, Pham H, Longaker MT, Chang J. Differential expression of transforming growth factor-beta receptors in a rabbit zone II flexor tendon wound healing model. Plast Reconstr Surg 2001;108:1260–1267.
Oliva F, Zocchi L, Codispoti A, et al. Transglutaminases expression in human supraspinatus tendon ruptures and in mouse tendons. Biochem Biophys Res Commun 2009;20:887–891.
Petersen W, Pufe T, Zantop T, Tillmann B, Mentlein R. Hypoxia and PDGF have a synergistic effect that increases the expression of the angiogenetic peptide vascular endothelial growth factor in Achilles tendon fibroblasts. Arch Orthop Trauma Surg 2003;123:485–488.
Popova SN, Rodriguez-Sánchez B, Lidén A et al. The mesenchymal alpha11beta1 integrin attenuates PDGF-BB-stimulated chemotaxis of embryonic fibroblasts on collagens. Dev Biol 2004;15:427–442.
Potenza AD. Tendon healing within the flexor digital sheath in the dog. J Bone Joint Surg Am 1962;44:49–64.
Premdas J, Tang JB, Warner JP, Murray MM, Spector M. The presence of smooth muscle actin in fibroblasts in the torn human rotator cuff. J Orthop Res 2001;19:221–228.
Provenzano PP, Alejandro-Osorio AL, Grorud KW, et al. Systemic administration of IGF-I enhances healing in collagenous extracellular matrices: evaluation of loaded and unloaded ligaments. BMC Physiol 2007;7:2.
Pufe T, Petersen W, Tillmann B, Mentlein R. The angiogenic peptide vascular endothelial growth factor is expressed in foetal and ruptured tendons. Virchows Arch 2001;439:579–585.
Randelli PS, Arrigoni P, Cabitza P, Volpi P, Maffulli N. Autologous platelet rich plasma for arthroscopic rotator cuff repair. A pilot study. Disabil Rehabil. 2008;30:1584–1589.
Reddy GK, Stehno-Bittel L, Enwemeka CS. Matrix remodeling in healing rabbit Achilles tendon. Wound Repair Regen 1999;7:518–527.
Rodeo SA. Biologic augmentation of rotator cuff tendon repair. J Shoulder Elbow Surg 2007;16:191–197.
Rompe JD, Nafe B, Furia J, Maffulli N. Eccentric loading, shock wave treatment, or a wait-and-see policy for tendinopathy of the main body of tendo Achillis: a randomized controlled trial. Am J Sports Med 2007;35:374–383.
Sanchez M, Anitua E, Azofra J, et al. Comparison of surgically repaired Achilles tendon tears using platelet-rich fibrin matrices. Am J Sports Med 2007;35:245–251.
Seeherman HJ, Archambault JM, Rodeo SA, et al. rhBMP-12 accelerates healing of rotator cuff repairs in a sheep model. J Bone Joint Surg Am 2008;90:2206–2219.
Selvanetti A, Cipolla M, Puddu G. Overuse tendon injuries: basic science and classification. Oper Tech Sports Med 1997;5:110–117.
Shah M, Foreman DM, Ferguson MW. Neutralisation of TGF-β1 and TGF-β2 or exogenous addition of TGFβ3 to cutaneous rat wounds reduces scarring. J Cell Sci 1995;108:985–1002.

Sharma P, Maffulli N. Biology of tendon injury: healing, modelling and remodelling. J Muscoloskelet Neuronal Interact 2006;6:181–190.
Skutek M, Van Griensven M, Zeichen J, Brauer N, Bosch U. Cyclic mechanical stretching modulates secretion pattern of growth factors in human tendon fibroblasts. Eur J Appl Physiol 2001;86:48–52.
Stein LE. Effects of serum, fibroblast growth factor, and platelet-derived growth factor on explants of rat tail tendon: a morphological study. Acta Anat (Basel) 1985;123:247–252.
Takahasih S, Nakajima M, Kobayashi M et. al. Effect of recombinant basic fibroblast growth factor (bFGF) on fibroblast-like cells from human rotator cuff tendon. Tohoku J Exp Med 2002;198:207–214.
Tallon C, Maffulli N, Ewen SW. Ruptured Achilles tendons are significantly more degenerated than tendinopathic tendons. Med Sci Sports Exerc 2001;33:1983–1990.
Thomopoulos S, Harwood FL, Silva MJ, Amiel D, Gelberman RH. Effect of several growth factors on canine flexor tendon fibroblast proliferation and collagen synthesis in vitro. J Hand Surg [Am] 2005;30:441–447.
Thomopoulos S, Zaegel M, Das R, et al. PDGF-BB released in tendon repair using a novel delivery system promotes cell proliferation and collagen remodeling. J Orthop Res 2007;25:1358–1368.
Trippel SB, Wroblewski J, Makower A, et al. Regulation of growth-plate chondrocytes by insuline-like growth-factor and basic fibroblast growth factor. J Bone Joint Surg Am 1993;75:177–189.
Tsubone T, Moran SL, Amadio PC, Zhao C, An KN. Expression of growth factors in canine flexor tendon after laceration in vivo. Ann Plast Surg 2004;53:393–397.
Tsubone T, Moran SL, Subramaniam M, et al. Effect of TGF-beta inducible early gene deficiency on flexor tendon healing. J Orthop Res 2006;24: 569–575.
Tsuzaki M, Brigman BE, Yamamoto J, et al. IGF-I is expressed by avian flexor tendon cells. J Orth Res 2000;8:546–556.
Uggen JC, Dines J, Uggen CW, et al. Tendon gene therapy modulates the local repair environment in the shoulder. J Am Osteopath Assoc 2005;105:20–21.
Wang XT, Liu PY, Tang JB. Tendon healing in vitro: genetic modification of tenocytes with exogenous PDGF gene and promotion of collagen gene expression. J Hand Surg [Am] 2004;29:884–890.
Wang XT, Liu PY, Tang JB. Tendon healing in vitro: modification of tenocytes with exogenous vascular endothelial growth factor gene increases expression of transforming growth factor beta but minimally affects expression of collagen genes. J Hand Surg [Am] 2005;30:222–229.
Wolfman NM, Hattersley G, Cox K, et al. Ectopic induction of tendon and ligament in rats by growth and differentiation factors 5,6, and 7, members of the TGF-beta gene family. J Clin Invest 1997;100:321–330.
Würgler-Hauri CC, Dourte LM, Baradet TC, Williams GR, Soslowsky LJ. Temporal expression of 8 growth factors in tendon-to-bone healing in a rat supraspinatus model. J Shoulder Elbow Surg 2007;16: 198–203.
Yalamanchi N, Klein MB, Pham HM, Longaker MT, Chang J. Flexor tendon wound healing in vitro: lactate up-regulation of TGF-beta expression and functional activity. Plast Reconstr Surg 2004;113:625–632.
Yamaguchi K, Ditsios K, Middleton WD, et al. The demographic and morphological features of rotator cuff disease. A comparison of asymptomatic and symptomatic shoulders. J Bone Joint Surg Am 2006;88:1699–1704.
Yoshikawa Y, Abrahamsson SO. Dose-related cellular effects of platelet-derived growth factor-BB differ in various types of rabbit tendons in vitro. Acta Orthop Scand 2001;72: 287–292.
Yu Y, Bliss JP, Bruce WJ, Walsh WR. Bone morphogenetic proteins and Smad expression in ovine tendon-bone healing. Arthroscopy 2007;23: 205–210.
Zhang AY, Pham H, Ho F, et al. Inhibition of TGF-beta-induced collagen production in rabbit flexor tendons. J Hand Surg [Am] 2004;29:230–235.
Zhang J, Cao R, Zhang Y, et al. Differential roles of PDGFR-α and PDGFR-β in angiogenesis and vessel stability. FASEB J 2009;23:153–163.

Chapter 16 Rotator cuff orthobiologics

Raffaele Garofalo, Stephen J. Snyder, Marco Conti, Alessandro Castagna

KEY FEATURES

- Orthobiologics are currently an enormous area of interest in shoulder surgery.
- The use of scaffolds has yielded mixed results depending on the scaffold used.
- Dermal matrix seems to provide better results in terms of reduced adverse reaction and improved clinical outcome, but there are no randomized clinical trials to support these findings.
- Placing and securing the patch graft arthroscopically is technically difficult, and implies longer surgical time and potential additional morbidity, without well-defined clinical benefits. Traditional open rotator cuff repair techniques are more reproducible, but there are concerns about deltoid detachment.
- The use of extracellular matrix patches cannot reverse muscular atrophy, and cannot re-establish the normal muscle–tendon function.

INTRODUCTION

Orthobiologics include an array of biologically active materials that influence tissue healing in orthopedic surgery. Some of these new biological products include biological scaffolds and reinforcement patches, methods for cell seeding, growth factor production and delivery, or a combination of these approaches. The use of orthobiologics in shoulder surgery is currently an enormous area of interest because the successful treatment of chronic, degenerative, full-thickness rotator cuff tear remains an unsolved surgical challenge (Boileau et al. 2005; Castagna et al. 2008).

Rotator cuff tears in the general population are very common: up to 30% of patients over the age of 70 years have rotator cuff tears. In addition, 35% of patients with a full-thickness rotator cuff tear on one shoulder will eventually develop a full-thickness tear on the other side. With increased longevity and improved lifestyle there is a corresponding increasing demand for a painless, functional rotator cuff mechanism. However, even with the many improvements in rotator cuff repair techniques and materials, including high-strength sutures, reliable anchors, improved knot tying, and advanced surgical ability, the rates of reported failure of cuff repairs ranges from 11% to 94%.

Several important non-controllable variables that consistently influence healing include tear size, the degree of tendon degeneration, fatty infiltration of the muscles, the patient's age, delamination and retraction of tendon, loss of tendon tissue, and chronicity of the tear (Lee et al. 2007; Tajana et al. 2009).

The high incidence of failed rotator cuff healing and recurrent rotator cuff tears has engendered great interest in developing methods to biologically augment and positively influence tendon repairs. Revision procedures and imaging studies usually confirm that the usual site of failure is at the tendon–suture interface. This occurs despite modifications of suture configuration and orientation and improved surgical technique intended to reduce the tension of rotator cuff during repair (such as placing the anchors along the articular margin) (Castagna et al. 2008). Historically, it was assumed that good clinical outcomes could be achieved despite the persistence of a rotator cuff defect. In fact, the failure to heal or a re-tear smaller than the original may well be tolerated especially in older, low-demand patients (Jost et al. 2000). However, this is not a consistent outcome as at times the re-rupture may be larger than the original tear, or more medial at the level of the musculotendinous junction, as often seen in double-row repair failures (Trantalis et al. 2008). Furthermore, outcomes that evaluate patient strength, pain, and functional recovery are better when the repaired cuff is completely healed (Boileau et al. 2005).

Considering an appropriate biological treatment that will reliably improve rotator cuff healing and thus shoulder function, it is essential to understand the etiopathology of rotator cuff tear and the process of healing. Although the precise pathogenesis and cellular and molecular changes associated with rotator cuff disease are still inconclusive, research seems to indicate that cuff tears result from a combination of extrinsic impingement from structures surrounding the cuff and intrinsic gradual degeneration and apoptosis within the tendon itself. The pathological effects of overuse seem to play a role in the development of rotator cuff wear. Overuse can cause an imbalance between the tendon wear and repair process, resulting in overproduction of matrix metalloproteases (MMPs) and tenocyte apoptosis.

MMPs play an important role in tissue remodeling after injury, but their overactivity can lead to progressive weakening of the extracellular matrix (ECM) of tendons. In healthy tendons, the activity of endogenous MMPs is contrasted by endogenous tissue inhibitors of MMPs (TIMPS), and the relative balance between MMPs and TIMPS plays an essential role in morphogenesis, homeostasis of normal tendon, healing, and remodeling. An increase in MMP synthesis and the resulting MMP-mediated alterations in the ECM of tendons have been implicated in the pathogenesis of rotator cuff wear (Bedi et al. 2010).

On the other hand, rotator cuff tears can also occur from a gradual degeneration of the bone-to-tendon interface. The tendon changes involve not just the tear margins, but also the more medial intact tendon, thus demonstrating that the failed healing response is not limited only to the margin of the torn tendon (Longo et al. 2008). When we consider the biology of the rotator cuff healing, there are two critical factors in the repair process to consider: the quality of tendon tissue and the restoration of the tendon-to-bone junction.

BIOLOGICAL AUGMENTATION OF ROTATOR CUFF REPAIR

Biological scaffolds and extracellular matrices have recently been developed for use in orthopedic soft-tissue applications because the poor structural and mechanical quality of the remaining native tissue associated with most chronic massive rotator cuff tears mandates a better method to augment repairs and stimulate healing. The most common method to biologically enhance the healing of rotator cuff repair is the use of ECMs.

An ECM is a complex structure consisting of structural proteins (collagen), specialized proteins (fibrillin, fibronectin), and various proteoglycans. The theoretical rationale is that these ECMs, when used as patches to reinforce soft-tissue repair during rotator cuff surgery, will reinforce and augment the repair and mediate the normal healing response. In addition, as the ECMs resemble the native structure of the human body, they might function as a valuable biological scaffold which might induce tenocytes to grow and remodel, thus improving the quality of repair. Scaffolds provide a well-defined geometrical structure for new tendon construction, and act as a tissue bridge between tendon and bone.

Requirements for scaffolding include biocompatibility, hemocompatibility, and the use of non-toxic materials that are durable, functional, and able to support cell attachment and ingrowth.

General considerations of biological patches

Rotator cuff ECMs patches have been engineered to contain purified collagen, primarily type I, as a scaffold from a variety of human (allograft) or animal (xenograft) sources. Concerns with the use of processed human and animal collagen, relating to infection (viral) transmission and inflammatory reaction, still exist, but some of the problems of graft rejection have been minimized by using acellular material. To our knowledge, there have been no xenograft- or allograft-associated infections related to the uses of rotator cuff ECMs.

An ideal rotator cuff scaffold should have several important features:

- A negligible risk of disease transfer or rejection
- Minimal inflammatory response
- Robust initial strength, mechanical properties sufficient to provide reinforcement of repair
- Supportive of biological incorporation, resorption, and remodeling of the matrix into host tissue
- Moderate elastic nature to prevent stress shielding and avoid suture cutout
- Favorable handling characteristics (not too stiff or rigid)
- Reasonable cost
- Encourage rapid repopulated and appropriate host cells (blood vessels, fibroblasts, etc.)
- Extended shelf-life and thus readily available for surgical use when needed
- Suitable for arthroscopic insertion.

Different laboratory processes are necessary to obtain an ECM scaffold. Techniques for cell removal are categorized into physical, chemical, and enzymatic. A complete decellularization of an allograft or xenograft will often include one or more approaches. The physical approach uses snap freezing or mechanical agitation to lyse the cells in the harvested tissue. The chemical approach lyses cells using hypotonic solutions or detergents; the cellular remnants are then solubilized and removed from the extracellular matrix by sequential washing. Enzymatic decellularization uses trypsin to degrade cellular material and can be used together with a solubilizing detergent.

The human source for rotator cuff ECMs is usually human dermal tissue, whereas animal sources include porcine small intestine submucosa (SIS), porcine dermis, and equine pericardium.

With any implanted allograft or xenograft tissue, there is a concern about the inflammatory reaction, tissue reorganization, and safety. Indeed, all the ECM scaffolds are associated with host cellular immune response. The amount of acceptable inflammation after ECM implant is unknown. The process of chemical (usually glutaraldehyde or peracetic acid) collagen cross-linking seems to have a central role in inciting soft-tissue reaction. In fact, chemical cross-linking diminishes surface recognition of epitopes and the subsequent graft degradation by the host environment (Badylak et al. 2004).

ECM scaffolds that are not cross-linked undergo a more rapid tissue degradation secondary to a very important host immune response. The degradation products of non-chemically cross-linked ECM patches act as chemoattractants and are responsible for important sequential phases, including vascular recruitment, mononuclear cell infiltration, and tissue remodeling during healing of rotator cuff repair. A recent study compared chemically cross-linked porcine dermis with non-cross-linked porcine SIS scaffolds in a primate body wall model, and showed that a more robust cellular infiltrate for different individual ECM scaffolds elicits distinct histological and morphological responses, which depend on the species and tissue of origin, processing methods, type of terminal sterilization, and mechanical loading environment (Sandor et al. 2009). However, regardless of the source of the ECM, chemical cross-linking is associated with an unfavorable host response.

The chemistry of a particular scaffold material influences the rate and degree of degradation and remodeling. Scaffolds derived from non-cross-linked SIS are rapidly remodeled and replaced by new host tissue, whereas scaffolds derived from dermis undergo slower remodeling, and may be incorporated by the host to some degree rather than completely replaced. It is likely that, during the process of partial or complete scaffold degradation, different growth factors can influence processes such as neovascularization, cell recruitment, and cell division (Reing et al. 2009). Recently, a published histological assessment of a human non-cross-linked dermal scaffold used to augment a rotator cuff repair demonstrated no calcification, infection, or inflammatory response at 3 months after surgery. The graft material was intact and identified by numerous dermal elastic fibers.

Extensive host cellular infiltration was evident along the margins of the graft, with the more central regions sparsely populated. Collagen bundles were well aligned and little blood vessel ingrowth was observed, indicating early organization of new tissue (Snyder et al. 2009). Obviously, degradation and remodeling of a scaffold device are associated with changes in its mechanical properties. Nevertheless, the temporal sequence of remodeling events, including the rate and extent of scaffold degradation and incorporation, is not yet established for most ECM products.

Allograft

Acellular non-cross-linked human dermal matrix

The acellular non-cross-linked human dermal matrix (GJA, GraftJacket Matrix, Wright Medical Technology, Inc., Arlington, TN) is a decellularized and cryopreserved, human dermal tissue, processed using a patented technique to remove epidermis, and to maintain an intact collagen and structure while avoiding intentional artificial cross-linking. The manufacturer states that collagen types I, III, IV, and VII are retained. In addition to the collagen, this ECM contains elastin and the proteoglycan fibronectin and preserved blood vessel channels.

GraftJacket requires rehydratation before use. The material is a single layer and is provided at various thicknesses (0.5–2.4 mm) and sizes for the different surgical indications. The GraftJacket has been well studied in terms of rotator cuff repair augmentation. In an in vitro biomechanical model, Barber et al. (2009) demonstrated a significant increase in the strength of a supraspinatus tendon repair when augmented with GJA compared with a non-augmented repair.

Fini et al. (2007) compared the effect of tenocytes on SIS and GJA, and demonstrated that GJA was able to support ECM synthesis better by maintaining higher levels of transforming growth factor β1 (TGF-β1), matrix proliferation, and lower inflammatory cell counts compared with SIS, although both supported ECM integration. GJA has been studied extensively in terms of rotator cuff repair augmentation. Adams et al. (2006) studied the use of GJA in a canine model of full-thickness infraspinatus tear.

At 6 weeks, there was normal chronic inflammation consistent with surgery and repair. By 6 months, the tendon–bone interface contained Sharpey's fibers, and a robust, remodeled tendon-like structure that still contained elastin fibers from the graft. Ide et al. (2009) found that rotator cuff tears repaired with GJA augmentation had higher tendon maturing scores than an untreated control defect group. They demonstrated greater mean ultimate force to failure than the non-augmented defect group, and performed better histologically and mechanically at every point in the study. Bond et al. (2008) reported the preliminary results of 16 patients with massive non-repairable rotator cuff tears treated arthroscopically, with GJA rotator cuff bridging replacing the missing tissue. At a mean follow-up of 26.8 months, 15 of 16 patients were satisfied with their procedure, 13 patients had full incorporation of the graft into native tissue as documented on magnetic resonance imaging (MRI), and 3 patients (19%) showed evidence of at least partial graft failure at 1 year.

Dopirak et al. (2007) reported on the use of GJA as an interposition graft in 16 patients with massive, contracted immobile rotator cuff tears. At more than 2 years after surgery, 75% of patients were satisfied with their result. MR scans at 3 and 12 months indicated three failures, two occurring in the first 3 months. There were no reported complications. Burkhead et al. (2007) evaluated 17 patients treated with the GJA graft augmentation in massive rotator cuff tears >5 cm in size and involving 2, 3, or 4 tendons. After an average of 1.2 years, 3 smaller recurrent tears were noted from 11 postoperative MR scans and a computed tomography (CT) arthrogram. Patients had significant improvement in postoperative UCLA scores with improvements in pain and function. Overall, 14 of the 17 patients were satisfied with their results.

Xenograft

Small intestine submucosa

SIS is derived from the tunica submucosa of porcine jejunum after removing several layers of the intestine (tunica mucosa, serosa, and muscularis), and is an acellular, collagen-based, resorbable biomaterial. The heterogeneous nature of SIS is due to the different areas of intestinal graft harvest, and this factor limits graft homogenicity. Not all SIS harvests sites were homogeneous, and consequently the biomechanical property is variable, e.g., samples harvested from the distal portion of the intestine are more elastic and less permeable than samples taken proximally.

Dejardin et al. (2001) examined the ability of SIS to induce healing and regeneration by replacing a 2-cm segment of the infraspinatus tendons in a canine shoulder model. Sixteen adult dogs underwent bilateral resection of the infraspinatus tendons. One side was sutured back in place while the other tendon was replaced by an SIS implant. The tissue was harvested at 3 and 6 months for histological and biomechanical analysis. Five additional cadavers underwent this procedure for time zero analysis, and four more were used as unoperated controls. Mechanically, the non-augmented shoulders had significantly greater cross-sectional areas than the regenerated tendon. Histologically, the graft integrated with the infraspinatus tendon.

Schlegel et al. (2006) produced a full-width infraspinatus injury and repair in a sheep. They placed a patch of SIS over the superficial aspect of the repaired tissue. The control was tendon repair without a graft. The investigators did not study the biomechanical benefit of using the graft devices at time zero.

At 3 months, repairs augmented with SIS were significantly stiffer (39%) than non-augmented repairs, and stiffness was 40% of a normal tendon. Zalavras et al. (2006) similarly examined SIS's regenerative capabilities in a rat model. A midsubstance supraspinatus tendon defect was produced in 40 animals. Twenty defects were repaired with a SIS patch and the others were left unrepaired to evaluate the spontaneous healing capacity of large defects as a control. Rats were sacrificed at 6 and 16 weeks for histological and biomechanical analysis. The regenerated tendons exhibited neovascularization and tenocytes oriented along the direction of greater mechanical stress, with no evident foreign body reactions. Mechanically, the regenerated tendons had higher tensile strength and stiffness compared with the tendons with full defects, but only reached approximately 75% of the normal tendon.

In a sheep rotator cuff repair, Nicholson et al. (2007) performed a partial-width infraspinatus injury and repair, investigating the effect of repair augmentation with SIS or cross-linked porcine dermis grafts. They reported little to no difference in ultimate load between augmented and non-augmented repairs at 9 or 24 weeks of healing. However, at 9 weeks, most SIS patches were completely resorbed, and fibroblasts and macrophages had invaded the area. In an SIS patch, there is a well-documented temporal course of cellular responses, which is affected by tissue processing.

In the first 3 weeks, a florid host cellular response is noted, with proliferation of mononuclear cells in the first 72 hours. Some studies also show that 80–90% of the ECM patch is removed by 1 month and is replaced by host tissue. SIS is available through several manufacturers, each with a proprietary processing and sterilization process. Among the available SIS materials there is the Restore soft-tissue implant (Ortobiologic Soft Tissue Implant, Depuy Orthopaedics, Inc., Warsaw, IN), which is composed of 10 *non-cross-linked* layers of SIS processed with peracetic acid and ethanol to remove cellular or immune response-inducing DNA components. This device contains predominately type I collagen, fibronectin, chondroitin sulfate, heparin, hyaluronate, and some growth factors. The implant is terminally sterilized using electron beam radiation, and is packaged dry. It requires rehydration before implantation.

The use of xenograft ECMs in rotator cuff repairs yielded mixed results in clinical trials. Malcarney et al. (2005) published their experiences in 25 patients. In four patients, an overt sterile inflammatory reaction at a mean of 13 days after surgery required débridement and removal of the graft. In a report by Zheng et al. (2005), similar sterile swelling and painful inflammatory response were observed. These adverse outcomes may have arisen because of the presence of porcine cellular and DNA elements in the Restore device. Iannotti et al. (2006) performed a randomized controlled trial to compare SIS augmentation with non-augmented cuff repairs in two groups of patients with tears of two tendons of the rotator cuff; 4 of 15 augmented shoulders healed in the SIS group compared with 9 of the 15 in the control group. Moreover, in the augmentation group, there was one event of erythema and spontaneous drainage, one case of swelling and pain, and one case of erythema and increased skin temperature. The authors did not recommend further use of SIS in human repairs.

On the other hand, Metcalf et al. (2002) also investigated the clinically efficacy of Restore for rotator cuff repairs in 12 patients who underwent arthroscopic repair of massive chronic rotator cuff tears. The Restore was used as an augmentation device. Postoperative MRI showed significant thickening of the cuff tendon with incorporation of the SIS graft in 11 patients. In 1 of the 12 patients, clinical failure was observed within 3 months with complete resorption of the graft.

There was no evidence of local or systemic rejection or infection in any patient. This study showed improved postoperative outcomes for patients treated with Restore graft augmentation compared with their preoperative condition.

Sclamberg et al. (2004) evaluated the use of Restore in 11 patients undergoing open repair of large or massive rotator cuff tears. The device was used as an augmentation graft in four patients and as an interpositional graft in seven patients. MR scans were obtained between 6 and 10 months postoperatively, and showed that 10 of the 11 patients exhibited large re-tears. Walton et al. (2007) initiated a prospective study comparing Restore with a non-augmented control. This study was stopped when 4 of 19 patients treated with SIS displayed an inflammatory response. Furthermore, patients whose rotator cuffs had been repaired with the Restore device experienced decreased post-repair strength, increased shoulder impingement, slower pain resolution after activity, and no decrease in re-tear rate when compared with patients whose rotator cuff tears had been repaired using standard surgical techniques.

The other available SIS is CuffPatch (Bioengineered Soft Tissue Reinforcement, Arthrotek, Biomet Sports Medicine, Inc., Warsaw, IN) an eight-layer acellular, lightly *cross-linked* SIS device. A non-detergent, non-enzymatic, chemical cleaning protocol is used to remove cells and cellular debris without damaging the native collagen structure. The implant is packaged hydrated and is terminally sterilized by gamma irradiation. CuffPatch is approximately 0.6 mm thick. Valentin et al. (2006), in a histological study comparing different xenografts and allografts used to augment rotator cuff repairs, demonstrated that rotator cuff repaired with CuffPatch experienced substantial inflammation when compared with other grafts.

Bovine dermis

The only available bovine dermis is an acellular, non-denatured, non-cross-linked collagen membrane. TissueMend (Soft Tissue Repair Matrix, Stryker Corp., Mahwah, NJ) is a single layer of fetal bovine dermis processed to remove cells, lipids, and carbohydrates, and terminally sterilized with ethylene oxide. The device is approximately 1 mm thick, and is composed primarily of type I and type II collagen. It is lyophilized and packaged dry. To date there is little clinical information using this implant. Seldes et al. (2006) did publish a technique for arthroscopic rotator cuff augmentation using this graft. A study comparing rotator cuff repairs augmented with patches demonstrated, however, that TissueMend had higher levels of DNA embedded in the ECM when compared with other xenograft materials (Derwin et al. 2006).

Porcine dermal collagen

Three types of porcine dermal collagen are available as scaffolds for rotator cuff surgery. Permacol (Zimmer Collagen Repair Patch, Zimmer Inc., Warsaw, IN; Tissue Science Laboratories, PLC, Aldershot, Hampshire, UK) is an acellular, porcine dermal collagen matrix. Organic and enzymatic extraction methods are used to remove fat, cellular materials, and proteins. This scaffold is cross-linked with diisocyanate, and thus resistant to enzymatic degradation. It is one layer and approximately 1.5 mm thick. It is packaged hydrated and terminally sterilized via gamma irradiation. In a number of preclinical studies, Permacol was reported to have been well tolerated as a subcutaneous implant. There was an absence of cellular infiltration and limited vascular ingrowth into the scaffold. Gilbert et al. (2009), in a study comparing the different commercially available biological ECMS, noted that Permacol had no detectable DNA in its matrix.

In a relatively recent prospective clinical study of 10 patients, Badhe et al. (2008) reported on a 4.5-year follow-up after augmented repair of rotator cuff using Permacol. All the patients had tears at least 5 cm in size involving the supra- and infraspinatus tendons. Imaging (MRI and ultrasonography) identified intact grafts in eight patients and graft disruption in two. There were no adverse side effects attributed to the Permacol graft during the study period.

In contrast, Soler et al. (2007) investigated the use of Permacol as a bridging device to repair massive rotator cuff defects. The graft device failed in all four patients within 6 months of treatment. All the four bridging cases had signs of inflammation, and two were revised to total shoulder replacement.

Another available porcine dermal collagen is Conexa (Tornier Edina, MN). It is an acellular, non-cross-linked scaffold. It is sterilized via a patented technique and further prepared by removal all the cellular components, and -galactose (α-Gal) residues to minimize human immunological reaction. Both primates and human have natural pre-existing antibodies to the α-Gal antigen. The reduction of the α-Gal antigen can minimize the immune response to xenograft tissues. The intact ECM supports tissue regeneration. Conexa is ready to use after a 2-minute rinse. This device is available in thicknesses of 1 and 2 mm, and in various sizes designed to meet the needs of specific orthopedic procedures and indications.

In a recent laboratory study performed to evaluate the response of human tenocytes in culture to seven commercially available ECM patches, it was noted that Conexa and GraftJacket Allograft evoked the most favorable responses. Furthermore, this study supports the clinical observations that high rates of failure and severe inflammatory response were observed with cross-linked dermal grafts or SIS (Shea et al. 2010). To date, however, there are no published clinical studies on the use of Conexa xenograft.

Biotape is the third porcine xenograft material (Wright Medical Technology, Inc., Arlington, TN). It is a terminally sterile, acellular, porcine dermal matrix. The collagen scaffold is preserved intact during processing, much like the GraftJacket allograft, and is not cross-linked. To date there are no clinical studies reporting the results of use of Biotape in the shoulder.

Equine pericardium

The OrthADAPT bioimplant (Pegasus Biologics, Irvine, CA) is the only ECM derived from equine pericardium. It is a decellularized, cross-linked, terminally sterilized, type I collagen matrix. This product is a very thin (<1 mm) and pliable scaffold. The OrthADAPT material has three subtypes that differ in the degree of cross-linking of collagen strands. The three products are named FX, PX, and MX in order of the degree of collagen cross-linking, with FX being most dense in cross-linking and hence most durable. A recent biomechanical study found that, in both tensile and suture pull-out strength tests, the products FX and MX had mechanical properties that were comparable with CuffPatch, whereas the mechanical strength of PX was significantly inferior to FX and CuffPatch in tensile strength test (Johnson et al. 2007). To date, however there have been no clinical reports using this material in rotator cuff. **Table 16.1** summarizes the main features of the current biological scaffold available for rotator cuff surgery.

Indications and contraindications

The current use of ECM patches in rotator cuff surgery occurs in two different settings: augmentation of repair of severely damaged tissue or bridging a non-repairable defect (**Figs 16.1** and **16.2**). The clinical indications for patch use are, however, still being refined because there are few clinical data supporting its different uses. For many young active patients with irreparable cuff tears, the only surgical options available are debridement and/or decompression, reverse total shoulder arthroplasty, latissimus dorsi or other muscle transfer, or glenohumeral joint arthrodesis.

Table 16.1 The main features of the biological scaffold

Product name	Manufacturer	Material source	Cross-link	Sterilization	Size
GraftJacket (allograft)	Wright Medical Technology, Inc.	Human dermis	No	Aseptic processing	Multiple
Restore (xenograft)	Orthobiologic Soft Tissue Implant; Depuy Orthopaedics	Small intestine Submucosa	No	E-beam	6 × 2 cm
CuffPatch (xenograft)	Arthrotek, Biomet Sports Medicine, Inc.	Small intestine Submucosa	Yes	Gamma irradiation	6.5 × 9 cm
TissueMend (xenograft)	Stryker Corporation	Fetal bovine dermis	No	Gamma irradiation	5 × 6 cm
Permacol ZCR Patch (xenograft)	Zimmer Inc.	Porcine dermal collagen	Yes	Gamma irradiation	5 × 5 cm
Conexa (xenograft)	Tornier Inc.	Porcine dermal collagen	No	Patented technique	Multiple
Biotape (xenograft)	Wright Medical Technology, Inc.	Porcine dermal collagen	No	Terminally sterile	4 × 7 cm 6 × 8 cm
OrthADAPT (xenograft)	Pegasus Biologics, Inc	Native equine pericardium	Yes	Terminally sterile	Multiple

ZCR, Zimmer Collagen Repair.

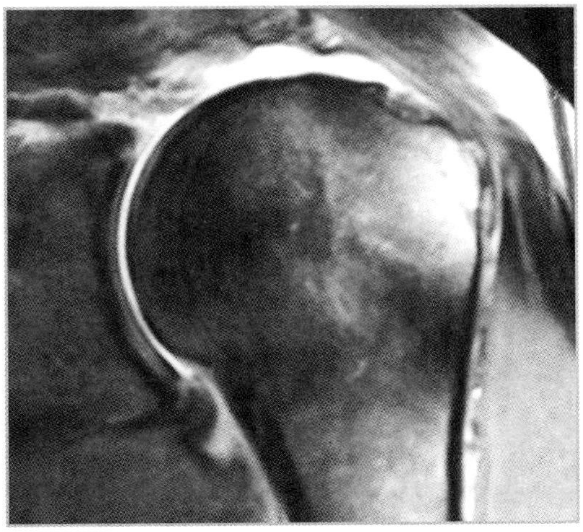

Figure 16.1 MRI of a male patient aged 46 years with a massive irreparable rotator cuff tear.

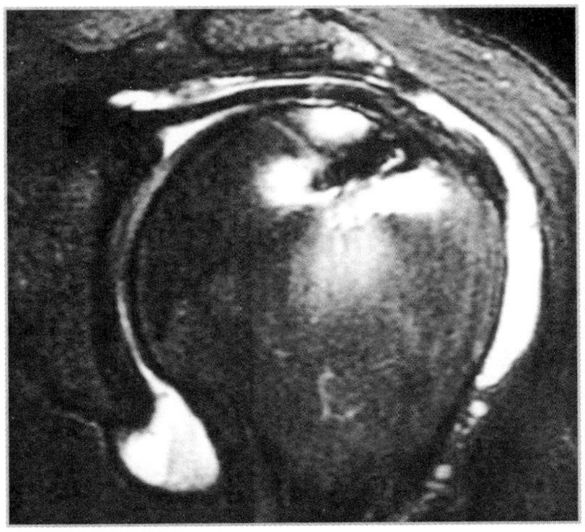

Figure 16.2 MRI at 2 years of follow-up after an arthroscopic repair using a biological scaffold as bridging tissue and suture anchors.

Most patients below the age of 60 with massive irreparable rotator cuff tears would be potential candidates to use the patch as a bridging device. Older patients are still potential candidates, but better incident-free outcomes are reported in patients aged <60 years, possibly from the more active healing response (Bond et al. 2008).

Advanced glenohumeral osteoarthritis and rotator cuff tear arthropathy are a relative contraindication, because these patients may develop stiffness and inadequate pain relief. Immunocompromised patients and heavy smokers are also relatively contraindicated and should be counseled.

The best patients are motivated, younger people with unacceptable pain, and well-maintained active motion. An intact biceps tendon is thought to be beneficial because the graft can be sewn to it, thus providing a robust anchor point along the anterior border. This method of graft anchor anteriorly has not been shown to adversely affect outcome (Snyder et al. 2009). However, we believe that in some cases, in which an irreparable cuff tear has associated severe (grade IV) muscle atrophy, especially with limited active motion, the use of patch as bridging is likely to be successful.

Rotator cuff revision surgery without a severe grade of muscle atrophy is considered a possible indication for ECM patches used for either bridging or augmentation, although there are currently no adequate clinical data supporting this indication.

The use of ECMs for augmentation has been shown to be helpful in patients in whom the repaired rotator cuff has a high likelihood of re-tear. This group may include those cases in which the repair is under some tension, the muscle has fatty degeneration or poor tissue quality, or cannot be repaired without a residual defect.

CONCLUSION

The use of an ECM in the management of shoulder rotator cuff tendon disorders continues to expand. The use of scaffolds as a support and direct tenocyte and collagen synthesis has yielded mixed results depending on the scaffold used.

Porcine SIS, although once promising, now appears a poor material as a scaffold. Dermal matrix seems to effect better results in terms of reduced adverse reaction and improved clinical outcome. However, these ECMs have limited evidence in their favor in rotator cuff repairs, and have not been studied in a randomized clinical trial. Advances in tissue engineering may provide better graft options with improved regenerative capacities.

Another important point to consider is the potential benefits that might accrue from adding additional growth factors or other biological enhancements to the ECM during the repair. Placing and securing the patch graft arthroscopically is technically difficult. The longer surgical time might add additional morbidity without well-defined clinical benefits. To place the graft patch using the traditional open rotator cuff repair technique would be more reproducible, but exposes the patient to the added morbidity of deltoid detachment.

An additional point of concern for patients with large irreparable rotator cuff tears is the severe fatty infiltration of muscle tissue that is often associated with them. Repair of this tendon even with an ECM patch cannot reverse the muscular atrophy, and hence this repair cannot re-establish the normal muscle–tendon function.

REFERENCES

Adams JE, Zobitz ME, Reach JS Jr, An KN, Steinmann SP. Rotator cuff repair using an acellular dermal matrix graft: an in vivo study in a canine model. Arthroscopy 2006;22:700–709.

Badhe SP, Lawrence TM, Smith FD, Lunn PG. An assessment of porcine dermal xenograft as an augmentation graft in the treatment of extensive rotator cuff tears. J Shoulder Elbow Surg 2008;17:35S–39S.

Badylak SF. Xenogeneic extracellular matrix as a scaffold for tissue reconstruction.Transpl Immunol 2004;12:367–377.

Barber FA, Aziz-Jacobo J. Biomechanical testing of commercially available soft-tissue augmentation materials. Arthroscopy 2009;25:1233–1239.

Bedi A, Kovacevic D, Hettrich C, et al. The effect of matrix metalloproteinase inhibition on tendon-to-bone healing in a rotator cuff repair model J Shoulder Elbow Surg 2010;19:384–391.

Boileau P, Brassart N, Watkinson DJ, et al. Arthroscopic repair of full-thickness tears of the supraspinatus: does the tendon really heal? J Bone Joint Surg Am 2005;87:1229–1240.

Bond JL, Dopirak RM, Higgins J, et al. Arthroscopic replacement of massive, irreparable rotator cuff tears using a GraftJacket allograft: technique and preliminary results. Arthroscopy 2008;24:403–409.

Burkhead W, Schiffern S, Krishnan S. Use of graft jacket as an augmentation for massive rotator cuff tears. Semin Arthrosc 2007;18:11–18.

Castagna A, Conti M, Markopoulos N, et al. Arthroscopic repair of rotator cuff tear with a modified Mason–Allen stitch: mid-term clinical and ultrasound outcomes. Knee Surg Sports Traumatol Arthrosc 2008;16:497–503 .

Dejardin LM, Arnoczky SP, Ewers BJ, et al. Tissue-engineered rotator cuff tendon using porcine small intestine submucosa. Histologic and mechanical evaluation in dogs. Am J Sports Med 2001;29:175–84.

Derwin KA, Baker AR, Spragg RK, Leigh DR, Iannotti JP. Commercial extracellular matrix scaffolds for rotator cuff tendon repair—biomechanical, biochemical, and cellular properties. J Bone Joint Surg Am 2006;88:2665–2672.

Dines JS, Grande DA, Dines DM. Tissue engineering and rotator cuff tendon healing. J Shoulder Elbow Surg 2007;16(5 suppl):S204–S207.

Dopirak R, Bond JL, Snyder SJ. Arthroscopic total rotator cuff replacement with an acellular human dermal allograft matrix. Int J Shoulder Surg 2007;1:7–15.

Fini M, Torricelli P, Giavaresi G, et al. In vitro study comparing two collageneous membranes in view of their clinical application for rotator cuff tendon regeneration. J Orthop Res 2007;25:98–110.

Gilbert TW, Freund JM, Badylak SF. Quantification of DNA in biologic scaffold materials. J Surg Res 2009;152:135–139 .

Iannotti JP, Codsi MJ, Kwon YW, et al. Porcine small intestine submucosa augmentation of surgical repair of chronic two-tendon rotator cuff tears (a randomized, controlled trial). J Bone Joint Surg Am 2006;88:1238–1244.

Ide J, Kikukawa K, Hirose J, et al. Reconstruction of large rotator-cuff tears with acellular dermal matrix grafts in rats. J Shoulder Elbow Surg 2009;18:288–295.

Johnson W, Inamasu J, Yantzer B, et al. Comparative in vitro biomechanical evaluation of two soft tissue defect products. J Biomed Mater Res B Appl Biomater 2007;Apr 5. [Epub ahead of print]

Jost B, Pfirrmann CW, Gerber C, Switzerland Z. Clinical outcome after structural failure of rotator cuff repairs. J Bone Joint Surg Am 2000;82:304–314.

Lee E, Bishop JY, Braman JP, et al. Outcomes after arthroscopic rotator cuff repairs. J Shoulder Elbow Surg 2007;16:1–5.

Longo UG, Franceschi F, Ruzzini et al. Histopathology of the supraspinatus tendon in rotator cuff tears. Am J Sports Med 2008;36:533–538.

Malcarney HL, Bonar F, Murrell GA. Early inflammatory reaction after rotator cuff repair with a porcine small intestine submucosal implant: A report of 4 cases. Am J Sports Med 2005;33:907–911.

Metcalf MH, Savioe FH, Kellum B. Surgical technique for xenograft (SIS) augmentation of rotator-cuff repair. Oper Tech Orthop 2002;12:204–208.

Nicholson GP, Breur GJ, Van SD, et al. Evaluation of a cross-linked acellular porcine dermal patch for rotator cuff repair augmentation in an ovine model. J Shoulder Elbow Surg 2007;16(suppl):S184–S190.

Reing JE, Zhang L, Myers-Irvin J, et al. Degradation products of extracellular matrix affect cell migration and proliferation. Tissue Eng Part A 2009;15:605–614.

Sandor M, Xu H, Connor J, et al. Host response to implanted porcine-derived biologic materials in a primate model of abdominal wall repair. Tissue Eng Part A 2009;14:2021–231.

Schlegel TF, Hawkins RJ, Lewis CW, et al. The effects of augmentation with Swine small intestine submucosa on tendon healing under tension: histologic and mechanical evaluations in sheep. Am J Sports Med 2006;34:275–280.

Sclamberg SG, Tibone JE, Itamura JM, Kasraeian S. Six-month magnetic resonance imaging follow-up of large and massive rotator cuff repairs reinforced with porcine small intestinal submucosa. J Shoulder Elbow Surg 2004;13:538–541.

Seldes RM, Abramchayev I. Arthroscopic insertion of a biologic rotator cuff tissue augmentation after rotator cuff repair. Arthroscopy 2006;22:113–116.

Shea KP, McCarthy MB, Ledgard F, et al. Human tendon cell response to 7 commercially available extracellular matrix materials: an in vitro study. Arthroscopy 2010;26:1181–1188.

Snyder SJ, Arnoczky SP, Bond JL, Dopirak R. Histologic evaluation of a biopsy specimen obtained 3 months after rotator cuff augmentation with GraftJacket matrix. Arthroscopy 2009;25:329–333.

Soler JA, Gidwani S, Curtis MJ. Early complications from the usebof porcine dermal collagen implants (Permacol) as bridging constructs in the repair of massive rotator cuff tears: a report of 4 cases. Acta Orthop Belg 2007;73:432–436.

Tajana MS, Murena L, Valli F, et al. Correlations between biochemical markers in the synovial fluid and severity of rotator cuff disease. Chir Organi Mov 2009;93(suppl 1):S41–S48.

Trantalis JN, Boorman RS, Pletsch K, Lo IK Medial rotator cuff failure after arthroscopic double-row rotator cuff repair. Arthroscopy 2008;24:727–731.

Valentin JE, Badylak JS, McCabe GP, Badylak SF. Extracellular matrix bioscaffolds for orthopaedic applications. A comparative histologic study. J Bone Joint Surg Am 2006;88:2673–2686.

Walton JR, Bowman NK, Khatib Y, Linklater J, Murrell GA. Restore orthobiologic implant: not recommended for augmentation of rotator cuff repairs. J Bone Joint Surg Am 2007;89:786–791.

Zalavras CG, Gardocki R, Huang E, et al. Reconstruction of large rotator cuff tendon defects with porcine small intestinal submucosa in an animal model. J Shoulder Elbow Surg 2006;15:224–231.

Zheng MH, Chen J, Kirilak Y, et al. Porcine small intestine submucosa (SIS) is not an acellular collagenous matrix and contains porcine DNA: possible implications in human implantation. J Biomed Mat Res B Appl Biomater 2005;73:61–67.

Chapter 17 Augmentation of massive rotator cuff tears

Umile Giuseppe Longo, Alfredo Lamberti, Nicola Maffulli, Vincenzo Denaro

KEY FEATURES

- Tendon transfers and shoulder arthroplasty as a treatment for rotator cuff arthropathy have had mixed results.
- Scaffold augmentations are currently available in three forms: xenograft, allograft, and synthetic extracellular matrices.
- To date, allografts seem to provide better results than xenografts, but most of the published evidence is limited to cellular and animal studies.
- Ideal candidates are younger people with disabling pain and massive rotator cuff tear, but intact biceps tendons and functioning subscapularis.
- The full impact of these novel technologies needs to be critically evaluated in controlled clinical trials.

INTRODUCTION

Management of patients with massive rotator cuff tears is challenging (Franceschi et al. 2007a–c, 2008a,b; Longo et al. 2007, 2008). They are difficult to repair and the failure rate is unacceptably high (Gartsman et al. 1998; Burkhart et al. 2001; Jones et al. 2003; Lo et al. 2004; Hanusch et al. 2009). The approach to massive rotator cuff tears requires a careful assessment of the needs of the patient and the extent of rotator cuff degeneration in order to determine the appropriate treatment (Hattrup 1995; Grondel et al. 2001; Chen et al. 2003; Lo et al. 2004; Cohen et al. 2006). Tendon transfers and shoulder arthroplasty have had mixed results (Wong et al. 2010). Excessive re-tear rates and poor clinical outcome after standard repair have led to alternative methods of treatment (Longo et al. 2012a–f).

Recently, there has been heightened interest in the development of scaffolds to bridge massive rotator cuff tears (Nho et al. 2010). These augmentations are currently available in three forms: xenograft, allograft, and synthetic extracellular matrices (Longo et al. 2010b).

The US Food and Drug Administration (FDA) has approved several scaffolds for rotator cuff repair in human patients. Currently, there are eight devices derived from extracellular matrix (ECM) (**Table 17.1**), and two synthetic devices available for clinical use in the USA (**Table 17.2**) (Longo et al. 2010b).

Xenografts

Several studies have been performed using xenogenic extracellular matrices for rotator cuff repairs, providing mixed results. The Restore graft (DePuy Orthopaedics, Warsaw, IN) is a circular implant consisting of 10 non-cross-linked layers of porcine small intestine submucosa (SIS) obtained from specific pathogen-free swine, 0.8–1 mm thick and with a 63 mm diameter. The Restore graft is made of 90% collagen with approximately 5–10% lipids and a small amount of carbohydrate (Barber et al. 2006; Coons et al. 2006).

Iannotti et al. (2006), in a randomized control trial, showed no improvement in patients with Restore augmentation compared with patients undergoing the same procedure without xenograft addition. Walton et al. (2007) reported decreased post-repair strength, increased shoulder impingement, slower pain resolution after activity, and no decrease in re-tear rate in patients whose rotator cuffs had been repaired with the Restore patch, compared with patients whose rotator cuff tears had been repaired using standard surgical techniques. The authors did not recommend use of this implant, due to a high proportion of patients with a severe inflammatory reaction to the xenograft.

Zimmer's Collagen Repair patch, marketed as Permacol (Tissue Science Laboratories, Covington, GA, licensed to Zimmer) is a single-layer porcine skin xenograft. It is an acellular cross-linked collagen sheet of cross-linked porcine dermis, 1.5 mm thick on average (Longo et al. 2010b).

A retrospective analysis of rotator cuff repair using Permacol showed improved functional scores by 50% at 4.5 years post-repair (Barber et al. 2008). Another study investigated the use of Permacol in bridging gaps in massive rotator cuff tears (Soler et al. 2007): re-tear

Table 17.1 Extracellular matrix scaffold FDA approved for rotator cuff repair

Product name	Source	Type	Company
Restore	Porcine	SIS	DePuy Orthopedics (IN)
CuffPatch	Porcine	SIS (cross-linked)	Arthrotek (IN)
GraftJacket	Human	Dermis	Wright Medical (TN)
Conexa	Porcine	Dermis	Tornier (MN)
TissueMend	Bovine	Dermis (fetal)	Stryker Orthopedics (N)
Permacol	Porcine	Dermis (cross-linked)	Zimmer (IN)
Bio-Blanket	Bovine	Dermis (cross-linked)	Kensey Nash Corp. (PA)
OrthADAPT Bioimplant	Equine	Pericardium (cross-linked)	Pegasus Biologic, Inc. (CA)

FDA, US Food and Drug Administration.

Table 17.2 Synthetic scaffold FDA approved for rotator cuff repair

Product name	Material	Company
SportMesh	Poly(urethane urea)	Biomet Sports Medicine (IN)
X-Repair	Poly-L-lactide	Synthasome (CA)

FDA, US Food and Drug Administration.

rates were no lower than for massive rotator cuff repairs performed without augmentation.

TissueMend (TEI Biosciences, Boston, MA, licensed to Stryker Howmedica Osteonics, Kalamazoo, MI) is a single-layer acellular, non-denatured collagen membrane derived from fetal bovine dermis, nominally 1 mm thick. The product is 99% non-denatured fetal bovine collagen, which is not artificially cross-linked. It is available as a rectangular 5 × 6 cm implant and was tested in two thicknesses: 1.1 and 1.2 mm. It is lyophilized and packaged dry (Longo et al. 2010b).

CuffPatch (Organogenesis, Canton, MA, licensed to Arthrotek) has eight layers of porcine SIS. It is composed of 97% collagen and 2% elastin and is acellular. It is nominally 0.6 mm thick and provided in a 6.5 × 9 cm sheet (Barber et al. 2006).

A study comparing rotator cuff repairs augmented with Restore, Cuffpatch, TissueMend, Permacol, and GraftJacket (Wright Medical Technology, Arlington, TN) demonstrated that rotator cuff repairs augmented with CuffPatch experienced substantial inflammation when compared with the other grafts (Valentin et al. 2006). A similar study demonstrated that TissueMend had higher levels of DNA embedded in the ECM when compared with other xenograft materials (Derwin et al. 2009).

Allografts

Allogeneic extracellular matrices have been developed via decellularization of cadaveric material. To date, two commercially available allogeneic ECMs have been studied, namely Allopatch and GraftJacket. The two graft materials are comparable in terms of stiffness, strength, and tissue retention (Barber and Aziz-Jacobo 2009).

Allopatch (Musculoskeletal Tissue Foundation, Edison, NJ) is derived from human allograft skin processed using proprietary procedures developed by the Musculoskeletal Transplant Foundation. GraftJacket (Wright Medical Technology, Inc.) is an acellular dermal matrix obtained from tissue bank human skin. It is in compliance with the American Association of Tissue Banks' guidelines for allograft material, and it is classified as human tissue for transplantation.

The GraftJacket is composed of collagen types I, III, IV, and VII, and elastin, chondroitin sulfate, proteoglycans, and fibroblast growth factor. It has an intact basement membrane complex and preserved vascular channels to allow rapid infiltration of fibroblasts and vascular tissue, with minimal host inflammatory response (Adams et al. 2006; Coons et al. 2006; Derwin et al. 2006). It is commercially available in several forms. With an average thickness of 1.0 mm, it is available in 5 × 5 and 5 × 10 cm sheets. With an average thickness of 1.5 mm, it is available in 4 × 7 or 5 × 5 cm sizes. With an average thickness of 2.0 mm, it is available in a 4 × 7 mm size (Coons et al. 2006).

GraftJacket has been studied extensively in terms of rotator cuff repair augmentation (Coons et al. 2006). Compared with other grafts, GraftJacket had a higher load to failure than Permacol, TissueMend, Restore, and CuffPatch, but was notably weaker than autologous tendon (Derwin et al. 2009). Ide et al. (2009) found that rotator cuff tears repaired with GraftJacket augmentation had higher tendon maturing scores than an untreated control defect group, demonstrating greater mean ultimate force to failure than the defect group, and performed better histologically and mechanically at every point in the study.

Cadaveric studies comparing rotator cuff repairs with or without GraftJacket augmentation showed that the use of human dermal allograft increased the strength of the repaired tendon; the mean failure strengths were 325 ± 74 N with allogeneic ECM and 273 ± 116 N without allogeneic ECM (Barber et al. 2008). There are, however, limited human data comparing repair with allogeneic augmentation to repair of comparable tears without allogeneic augmentation.

Bond et al. (2008) showed that repairing massive rotator cuff tears with GraftJacket yielded a failure rate of 19%. This rate is lower than the 38–95% failure rate demonstrated in several studies evaluating unaugmented massive rotator cuff repairs (Gerber et al. 2000; Bishop et al. 2006; Galatz et al. 2006; Zumstein et al. 2008).

A histological assessment of one patient's augmented rotator cuff repair with GraftJacket demonstrated no calcification, infection, or inflammatory response at 3 months. It has been hypothesized that good alignment of collagen and little blood vessel ingrowth demonstrated improved bone-to-tendon healing with allograft ECM augmentation (Snyder et al. 2009).

Recently GraftJacket has also been used to resurface the arthritic glenoid, together with arthroscopic debridement, in a middle-aged population (de Beer et al. 2010) providing pain relief, functional improvement, and patient satisfaction in approximately two-thirds (72%) of the patients in the intermediate term (over 2–4 years).

However, allogeneic ECMs are not lacking in problems. The devices can still contain some DNA from their allogeneic source and may induce inflammatory responses in the host (Gilbert et al. 2009). These inflammatory responses can cause pain and edema at the site of repair and may increase the degeneration of the rotator cuff repair that has been documented in the initial degenerative process of the rotator cuff (Zheng et al. 2005). They are also less elastic than autogenic tendon, which may result in comparably increased re-tear rates due to decreased load-carrying abilities (Derwin et al. 2006).

Synthetic ECM grafts

As allograft materials may create inflammatory responses in the host, there is great interest in developing synthetic ECM grafts for surgical use. Synthetic ECMs may still serve as an adequate scaffold for cellular and fibrotic growth, while running a smaller risk of provoking an inflammatory response than allograft ECMs. Several animal studies have investigated the benefit of augmenting rotator cuff repair with synthetic ECMs.

Yokoya et al. (2008) used a polyglycolic acid (PGA) sheet to augment rotator cuff repairs of infraspinatus tendons in Japanese white rabbits, showing histological improvement in fibrocartilage layering but only a slight improvement in tensile strength when compared with control tendons augmented with another slowly absorbing synthetic material (Yokoya et al. 2008).

In a similar study, Funakoshi et al. (2006) demonstrated increased fibroblast presence and collagen formation when synthetic ECM was surgically applied to rotator cuff tears. In this experiment, a 10-mm surgical defect was performed at the humeral insertion of the infraspinatus tendon in 21 Japanese white rabbits. In one shoulder, the 10-mm defect was covered with chitin, a biodegradable polymer, sutured into the bone trough and attached to the free end of the infraspinatus tendon. The contralateral shoulder was left untreated as a control. Throughout the experiment, tendon-to-bone junctions covered with chitin fabric demonstrated greater cell numbers, better collagen fiber alignment, and greater mechanical strength than the tendon-to-bone junctions left free as controls (Funakoshi et al. 2006).

In another study, MacGillivray et al. (2006) used polylactic acid patches in goats, showing no observable difference between the treated and control groups. A similar experiment, using a woven poly-L-lactide device, was performed by Derwin et al. (2009) in a dog model. The superior two-thirds of each infraspinatus tendon were removed from the rotator cuff and then repaired in both shoulders.

In one shoulder, a woven poly-L-lactide device was placed over the repair. In the contralateral shoulder, the repair was left unaugmented. The augmented rotator cuff repair resulted in fewer tendon retractions, greater strength, and increased stiffness when compared with the contralateral untreated, rotator cuff repairs. A recent study demonstrates that the application of the X-Repair device significantly increased the yield load and ultimate load of rotator cuff repairs in a human cadaveric model and altered the failure mode, but did not affect initial repair stiffness (McCarron et al. 2010).

ECM scaffold for autogenic cells

Several studies recently reported on the use of ECMs as a scaffold for autogenic cells in vitro, as well as in rotator cuff repair. First, autologous cells are harvested from undamaged sites on the host such as patellar ligaments, fascia lata, or other tendinous structures by a small biopsy punch. When the cells have been appropriately purified, they are cultured in incubation flasks alone for several days and then cultured with the ECM for up to 5 days to appropriately seed the matrix in vitro (Chen et al. 2007).

This construct of allogeneic, xenogenic, or synthetic ECM and autogenic cells has several potential applications. ECM autogenic cell constructs can be incubated in appropriate media and result in engineered autogenic tendons. These tendons have been investigated as augmentation materials in the repair of rotator cuff tears.

Chen et al. (2007) modeled the effect of using such engineered tendons to augment rotator cuff tears in Japanese white rabbits. Tenocytes were harvested from patellar ligaments, purified using markers for types I and III collagen expression, and then implanted on to xenogenic and synthetic ECMs. Fibers were cultured for 5 days to allow for appropriate tenocyte matrix formation. Rotator cuff tears were performed in the infraspinatus tendon and then repaired with genetically engineered tendon, ECM, or autologous tendon. When compared with ECM augmentation alone, augmentation with engineered autologous tendon resulted in increased type I and III collagen deposition, decreased immunological response, and improved absorption into the host tendon. Augmentation with engineered autologous tendon was comparable to the autogenic cellular augmentation performed as a control.

ECM autogenic cell constructs can also be manipulated via gene therapy. Dines et al. (2007) investigated repair of rotator cuff tears using interposed genetically engineered autologous tendon in Sprague Dawley rats. Tenocytes were isolated from the rotator cuff and then transduced with the genes for platelet-derived growth factor B (PDGF-B) or insulin-like factor 1 (IGF-1), two factors that promote fibroblast proliferation and minimize inflammation. The transduction was performed using a retroviral vector. Successfully transduced cells were again isolated, seeded on to PGA, and used to augment rotator cuff repair. When incorporated into rotator cuff repair, the tendons transduced with PDGF-B showed no improvement over controls augmented with PGA matrix alone or simple repair. However, the fibroblastic cells transduced to express IGF exhibited an improvement in both toughness and maximum load.

The growth factors that Dines et al. (2007) chose to transpose represent only two of a handful of known growth factors involved in new tendon formation and wound healing. It appears that gene therapy in genetically engineered autogenous tendons is a promising delivery system for growth factors required for appropriate tendon healing, and further investigation here is merited.

INDICATIONS AND CONTRAINDICATIONS

To date there are no clear indications or contraindications for the use of grafts to augment massive rotator cuff tears.

Indications

Some authors have suggested that the ideal candidates are younger people with disabling pain but intact biceps tendons, and well-maintained active motion with a functioning subscapularis (Wong et al. 2010). Younger patients with an intact deltoid can often compensate for dysfunctional rotator cuffs and maintain adequate motion.

Metcalf et al. (2002) selected patients with significant atrophy of supraspinatus and infraspinatus muscles and tendons, as measured by preoperative MRI.

Older patients with little pain, poor motion, and arthritis are less likely to fully benefit from the procedure and are often better candidates for reverse total shoulder arthroplasty or non-surgical care (Bond et al. 2008).

Contraindications

Glenohumeral arthritis is a relative contraindication because significant stiffness may develop in these patients with inadequate pain relief. Immunocompromised patients and people who are heavy smokers are also relatively contraindicated. Fatty infiltration, muscle atrophy, muscle retraction, humeral head position, and prior surgery are acceptable variables for inclusion (Wong et al. 2010).

DESCRIPTION OF TECHNIQUE

In our clinical practice, we perform augmentation grafting of rotator cuff tears as described by Snyder's group (Bond et al. 2008; Wong et al. 2010).

Patients undergo brachial plexus block, and are placed in a lateral decubitus position. The arm is suspended at approximately 45° abduction and 20° forward flexion. Distraction of the shoulder joint is accomplished with 4.5–6.5 kg of traction. Four to six portals are used.

A posterior portal is created, and the arthroscope is inserted into the glenohumeral joint. A diagnostic arthroscopy is then performed to evaluate the extent of the rotator cuff tear, any lesions of the biceps tendon, and other associated lesions.

The main subacromial portals are the posterolateral viewing, and the anterolateral and lateral working portals. To control subacromial bleeding, we used radiofrequency and epinephrine admixture to the irrigation fluid, and asked the anesthesiologist to lower the systolic blood pressure to 90 mmHg if possible. An arthroscopic pump maintains fluid pressure at 40 mmHg, increasing it temporarily on demand.

A spinal needle is introduced percutaneously to determine the precise location for placement of the anterolateral portal produced approximately 2–3 cm anterior and lateral to the anterolateral corner of the acromion. The lateral portal is used to mobilize the rotator cuff back to its bony insertion. The mobility of the rotator cuff is assessed. Using a burr through the lateral portal, the footprint of the greater tuberosity is abraded.

The cuff tear is closely evaluated for size, tissue quality, and mobility. A 7-mm cannula is placed in both the standard posterior and anterior portals and an 8.2-mm cannula in the midlateral portal.

Short-tailed interference knotted (STIK) sutures are prepared on the back table by tying mulberry-type knots on the end of a no. 2 suture. The graft is rehydrated and then cut to the proper size as measured with the knotted suture tool. The midline of the graft on the lateral edge is marked with a surgical marker. The STIK sutures are placed around the anterior, medial, and posterior grafts, 3 mm from the edge and 4 mm apart using a Keith needle. Four or five STIK sutures are placed along the medial edge of the graft, and two or three STIK sutures along the anterior and posterior borders, ensuring that the knotted end is located on the smooth or "basement membrane" surface of the graft. The graft is then sutured to the edge of the rotator cuff (Bond et al. 2008; Wong et al. 2010).

POSTOPERATIVE MANAGEMENT

As for surgical indications and contraindications, there is no specific postoperative rehabilitation program for augmented repairs of massive rotator cuff tears.

For massive rotator cuff tears surgically repaired and augmented with GraftJacket, Snyder and colleagues (Bond et al. 2008; Wong et al. 2010) applied a rehabilitation program of 6 months, in which the patients supported the arm in an Ultra-Sling for 6 weeks, removing it daily for scapular mobilization, as well as elbow, wrist, and hand exercises, and initiated pendulum exercises at 1 week and active assisted elevation at 12 weeks, allowing progressive resistance exercises at 4 months.

For massive rotator cuff tears surgically repaired and augmented with Restore, Walton et al. (2007) provided the patients with a sling for 4 weeks and passive range of motion exercises, starting with graduated active range-of-motion and strengthening exercises after 4 weeks.

Metcalf et al. (2002) immobilized the shoulder in a sling for 3 weeks, allowing its removal for dressing and bathing and pendulum exercises during the first 3 weeks, starting active assisted range of motion from 3 weeks to 6 weeks, and strengthening exercises when range of motion was obtained, typically at 8–12 weeks.

Iannotti et al. (2006) immobilized the shoulder in a sling for 1 week postoperatively, allowing only passive forward flexion and external rotation for 8 weeks. The patient then progressed to active shoulder motion. Strengthening was started at 10–12 weeks postoperatively. Malcarney et al. (2005) provided the patients with a sling and passive range-of-motion exercises for 1 week, after which the patient was encouraged to progress to active assisted exercises as tolerated until the anticipated next office visit at 6 weeks after the rotator cuff repair.

CONCLUSION

Massive rotator cuff tears give rise to significant morbidity. A better understanding of tendon pathology, function, and healing will allow specific treatment strategies to be developed. Several interesting techniques are being pioneered (Lippi et al. 2010; Longo et al. 2010a,c). The optimization strategies discussed in this chapter are currently at an early stage of development. Although these emerging technologies may develop into substantial clinical treatment options, their full impact needs to be critically evaluated in a scientific fashion.

REFERENCES

Adams JE, Zobitz ME, Reach JS Jr, An KN, Steinmann SP. Rotator cuff repair using an acellular dermal matrix graft: an in vivo study in a canine model. Arthroscopy 2006;22:700–709.

Barber FA, Aziz-Jacobo J. Biomechanical testing of commercially available soft-tissue augmentation materials. Arthroscopy 2009;25:1233–1239.

Barber FA, Herbert MA, Coons DA. Tendon augmentation grafts: biomechanical failure loads and failure patterns. Arthroscopy 2006;22:534–538.

Barber FA, Herbert MA, Boothby MH. Ultimate tensile failure loads of a human dermal allograft rotator cuff augmentation. Arthroscopy 2008;24:20–24.

Bishop J, Klepps S, Lo IK, et al. Cuff integrity after arthroscopic versus open rotator cuff repair: a prospective study. J Shoulder Elbow Surg 2006;15:290–299.

Bond JL, Dopirak RM, Higgins J, Burns J, Snyder SJ. Arthroscopic replacement of massive, irreparable rotator cuff tears using a GraftJacket allograft: technique and preliminary results. Arthroscopy 2008;24:403–409, e401.

Burkhart SS, Danaceau SM, Pearce CE Jr. Arthroscopic rotator cuff repair: Analysis of results by tear size and by repair technique-margin convergence versus direct tendon-to-bone repair. Arthroscopy 2001;17:905–912.

Chen AL, Shapiro JA, Ahn AK, Zuckerman JD, Cuomo F. Rotator cuff repair in patients with type I diabetes mellitus. J Shoulder Elbow Surg 2003;12:416–421.

Chen JM, Willers C, Xu J, Wang A, Zheng MH. Autologous tenocyte therapy using porcine-derived bioscaffolds for massive rotator cuff defect in rabbits. Tissue Eng 2007;13:1479–1491.

Cohen DB, Kawamura S, Ehteshami JR, Rodeo SA. Indomethacin and celecoxib impair rotator cuff tendon-to-bone healing. Am J Sports Med 2006;34:362–369.

Coons DA, Alan Barber F. Tendon graft substitutes-rotator cuff patches. Sports Med Arthrosc 2006;14:185–190.

de Beer JF, Bhatia DN, van Rooyen KS, Du Toit DF. Arthroscopic debridement and biological resurfacing of the glenoid in glenohumeral arthritis. Knee Surg Sports Traumatol Arthrosc 2010;18:1767–1773.

Derwin KA, Baker AR, Spragg RK, Leigh DR, Iannotti JP. Commercial extracellular matrix scaffolds for rotator cuff tendon repair. Biomechanical, biochemical, and cellular properties. J Bone Joint Surg Am 2006;88:2665–2672.

Derwin KA, Codsi MJ, Milks RA, et al. Rotator cuff repair augmentation in a canine model with use of a woven poly-L-lactide device. J Bone Joint Surg 2009;91:1159–1171.

Dines JS, Grande DA, Dines DM. Tissue engineering and rotator cuff tendon healing. J Shoulder Elbow Surg 2007;16:S204–S207.

Franceschi F, Longo UG, Ruzzini L, et al. To detach the long head of the biceps tendon after tenodesis or not: outcome analysis at the 4-year follow-up of two different techniques. Int Orthop 2007a;31:537–545.

Franceschi F, Longo UG, Ruzzini L, et al. The Roman Bridge: a "double pulley–suture bridges" technique for rotator cuff repair. BMC Musculoskel Disord 2007b;8:123.

Franceschi F, Ruzzini L, Longo UG, et al. Equivalent clinical results of arthroscopic single-row and double-row suture anchor repair for rotator cuff tears: a randomized controlled trial. Am J Sports Med 2007c;35:1254–1260.

Franceschi F, Longo UG, Ruzzini L, et al. No advantages in repairing a type II superior labrum anterior and posterior (SLAP) lesion when associated with rotator cuff repair in patients over age 50: a randomized controlled trial. Am J Sports Med 2008a;36:247–253.

Franceschi F, Longo UG, Ruzzini L, et al. Soft tissue tenodesis of the long head of the biceps tendon associated to the Roman Bridge repair. BMC Musculoskel Disord 2008b;9:78.

Funakoshi T, Majima T, Suenaga N, et al. Rotator cuff regeneration using chitin fabric as an acellular matrix. J Shoulder Elbow Surg 2006;15:112–118.

Galatz LM, Sandell LJ, Rothermich SY, et al. Characteristics of the rat supraspinatus tendon during tendon-to-bone healing after acute injury. J Orthop Res 2006;24:541–550.

Gartsman GM, Khan, M, Hammerman SM. Arthroscopic repair of full-thickness tears of the rotator cuff. J Bone Joint Surg 1998;80:832–840.

Gerber, C, Fuchs, B, Hodler, J. The results of repair of massive tears of the rotator cuff. J Bone Joint Surg 2000;82:505–515.

Gilbert TW, Freund JM, Badylak SF. Quantification of DNA in biologic scaffold materials. J Surg Res 2009;152:135–139.

Grondel RJ, Savoie FH 3rd, Field LD. Rotator cuff repairs in patients 62 years of age or older. J Shoulder Elbow Surg 2001;10:97–99.

Hanusch BC, Goodchild L, Finn P, Rangan A. Large and massive tears of the rotator cuff: functional outcome and integrity of the repair after a mini-open procedure. J Bone Joint Surg Br 2009;91:201–205.

Hattrup SJ. Rotator cuff repair: relevance of patient age. J Shoulder Elbow Surg 1995;4:95–100.

Iannotti JP, Codsi MJ, Kwon YW, et al. Porcine small intestine submucosa augmentation of surgical repair of chronic two-tendon rotator cuff tears. A randomized, controlled trial. J Bone Joint Surg Am 2006;88:1238–1244.

Ide J, Kikukawa K, Hirose J, et al. Reconstruction of large rotator-cuff tears with acellular dermal matrix grafts in rats. J Shoulder Elbow Surg 2009;18:288–295.

Jones CK, Savoie FH 3rd. Arthroscopic repair of large and massive rotator cuff tears. Arthroscopy 2003;19:564–571.

Lippi G, Longo UG, Maffulli N. Genetics and sports. Br Med Bull 2010;93:27–47.

Lo IK, Burkhart SS. Arthroscopic revision of failed rotator cuff repairs: technique and results. Arthroscopy 2004;20:250–267.

Longo UG, Franceschi F, Ruzzini L, et al. Light microscopic histology of supraspinatus tendon ruptures. Knee Surg Sports Traumatol Arthrosc 2007;15:1390–1394.

Longo UG, Franceschi F, Ruzzini L, et al. Histopathology of the supraspinatus tendon in rotator cuff tears. Am J Sports Med 2008;36:533–538.

Longo UG, Fazio V, Poeta ML, et al. Bilateral consecutive rupture of the quadriceps tendon in a man with BstUI polymorphism of the ***COL5A1*** gene. Knee Surg Sports Traumatol Arthrosc 2010a;18:514–518.

Longo UG, Lamberti, A, Maffulli, N, Denaro, V. Tendon augmentation grafts: a systematic review. Br Med Bull 2010b;94:165–188.

Longo UG, Lamberti, A, Maffulli, N, Denaro, V. Tissue engineered biological augmentation for tendon healing: a systematic review. Br Med Bull 2010c;93:27–47.

Longo UG, Berton A, Papapietro N, Maffulli N, Denaro V. Epidemiology, genetics and biological factors of rotator cuff tears. Med Sport Sci 2012a;57:1–9. Epub 2011 Oct 4. PubMed PMID: 21986040.

Longo UG, Berton A, Papapietro N, Maffulli N, Denaro V. Biomechanics of the rotator cuff: European perspective. Med Sport Sci 2012b;57:10–17. Epub 2011 Oct 4. PubMed PMID: 21986041.

Longo UG, Franceschi F, Berton A, Maffulli N, Droena V. Conservative treatment and rotator cuff tear progression. Med Sport Sci 2012c;57:90–99. Epub 2011 Oct 4. PubMed PMID: 21986048.

Longo UG, Berton A, Marinozzi A, Maffulli N, Denaro V. Subscapularis tears. Med Sport Sci 2012d;57:114–121. Epub 2011 Oct 4. PubMed PMID: 21986050.

Longo UG, Franceschi F, Berton A, Maffulli N, Denaro V. Arthroscopic transosseous rotator cuff repair. Med Sport Sci 2012e;57:142–152. Epub 2011 Oct 4. PubMed PMID: 21986052.

Longo UG, Lamberti A, Rizzello G, Maffulli N, Denaro V. Synthetic augmentation in massive rotator cuff tears. Med Sport Sci 2012f;57:168–177. Epub 2011 Oct 4. PubMed PMID: 21986054.

McCarron JA, Milks RA, Chen X, Iannotti JP, Derwin KA. Improved time-zero biomechanical properties using poly-L-lactic acid graft augmentation in a cadaveric rotator cuff repair model. J Shoulder Elbow Surg 2010;19:688–696.

MacGillivray JD, Fealy, S, Terry MA, et al. Biomechanical evaluation of a rotator cuff defect model augmented with a bioresorbable scaffold in goats. J Shoulder Elbow Surg 2006;15:639–644.

Malcarney HL, Bonar F, Murrell GA. Early inflammatory reaction after rotator cuff repair with a porcine small intestine submucosal implant: a report of 4 cases. Am J Sports Med 2005;33:907–911.

Metcalf MH, Savoie FH, Kellum B. Surgical technique for xenograft (SIS) augmentation of rotator-cuff repairs. Oper Tech Orthop 2002;12:204–208.

Nho SJ, Delos D, Yadav H, et al. Biomechanical and biologic augmentation for the treatment of massive rotator cuff tears. Am J Sports Med 2010;38:619–629.

Snyder SJ, Arnoczky SP, Bond JL, Dopirak R. Histologic evaluation of a biopsy specimen obtained 3 months after rotator cuff augmentation with GraftJacket Matrix. Arthroscopy 2009;25:329–333.

Soler JA, Gidwani S, Curtis MJ. Early complications from the use of porcine dermal collagen implants (Permacol) as bridging constructs in the repair of massive rotator cuff tears. A report of 4 cases. Acta Orthop Belg 2007;73:432–436.

Valentin JE, Badylak JS, McCabe GP, Badylak SF. Extracellular matrix bioscaffolds for orthopaedic applications. A comparative histologic study. J Bone Joint Surg Am 2006;88:2673–2686.

Walton JR, Bowman NK, Khatib Y, Linklater J, Murrell GA. Restore orthobiologic implant: not recommended for augmentation of rotator cuff repairs. J Bone Joint Surg Am 2007;89:786–791.

Wong I, Burns J, Snyder S. Arthroscopic GraftJacket repair of rotator cuff tears. J Shoulder Elbow Surg 2010;19:104–109.

Yokoya S, Mochizuki Y, Nagata Y, Deie M, Ochi M. Tendon-bone insertion repair and regeneration using polyglycolic acid sheet in the rabbit rotator cuff injury model. Am J Sports Med 2008;36:1298–1309.

Zheng MH, Chen J, Kirilak Y, et al. Porcine small intestine submucosa (SIS) is not an acellular collagenous matrix and contains porcine DNA: possible implications in human implantation. J Biomed Mater Res B Appl Biomater 2005;73:61–67.

Zumstein MA, Jost B, Hempel J, Hodler J, Gerber C. The clinical and structural long-term results of open repair of massive tears of the rotator cuff. J Bone Joint Surg 2008;90:2423–2431.

Chapter 18 Platelet-rich plasma: does it help tendon healing?

Omer Mei-Dan, Michael R. Carmont

KEY FEATURES

- Platelet-rich plasma (PRP) injection is a controversial treatment thought to accelerate muscle and tendon healing.
- There is no agreement as to the best volume and frequency of the injections, the ideal period between multiple injections, or the mechanism of platelet activation and degranulation.
- Appropriately powered level I studies with adequate and relevant outcome measures and clinically appropriate follow-up are needed to further evaluate this emerging treatment alternative.

INTRODUCTION

Patients, physicians, and surgeons constantly search for new methods to promote healing and return to normal function after injury or degenerative pathology. Accelerating the healing process reduces the socioeconomic effects of injury and illness.

After acute trauma, injury results in bleeding and hematoma formation. There is an initial inflammatory response before the tissue becomes organized, heals, and matures. Conversely, microtrauma may occur without significant bleeding. This results in small tears, which, in some body sites, heal poorly and lead to the formation of weak and painful degenerated tissue.

New techniques have focused on the promotion of healing by the injection of blood and blood components at the site of injury. Early methods included the injection of pure autologous blood. Over time, these techniques have evolved to the administration of platelet-rich serum and, most recently, concentrations of serum specifically rich in the factors that are reputed to promote healing. Although there is growing evidence to confirm the efficacy of serum fractions, there is increased evidence that does not favor whole blood injections (De Vos et al. 2010b).

Platelets are cytoplasmic fragments of megakaryocyte leukocytes; they lack nucleoli but contain mitochondria, microtubules, and granules. They contain many biologically active factors, which promote hemostasis, the synthesis of new connective tissue, and revascularization. The alpha granules, numbering approximately 50–80/platelet, contain bioactive growth factors, proteins, which promote healing (Harrison and Cramer 1993).

Platelets and preparations rich in growth factors are obtained by the centrifugation of whole blood into its component fractions. The separation of platelet-rich plasma (PRP) from whole blood was first described in 1999 by a research group in Vitoria, Spain (Anitua et al. 1999).

The term "PRP" may be applied to any fraction of autologous blood that has a platelet concentration above that of the baseline (Marx et al. 1998; Alsousou et al. 2009). The centrifugation process removes the erythrocytes, which are not beneficial to the healing process, from the serum. The role of the leukocytes in healing is less clear. PRP preparations can be formulated with leukocytes either eliminated from the samples or concentrated in the samples. Neutrophils promote additional muscle damage after the original injury, and they do not play a beneficial role in muscle repair or regeneration (Sánchez et al. 2009).

Many production methods are available with differing preparation protocols, kits, centrifuges, and methods to trigger platelet activation. The cost of each injection varies. Understandably, there is variation between the volume and concentration of platelets and growth factors depending on the method of production used. Typically, 10% of the initial volume of autologous blood is yielded as PRP concentrate after centrifugation. It has been stated that a therapeutic dose of PRP would need to be at least three to six times higher than the normal baseline (Weibrich et al. 2004; Graziani et al. 2006). Higher concentrations have inhibitory effects (Anitua et al. 2006b).

A preparation rich in growth factors (PRGF) specifically refers to preparations made using the Vitorian method, currently marketed by BTI (Centro De Formacion BTI, Vitoria, Spain), which have a higher concentration of growth factors but without the presence of platelets. PRGF is only one of the PRP concentrates used worldwide.

Depending on the method of separation and concentration used, the composition of the constituents of PRP may vary. This variation means that preparations are unique in composition, which makes comparative research in the area of PRP and PRGF difficult. In addition the constituents of the serum obtained from a patient will also vary according to food consumed by the patient before venepuncture. To standardize constituents, patients are asked to fast before the blood samples are taken.

The serum yielded may be given by different means. PRP can be injected into and around tendons, or given via a fibrin scaffold during open or arthroscopic surgery.

The volume and timing of the application vary according to the concentration and activation of the platelet components themselves. After production, the sample of serum will coagulate over time and the platelets themselves will start secreting growth factors immediately (Marx 2001, 2004). Sodium citrate can be added to the serum to prevent clotting before clinical application. The administered platelets will synthesize and secrete additional growth factors for the remainder of their 7- to 10-day lifespan. This initial short-lived burst nevertheless has prolonged efficacy (Marx 2004; Sampson et al. 2008).

The main growth factors in the PRP concentrate are transforming growth factor β1 (TGFβ), platelet-derived growth factor (PDGF), vascular endothelial growth factor (VEGF), hepatocyte growth factor (HGF), and insulin-like growth factor 1 (IGF-1). These biologically active growth factors work using endocrine, paracrine, autocrine, and intracrine mechanisms by stimulating angiogenesis, epithelialization, cell differentiation–replication–proliferation, and the formation of extracellular matrix (Sánchez et al. 2007; Schnabel et al. 2007).

In one study involving human tenocytes, platelet-rich clot releasate led to an increase in total collagen, collagen gene expression, and cell proliferation. PRP might accelerate the catabolic demarcation of traumatically injured tendon matrices, and promote angiogenesis and the formation of fibrovascular callus (De Mos et al. 2008).

Individual growth factors have specific effects. PDGF is a powerful mitogen for connective tissue cells, TGFβ is implicated in collagen synthesis, IGF-1 is known to be critical for cell survival, growth, and metabolism, and VEGF and HGF induce endothelial cell proliferation leading to new blood vessel formation (Sánchez et al. 2009). IGF-1 has anti-inflammatory effects in sectioned tendon healing (Kurtz et al. 1999).

A review of the literature on the benefits of PRP on tendon healing has revealed little firm evidence, with most recommendations being expert opinion (Hall et al 2009; Engebretsen et al. 2010). However, further evidence is being gathered in both acute injury and tendon rupture and the chronic overuse states of tendinopathy.

With increasing research, the clinical benefits of growth factors are being increasingly appreciated. In sheep models, repeated injections of PRGF within Achilles tendon fascicles lead to increased cell number and angiogenesis but little fibrosis (Anitua et al. 2006a,b). There is increased evidence to support the effect of angiogenesis when significantly more neovascularization on color Doppler occurs in surgically treated lesions of the equine superficial digital flexor tendon (Bosch et al. 2010). Additional differentiation changes have been noted after the application of PRP to tenocyte stem cells. These stem cells became larger, and were well spread and elongated with the downregulation of nucleostemin expression after PRP application. There was also increased tenocyte-related gene expression, cell proliferation, and total collagen production (Zhang and Wang 2010).

In addition to the histological changes, improved biomechanical properties have been noted after PRP application. When transected Achilles tendons in rats were treated using percutaneous injections of PRP, the tendon callus strength and stiffness were 30% higher in those treated by PRP after 1 week. Mechanical testing showed improved callus maturation (Aspenberg and Virchenko 2004). Similar improvements in mechanical strength were observed in a rat patellar tendon-healing model. One group of specimens, with the most successful platelet concentrations, was noted to have a higher ultimate tensile load and energy to failure (Spang et al. 2011). Increased tendon regeneration and strength have been reported in repaired tendons after only one injection at 1 week after surgery in a laboratory model (Virchenko and Aspenberg 2006). Lyras' group (Lyras at al. 2010a,b) has performed a series of laboratory-controlled animal studies of tendon healing with the application of PRP gel at the time of tendon repair. They report faster healing of the PRP group compared with controls and histologically increased numbers of various cell types during the first 2 weeks of healing and increased IGF-1 in tenocytes, the epitenon, and endotenon, with cytoplasmic and nuclear expression during the later stages. They also reported an upregulation of TGFβ during the first 2 weeks and downregulation in the third and fourth weeks.

Although there are relatively few studies in human patients, cohort comparison studies in patients with ruptured Achilles tendons have shown accelerated functional recovery with the addition of PRGF injections. The PRGF group also demonstrated the surprising long-term consequence (>18 months) of decreased cross-sectional area in the healed tendon (Sánchez et al. 2007). We have conducted a level 1 study comparing percutaneous repair of the Achilles tendon biologically augmented with PRGF injections versus control tendons with repair only. Ultrasound examination with repeated follow-up has shown healing characteristics at early stages but with reduced scar formation and more normal looking tissue in the treated group. A prospective randomized study has been reported which shows no difference in the outcome after the application of PRP during Achilles tendon repairs (Schepull et al. 2007). In the treatment arm of this series relatively large volumes of PRP were injected into the paratenon following closure.

There is much more evidence relating to the role of PRP in the treatment of chronic tendon problems, i.e., tendinopathy. Traditional injection treatments such as corticosteroid injections may be problematic. The use of PRP is potentially a more beneficial treatment option (Sánchez et al. 2009).

Areas susceptible to tendinopathy are typically origin and insertional sites including the Achilles, patella tendon, and common wrist extensor origin. These sites are frequently related to microtrauma involved in running, jumping, and racquet sports, respectively.

Once again the evidence is scant. Gaweda et al. (2010) report significant improvement of the American Orthopedic Foot and Ankle Society Scores (Kitaoka et al. 1994) and improved imaging characteristics after the administration of PRP for patients with Achilles tendinopathy. Similarly, Volpi et al. (2007) performed single PRP injections on a small series of eight athletes with chronic patellar tendinopathy, and reported a significant improvement of 91% on VISA-P (Vitorian Institute of Sport Assessment – Patella) (Visentini et al. 1998) assessment. Magnetic resonance imaging (MRI) revealed a noticeable reduction in tendon irregularity of the affected tendon in 80% of the patients.

Mishra and Pavelko (2006) attempted a cohort study of the injection of PRP versus local anesthetic for chronic elbow tendinosis. Although 60% of patients reported an improvement in symptoms compared with 16% in the control group, three-fifths of the patients in the control group withdrew or sought other treatment, preventing definitive long-term comparisons. Peerbooms and co-workers (2010) compared PRP with corticosteroid injection for elbow lateral epicondylitis. Those patients who had received the PRP had reduced pain and improved function exceeding the effect of the corticosteroid injection.

Filardo et al. (2010a) and Kon et al. (2009) both reported prospective case series on PRP administered to patellar tendons for tendinopathy. The patients in both series improved notably, and in Filardo's series a statistically significant improvement in Tegner's and visual analog scores was shown. Neither series reported any complications. We have had a similar result with a large group of professional athletes with patellar tendinopathy.

A recent randomized controlled trial by De Vos et al. (2010a) is less convincing for the therapeutic benefits for Achilles tendinopathy. In a prospective randomized study of 53 patients, the mean Victorian Institute of Sport Assessment (VISA) Achilles scores improved in both treatment (eccentric exercises and PRP) and control (eccentric exercises only) groups without significant improvement in the treatment group. Of note, only one injection of PRP was performed whereas most retrospective cohort comparisons reporting improved outcome use a series of injections. Many surgeons suggest the minimum use of three injections to treat tendinopathic conditions, reserving a single PRP injection for the treatment of acute problems, e.g., muscle tears.

Given the lower limb predisposition for tendinopathy with the exemption of elbow epicondylitis, it is not surprising that there have been fewer studies on the upper limbs. When different forces are applied to the upper and the lower limbs, the effects reported on an upper limb tendinous structure may not be directly comparable with the lower limb. Conversely, the rotator cuff tendons exhibit a unique form of impingement, given the numerous biomechanical predisposing factors, which mostly relate to surrounding structures. This can lead to tears in the cuff tendons and subacromial bursitis as well as bicep tendon pathologies. Upper limb tendinopathy may present later, and the prognosis may be worse. Local anesthetic and steroid injections may settle subacromial bursal inflammation and alleviate the symptoms, but this injection will not improve the healing of partial rotator cuff microtears. Steroid injections also weaken tissue, causing long-term damage to the rotator cuff and possible tear promotion.

There have been a few papers published on human patients reporting the outcome after surgery with the addition of PRP. Procedures reported include treatment for subacromial pathology, open subacromial decompression, and rotator cuff surgery (Nho et al. 2010).

A retrospective cohort comparison has been performed for subacromial syndrome surgery comparing the outcome when PRP was applied to traditional, mini-open, and arthroscopic surgery versus previous patients. The authors reported a significant reduction in rehabilitation time and an early improvement in the pain score (Jimenez-Martin et al. 2009). The exogenous application of platelet leukocyte gel during open subacromial decompression has contributed to faster recovery, earlier return to daily activities, and less analgesic requirement (Everts et al. 2008).

PRP was used to augment arthroscopic cuff repair in a case series of 14 patients, leading to improved pain and functional outcome without any adverse events being reported (Randelli et al. 2008). The same research groups have recently published a level 1, prospective, randomized, double-blind, controlled study. Patients reported significantly less pain and improved strength in external rotation, Simple Shoulder Test, UCLA, and Constant scores at 3 months after surgery. No difference was shown in scores between the two groups at 6, 12, and 24 months after surgery. Imaging also did not show a difference in healing rate. For smaller tears (grades 1 and 2) with less retraction, there was significantly higher external strength at all stages after surgery (Randelli et al. 2010). A randomized controlled study completed by Castricini et al. (2011) has shown that there was no significant difference in Constant scores in small and medium-sized tears.

As research progresses, the benefits of PRP and PRGF injections are being increasingly appreciated. Although improved outcomes are difficult to prove conclusively, it is worth noting that there are no complications reported related to the use of PRP, which should be considered experimental in all aspects of sports medicine (Creaney and Hamilton 2008). The current lack of evidence is probably not a reason to withhold its use given the lack of recognized side effects. We encourage additional randomized studies to enable firm conclusions about its efficacy.

INDICATIONS FOR PRP APPLICATION IN TENDON HEALING

In general there are two major indications for use of PRP in tendon injuries. The most beneficial one, with the best results, would be acute tendon tears, while the other is long-standing tendinopathy.

Unlike steroid injections, which predispose the soft tissue to future injury, damage, and possible tear, PRP does not seem to weaken the tendon. The fact that the treatment is being prepared from the patient's own blood makes it safe and relatively easy.

Few centers around the world have experience with PRP application to numerous soft-tissue injuries, mainly muscle and tendon tears, and together with long-standing inflammatory conditions. Even fewer centers have presented their experience with top-level athletes, claiming to reduce their return to play time by up to 50% (Sánchez et al. 2009; Mei-Dan et al. 2010b). Unfortunately, there are no high-level evidence studies to confirm this belief. Professional athletes are unlikely to participate in any study where there is the possibility that they could be given a placebo or not given the treatment arm of a study. As a result, the evidence-based medicine for PRP treatment in professional athletes lags behind the clinical impression obtained from recreational athletes and the non-sporting population.

The following indications have been used in published series of PRP treatment and represent the more common tendon pathologies treated by this technique. It should be emphasized that, as long as an authorized, accepted, and safe technique is applied, this treatment can be performed for every tendon or muscle injury, regardless of its anatomical location. Put simply, we believe that, wherever rupture with bleeding occurs, PRP is likely to improve the outcome.

Acute tendon injuries

The relatively short worldwide experience with acute tendon injuries treated by PRP has shown promising results. The application of platelets, with their accompanying growth factors, may speed up the healing process initiated after an injury. The theory behind the encouraging clinical and laboratory results suggests that, by applying PRP to the injured site, we skip over a phase of the natural healing process. When a tendon, or muscle, is injured we expect it to go through the three known stages of the healing process: Inflammation/degeneration, regeneration, and fibrosis. Usually the platelets within the hematoma formed at the site of injury initiate this chemotactic cascade (Kajikawa et al. 2008) and attract the growth factor, which will take over the process. PRP reduces the steps in the healing cascade, and so may yield better quality tissue in a shorter period.

The application of PRP in acute tendon injuries occurs typically in two treatment scenarios.

Conservative treatment with the usage of PRP

PRP would be applicable for almost every musculotendinous junction injury in the body and to tendon mid-substance tears, acute or acute on chronic, which are not retracted. Examples include:

- Partial-thickness tear of rotator cuff tendons (Figs 18.1 to 18.3)
- Partial Achilles tendon tear
- Adductor tendon traumatic tears
- Peroneal or tibialis posterior tendon partial tears.

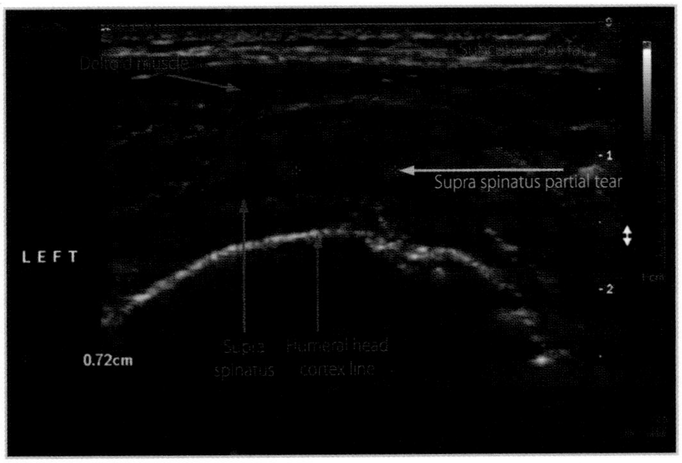

Figure 18.1 An axial ultrasound scan of a partial tear of supraspinatus (yellow arrow). The red arrows are pointing at the anatomical landmarks of the region. The pre-injection imaging of the supraspinatus tendon and the tear measurement are routinely performed in the longitudinal and axial planes. Given the anatomical characteristic of this area, the injection of the platelet-rich plasma is usually performed in the axial plane. Only the tip of the needle into the lesion can be seen in this projection.

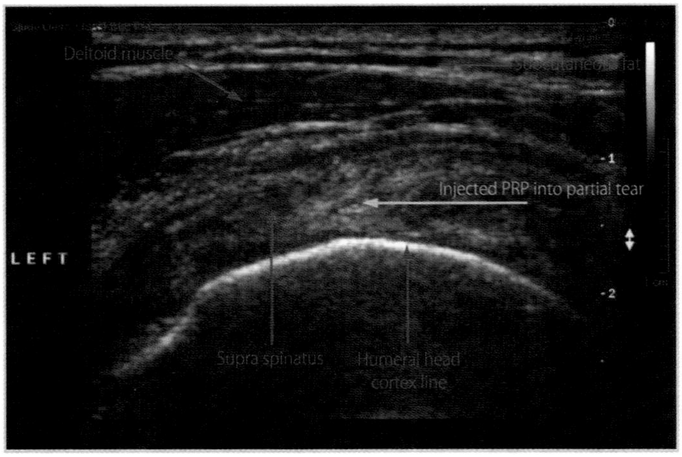

Figure 18.2 An axial ultrasound scan of a partial tear of supraspinatus after injection with platelet-rich plasma, seen as the white/hyperechoic area marked with a yellow arrow. Red arrows are pointing at the anatomical landmarks of the region.

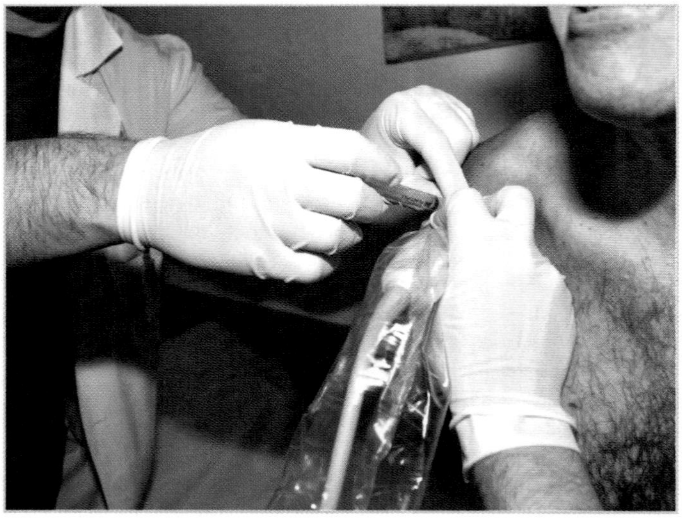

Figure 18.3 Ultrasound-guided injection.

PRP application after suture or repair of an injured tendon

In this case, the treatment is applied intraoperatively at the end of surgical repair or reattachment. Alternatively, injections may be applied after the initial hematoma has resolved or arthroscopic irrigation fluid has absorbed. Known examples are:

- After arthroscopic repair of the rotator cuff
- After Achilles tendon suture (when performed open the application is during surgery; when performed percutaneously, we recommend to apply PRP 3–5 days after the index procedure)
- After flexor tendon repairs.

Chronic tendon injuries and tendinopathies

The clinical picture of tendinopathy is pain and swelling associated with a failed healing response, and is an active tendon cell-mediated process. This involves increased turnover and remodeling, and gradual transformation in the quality and quantity of extracellular matrix that habitually precedes tendon rupture.

Few researchers have studied the influence of PRP on this very "hard to treat" entity. As opposed to acute tendon injuries, where the tendon is essentially normal, the variety of scenarios and presentations here is endless. Many of these patients have already been treated with a variety of methods and modalities before PRP treatment, and as a cohort they are often very chronic and have been resistant to all other forms of management. We can never compare the outcome of a patient with lateral epicondylitis of short duration, which was treated with PRP as a first-line treatment, with a 3-year-old resilient disease with chronic changes, which was treated with numerous steroid injections and shock wave therapy.

TECHNIQUES

PRP preparation process

The unique properties of PRPs have led to the commercial development of multiple systems that offer an easy and cost-effective strategy to obtain high concentrations of factors for tissue healing and regeneration in the clinical setting.

The process of PRP preparation is relatively straightforward, and can be performed in the clinic or the operating room. In most cases, it can be completed within minutes. The cost to both medical practitioners and patients varies widely depending on the method used to produce the PRP. A commercial kit yields a PRP concentrate at the cost of several hundred US$ (US$300–600). On the other hand, in-house manual techniques produce a PRP concentrate for around US$20.

For PRP preparation, peripheral blood is drawn from the patient under sterile conditions, with or without anticoagulants depending on the technique used. The plasma is prepared by centrifugation or filtration. The volume can be adapted to the clinical needs. The methods of producing PRPs determine the composition and concentration in terms of leukocytes, erythrocytes, and platelets in a given plasma volume. In the last few years, several semi-automatic machines have been developed for centrifugal separation of PRP for therapeutic use, but the most common, simple, and flexible (can be adjusted to the specific indication treated) is the manual one.

Methods of PRP preparation

- Double spinning methods using automated machines along with commercial kits
- Single spinning methods using conventional laboratory centrifuges followed by manual PRP separation (**Fig. 18.4**)
- Selective blood filtration using commercial available technology.

It should be emphasized that most of the commercial available PRP kits eliminate the need for manual separation because the endpoint of their process is a syringe with "ready to use" PRP. These kits will always contain white blood cells (WBCs) within the applied concentrate because gravity fraction separation after centrifugation cannot differentiate between the WBCs and the bottom plasma layer rich in growth factors.

Accordingly, platelet concentrates have been categorized in pure platelet-rich plasma (P-PRP), in which leukocytes are purposely eliminated from the PRP, and leukocyte and platelet-rich plasma (L-PRP), containing high concentration of leukocytes. Whether leukocytes have detrimental effects in particular orthopedic sport applications is controversial, but basic evidence points toward a deleterious effect of neutrophils, particularly in joint or muscle injuries. The improved

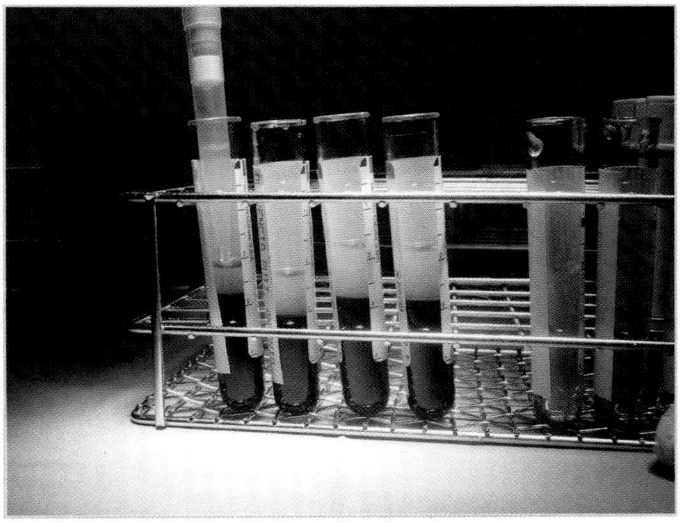

Figure 18.4 The tubes represent different fractions that a single centrifugation (preparation rich in growth factors or PRGF technique, 460 × g for 8 min) would yield in a 3.8% sodium citrate 4 mL tube. The technique uses a manual separation process that yields platelet-rich plasma.

homogeneity of P-PRP and its reduced donor-to-donor variability would support the view that some PRP production techniques are more reproducible and predictable than others.

There is little consensus about the dose of platelets, and growth factors, needed to obtain efficient clinical results. The clinical variability observed in scientific studies suggests that some techniques might not produce a sufficient number of functional platelets to produce the expected outcome. Similarly, there is frequently no consistency in the methods of application of this therapy, timing of treatment, the number of injections or volume of injection. This has precluded the establishment of the standards necessary to integrate the extensive relevant literature in basic and clinical science. Also, each method leads to a different product with different biological properties and potential uses. Currently, it is unclear whether these differences have any clinical relevance. Some authors have suggested that PRP preparations containing only moderately elevated platelet concentrations induce optimal biological benefit, whereas lower platelet concentrations produce suboptimal effects, and higher ones inhibitory effects. Further, the actual growth factor content does not correlate with the platelet count in whole blood or in PRP when leukocytes are present in the preparation, and there is no evidence that gender or age affects platelet count or growth factor concentrations. Age may influence the number of receptors of local cells interacting with the plasma signals.

Once the PRP is separated from the whole blood, it is stable for up to 8 hours, or for even longer periods. However, as these procedures are considered as an autograft by the regulatory organizations, the plasma should be prepared and immediately used at the point of care, and should not be stored.

Before application, platelets can be slowly activated by setting in motion the coagulation cascade with the addition of calcium chloride, a necessary cofactor for conversion of prothrombin into thrombin. Alternatively, coagulation and platelets can be instantly activated by adding to the PRP a standard solution of 1000 units/mL of bovine or human thrombin along with 10% calcium chloride. After plasma activation, the fibrin scaffold can be formed in vivo or ex vivo: the latter is suitable for implantation in surgery or in ulcer care, and provides a gradual release of growth factors in the area where it has been applied.

Injection technique

After appropriate clinical examination, imaging will assist in establishing the exact location and extent of the injury. As PRP is considered to best act when placed at the site of injured tissue, we recommend ultrasound guidance to verify accurate needle placement when treatment is not during a surgical procedure (see **Fig. 18.3**).

If application of PRP is to be planned for a day or two after a surgical procedure, a sterile port (such as a drainage hole), placed during the procedure, can serve as an accurate injecting measure. This is particularly helpful if ultrasound guidance is not available. It is assumed that application of the concentrate around and over the tendon would be sufficient and there is no need to try to infiltrate the tendon itself, avoiding possible damage to its inner structure.

One of the exceptions to the above is the common patellar tendinopathy (jumper's knee), which lies within the tendon substance and will usually require an intrasubstance tendon needle placement. In the presence of exudates or hematoma around the tendon, we suggest that this be evacuated before PRP is injected. In the physiological process of wound healing, platelets embedded within the blood clot serve as a primary source of biologically active factors. Typically, after muscle and tendon strain or contusion the hematoma that originates as a consequence of vessel disruption contains about 94% red blood cells, a small number of platelets (4%), and less than 1% leukocytes. The rationale for the use of PRP involves replacing the blood clot with PRP, thus minimizing the presence of red blood cells and increasing platelet concentration at the injury site. In doing so, we achieve supraphysiological concentrations of growth factors that accelerate the repair process by direct or indirect mechanisms, i.e., enhancing further synthesis of growth factors by local cells.

If PRP is administered at arthroscopy (**Figs 18.5a** to **d**), the injection should be performed after emptying the joint of arthroscopic fluid. Some intra-articular indications, such as meniscal repair, will enable accurate placement of an arthroscopic guidance needle, which theoretically yields better clinical results. In the case of open surgery, application of PRP can be undertaken using one of the gel and semi-solid forms just before closure or by infiltrating the concentrate at the desired area.

The concomitant use of local anesthesia with application of PRP may be disadvantageous. Many surgeons suspect that using local anesthetic will be detrimental to the final clinical outcome, given the changes in the pH of the tissue and interactions with the PRP concentrate. We therefore recommend avoiding local anesthetic when injecting PRP into a relatively superficial tissue. It is still possible to infiltrate the skin and subcutaneous tissue with local anesthetic when the PRP target is a deep soft-tissue construct (or joint), such as the origin of the hamstring tendons or the insertion of the supraspinatus tendon.

We recommend specific equipment that is available in any facility were PRP is used. The area to be injected should be prepared in a sterile fashion, similar to a lumbar puncture procedure. A sterile tray should be utilized. We use a 23 G size needle for every superficially located injection and a 18 G spinal needle for deep soft-tissue injections. When injecting a deep joint, such as the hip, we sometimes prefer to use a 22 G spinal needle when local anesthesia is not used.

It is crucial to always use a Luer-type syringe because on many occasions the tissue to be injected will produce a relative resistance that, if not using this type of syringe, would result in fluid backflow. We also recommend injecting the PRP in an easy and slow manner to make sure that the needle does not move, under ultrasound guidance

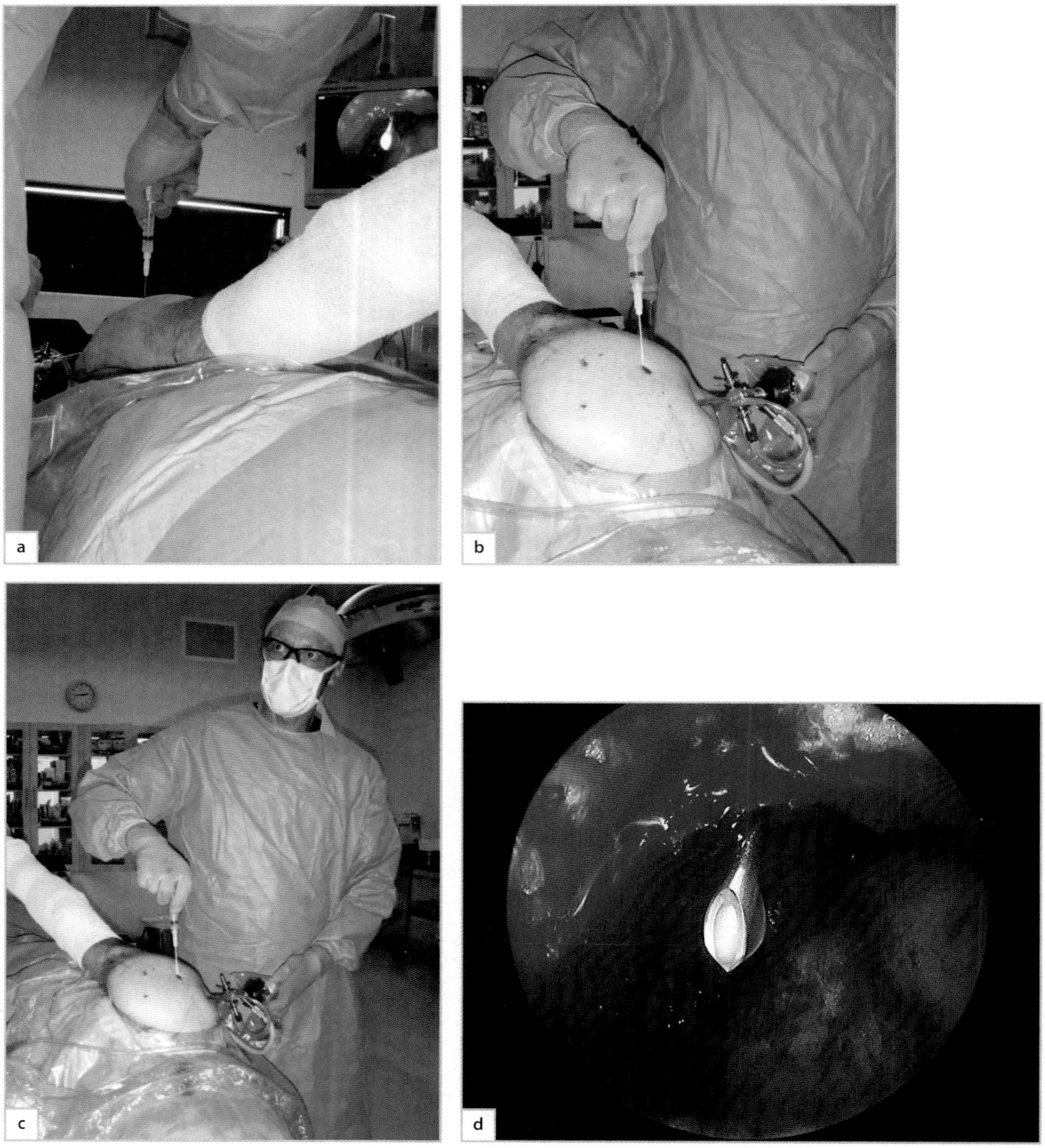

Figure 18.5 (a–c) Arthroscopic rotator cuff repair followed by injection of a preparation rich in growth factors over the repaired tendon via the subacromial joint. When platelet-rich plasma is administered at arthroscopy, the injection should be performed after emptying the joint of arthroscopic fluid. Once surgical procedure is complete, the appropriately placed needle can infiltrate the target tissues or spread around the repaired site, under dry vision. (d) After emptying the subacromial space from arthroscopic fluid, platelet-rich plasma is administered under direct vision, if possible.

if possible throughout the procedure, because even the greatest PRP concentrate would not yield any clinical results if placed away from the designated pathology.

Post-injection treatment

Platelets influence only the early phases of regeneration, but this allows mechanical stimulation to start the healing process (Virchenko and Aspenberg 2006). We advocate that PRP should be combined with an appropriate loading regimen to enhance extracellular matrix organization in the short term.

Indeed, in one study, injections of PRP 1 week postoperatively increased tendon regenerate strength after 4 weeks if combined with early therapy (Fufa et al. 2008).

Recently, a placebo-controlled experimental trial in six horses reported less inflammation and increased metabolic activity and maturation, higher strength at failure, and elastic modulus in tendons treated with PRP (Foster et al. 2009). As a result, many clinicians would speed up the standard and common rehabilitation processes.

We reported on an Olympic judoka who had completely torn his elbow medial complex (both medical collateral ligament and common flexor tendon origin) just 10 months before the Olympics. Surgery at that stage would have eliminated his chances to qualify for the games. He elected to be treated with PRP, followed by a tailored and accelerated rehabilitation protocol. The athlete's elbow was stable 6 weeks after his injury and two PRGF injections. The athlete went on to win a gold medal in a world cup tournament, 5.5 months past his injury (Mei-Dan et al 2010b).

Most of the published literature on accelerated return to play with professional athletes is anecdotal. Nevertheless, many doctors experienced with PRP generally favor a combined approach.

There is no general agreement on post-injection treatment and this will obviously depend on the specific indication treated. Most studies have allowed light exercises 2–5 days after tendinopathy-related injection. Patients should follow general recommendations after an injection with rest, ice, and limb elevation for 48 hours if the area is either in an acute injury phase or very inflamed. Depending on the site of treatment, and extent and duration of the condition, patients could follow an accelerated rehabilitation protocol under appropriate supervision.

For partial tendon and muscle acute tears, the authors recommend a single ultrasound-guided injection which would be followed by 24 hours of complete rest, enabling the tissues to absorb the concentrate, and avoiding additional stress and pain in the injected area. If the patient is completely non-tender, and pain is not an issue, and especially with professional athletes, we sometimes guide the team physical therapist to undertake very gentle superficial friction massage to the area a few hours after the injection. Day 2 and day 3 post-injection are usually pain free and local massage with full, open, kinetic chain, active and passive range of motion are advised. Cryotherapy should be followed at the end of each session, reducing the chance of excessive fluid production, including muscle seroma or reactive tenosynovitis.

With regard to the injured tissue anatomical location and size, and with respect to the experienced pain, light jogging and strengthening work can be initiated on days 3–4. We usually clear an athlete for high level sports training after full activity tests of the injected area, with no pain during or after the above. This subjective feeling must be followed with the evidence of newly formed scar tissue within the lesion, on follow-up sonography. That time frame can be as short as a week for some muscle tears in professional athletes.

An injection to a partial-thickness tear of supraspinatus in a recreational athlete, for example, would be followed by 24 hours of shoulder girdle rest. Although resting from activity, passive range of motion of the affected side every few hours and possible local massage and ice should be used. When local pain is improved, usually within 2–3 days, active assisted range of motion can be initiated in a very slow and easy manner.

There is disagreement about the use of concomitant non-steroidal anti-inflammatory drugs (NSAIDs) before the PRP treatment and during the first 2 weeks after its application. Although there are published data on the role of NSAIDs and the healing of various tissues such as bone, tendon, and muscle, there are no data on concomitant use with PRP. We recommend avoiding NSAIDs, when possible, at least 2 days before PRP application and throughout the treatment timeframe, usually up to 2 weeks post-injection.

APPLICATION DURING SURGERY

PRP and PRGF may be applied to an injured or operated area by two processes, either injection or direct application. Intraoperative injection can be performed under direct vision with the injection of the products of the centrifugation process directly into the repaired area. This has the advantage that specific fractions of serum with highly concentrated small volumes of PRP may be injected into repair sites. Rotator cuff and meniscal repairs are localized repairs suitable for this. Arthroscopic visualization allows a narrow-bore spinal needle, e.g., 22 G, to inject samples directly into the opposed tendon ends. If this occurs at the end of the procedure when minimal further movement is likely to occur, the injected solution is likely to remain within and around the repair site itself rather than being diluted by the irrigation fluid.

The application of PRP mesh has the benefit of ease of use but the timing of application is such that the initial release of growth factors may be missed during the coagulation process. This may be minimized by preparing two separate serum samples. The first may be allowed to coagulate and form the fibrin matrix. The second can be activated at a later stage and injected into this matrix to supplement the healing process.

A combination of both techniques may be used to provide local infiltration of the repair site with growth factors and the repair may then be covered with the growth factor-enriched fibrin matrix.

The application of PRP at any other time is likely to require ultrasound guidance to ensure that it is injected into the area of pathology. We have previously commented that most PRP treatments involve a series of injections. After the initial intraoperative injection, subsequent injections require image guidance. This enables the PRP to be placed exactly at the location of the repair. Given the importance of the centrifugation process to prepare the growth factor, it is essential to ensure that the optimal concentrations of factors are injected into the repair site.

POSTOPERATIVE MANAGEMENT

Given the current evidence of the benefits of growth factors to promote healing and strengthening of the tissue formed, the administration of growth factors should not alter the normal postoperative rehabilitation (Maniscalco et al. 2008; Conti et al. 2009). We currently believe that the PRP treatment method will allow injured or operated tissues to heal better and in a shorter time. The program of rehabilitation may consequently be increased with the accelerated recovery process. The current published literature reveals few studies to support this theory. High-level studies are currently under way.

In the Sánchez cohort comparison group for repair of the Achilles tendon, those participants who had received PRP recovered normal range mobility after 7 weeks rather than 11 weeks, and were able to return to play at 14 weeks compared with 22 weeks for the non-treated group (Sánchez et al. 2007). Both groups had their protective casts removed at 2–3 weeks after surgery and received the same range-of-movement and active strengthening rehabilitation program. Randelli et al.'s (2010) randomized study of biologically augmented repair used a standard postoperative regimen for both groups consisting of the introduction of passive exercises at day 10 after surgery. Once this was restored at 30 days after surgery, assisted active exercises were started with selective strengthening started at 2 months after the procedure. Our experience is that patients returned to activities of daily living and play sooner with an active strengthening regimen.

Other studies show similar outcomes. Berghoff et al. (2006) performed a randomized prospective study applying autologous platelet gel during closure of total knee arthroplasty. Treated patients were discharged from hospital earlier and had improved range of motion at 6 weeks. Improved range of motion at 6 weeks postoperatively has also been noted by others authors administering platelet gel during total knee replacement (Mooar et al. 2000).

For rotator cuff pathology, the repair may either be protected or have a moderate restriction depending on the size of the repair and the repaired tissue quality, as described by the surgeon. Given a program in which progression is based on the quality of the repaired tissue, it is likely that patients will progress rapidly through a rehabilitation regimen, and this can be tailored accordingly. Ultrasonography may also play a role in the decision to adopt an accelerated rehabilitation program. A typical rehabilitation protocol is outlined in **Table 18.1**.

Care should be taken with postoperative analgesia control. Most patients use a combination of analgesics and anti-inflammatory medication. However, the method of action of NSAIDs alters the normal process of healing by reducing platelet function. We therefore recommend the avoidance of NSAIDs whenever PRP is used to treat rotator cuff tendons.

CONCLUSION

The use of PRP improves healing when compared with standard healing times; however, there is currently a lack of prospective randomized studies in the literature. We believe that PRP injections after surgery will have a beneficial effect on the ongoing healing process of rotator cuff repairs and there have been no complications reported from its use. Obviously, additional prospective randomized trials are needed before any firm conclusions about the efficacy of PRP can be made.

Table 18.1 Typical rehabilitation timetable

	Grade 1 tear	Grade 2 tear	Grade 3 tear
Protection	0–2 weeks	0–3 weeks	0–4 weeks
Passive range of motion exercises	2–4 weeks	3–6 weeks	4–8 weeks
Flexion exercises	4–8 weeks	6–12 weeks	8–16 weeks
Strengthening exercises	8–12 weeks	12–16 weeks	16–24 weeks
Global resistance exercises	12–16 weeks	16 weeks	24 weeks

Grade 1 stands for a small tear with good quality tissue, grade 2 is a larger tear with good tissue or small tear with poor tissue, and grade 3 would stand for larger tear with poor tissue requiring maximal protection.

REFERENCES

Alsousou J, Thompson M, Huley P, Willet K. the biology of platelet rich plasma and its application in trauma and orthopaedic surgery. A review article. J Bone Joint Surg Br 2009;51:987.

Anitua E. Plasma rich in growth factors: preliminary results of use and preparation of sites for implants. Int J Oral Maxillofacial Implants 1999;14:529–535.

Anitua E, Sánchez M, Nurden AT, et al. Autolgous fibrin matrices: A potental source of biological mediators modulate tendon cell activities. J Biomater Res A 2006a;77:285–293.

Anitua E, Sánchez M, Nurden AT, et al. New insights into novel applications for platelet rich fibrin therapies. Trends Biotechnol 2006b;24:227–234.

Aspenberg P, Virchenko O. Platelet concentrate injection improves Achilles tendon repair in rats. Acta Orthop Scand 2004;75:93–99.

Berghoff WJ, Pietrzak WS, Rhodes RD. Platelet rich plasma application during closure following total knee arthroplasty. Orthopaedics 2006;29:590.

Bosch G, Moleman M, Barneveld A, Van Weeren PR, Van Schie HT. The effect of PRP on neovascularisation of surgically treated equine superficial flexor digital flexor tendon lesions. Scand J Med Sci Sports 2011;21:554–561.

Castricini R, Longo UG, De Benedetto M, et al. Platelet rich plasma augmentation for arthroscopic rotator cuff repair: a randomized controlled trial. Am J Sports Med 2011;3:258–265.

Conti M, Garofalo R, Delle Rose G, et al. Post operative rehabilitation after surgical repair of the rotator cuff. Chir Organi Mov 2009;93(suppl 1):S55–S63.

Creaney L, Hamilton B. Growth factor delivery methods in the management of sports injuries: state of play. Br J Sports Med 2008;42:314–320.

De Mos M, Van der Windt AE, Jahr H et al. Can platelet rich plasma enhance tendon repair? A cell culture study. Am J Sports Med 2008;36:1171–1178.

De Vos RJ, Weir A, van Schie HT, et al. Platelet-rich plasma injection for chronic Achilles tendinopathy: a randomized controlled trial. JAMA 2010a;303:144–149.

De Vos RJ, Van Veldhoven PL, Moen MH, et al. Autologous growth factor injections in chronic tendinopathy: a systematic review. Br Med Bull 2010b;95:63–77.

Engebretsen L, Steffen K, Alsousou J, et al. IOC consensus paper on the use of platelet rich plasma in sports medicine. Br J Sports Med 2010;44:1072–1081 .

Everts PA, Devilee RJ, Brown Mahoney C, et al. Exogenous application of platelet leucocyte gel during open subacromial decompression contributes to improved patient outcome. A prospective radomised double blind study. Eur Surg Res 2008;40:203–w10.

Filardo G, Kon E, Della Villa S, et al. Use of platelet-rich plasma for the treatment of refractory jumper's knee. Int Orthop 2010a;34:909–915.

Filardo G, Presti ML, Kon E, Marcacci M. Non operative biological treatment approach for partial Achilles tendon lesion. Orthopaedics 2010b;33:120–123.

Foster TE, Puskas BL, Mandelbaum BR, Gerhardt MB, Rodeo SA. Platelet rich plasma. From basic science to clinical applications. Am J Sport Med 2009;37:2259–72.

Fufa D Shealy B, Jacobsen M, et al. Activation of Platelet Rich Plasma using soluble type 1 collagen. J Oral Maxillofax Surg 2008;66:684–690.

Gaweda K, Tarczynska M, Krzyzanowski W. Treatment of Achilles tendinopathy with Platelet Rich Plasma. Int J Sports Med 2010;31:577–583.

Graziani F, Ivanovski S, Cei S, et al. The in vitro effect of different PRP concentrations of osteoblasts and fibroblasts. Clin Oral Implants Res 2006;17:212–219.

Hall MP, Band PA, Meislin RJ, Jazrawi LM, Cardone DA. Platelet rich plasma: current concepts and application in sports medicine. J Am Acad Orthop Surg 2009;17:602–608.

Harrison P, Cramer EM. Platelet alpha-granules. Blood Rev 1993;7:52–62.

Jimenez-Martin A, Angulo-Gutierrez A, Gonzalez-Herranz J, et al. Surgery of subacromial syndrome with application of plasma rich in growth factors. Int J Shoulder Surg 2009;3:28–33.

Kajikawa Y, Morihara T, Sakamoto H, et al. Platelet-rich plasma enhances the initial mobilization of circulation-derived cells for tendon healing. J Cell Physiol 2008;215:837–545.

Kitaoka H, Alexander IJ, Adelaar RS, et al. Clinical rating systems for the ankle-hindfoot, midfoot, halluz and lesser toes. Foot Ankle Int 1994;15:349–353.

Kon E, Filardo G, Delcogliano M, et al. Platelet-rich plasma: new clinical application: a pilot study for treatment of jumper's knee. Injury 2009;40, 598–603.

Kovacevic D, Rodeo SA. Biological augmentation of rotator cuff tendon repair. Clin Orthop Relat Res 2008;466:622–633.

Kurtz CA, Loebig TG, Anderson DD, DeMeo PJ, Campbell PG. Insulin-like growth factor 1 accelerates functional recovery from Achilles tendon injury in a rat model. Am J Sports Med 1999;27:363–369.

Lyras DN, Kazako K, Agrogiannis IG, et al. Experimental study of tendon healing in the early phase: is IGF 1 expression influenced by platelet rich plasma gel? Orthop Traumatol Surg Res 2010a;96:381–387.

Lyras DN, Kazakos K, Tryfonidis M, et al. Temporal and spatial expression of TGF Beta in Achilles tendon section model after application of PRP. Foot Ankle Surg 2010b;16:137–141.

Maniscalco P, Gambera D, Lunati A, et al. The "Cascade" membrane: new PRP device for tendon ruptures. Description and case report on rotator cuff tendon. Acta Biomed 2008;79:223–226.

Marx RE. Platelet rich plasma (PRP): What is PRP and what is not PRP? Implant Dent 2001;10:225–228.

Marx RE. Platelet rich plasma: Evidence to support its use. J Oral Maxillofac Surg 2004;62:489–496.

Marx RE, Carlson ER, Eichstaedt RM, et al. Platelet rich plasma. Growth factor enhancement for bone grafts. Oral Surg Oral Med Oral Pathol Oral Radiol Endod 1998;85:638–646.

Mei-Dan O, Mann G, Maffulli N. Platelet rich plasma: Any substance to it? Br J Sports Med 2010a;44:618–619.

Mei-Dan O, Carmont MR, Kots E, et al. Early return to play following complete rupture of the medial collateral ligament of the elbow using a preparation rich in growth factors: a case report. J Shoulder Elbow Surg 2010b;19:e1–e5.

Mishra A, Pavelko T. Treatment of chronic elbow tendinosis with buffered platelet rich plasma. Am J Sports Med 2006;34:1774–8.

Mooar PA, Gardner MJ, Klepchick PR, et al The efficacy of autologous platelet gel in total knee arthroplasty: an analysis of range of motion, haemoglobin and narcotic requirements. Presented at the American Academy of Orthopaedic Surgeons 6th Annual Meeting. American Academy of Orthopaedic Surgeons, 2000: 148.

Nho SJ, Delos D, Yadav H, et al. Biomechanical and biologic augmentation for the treatment of massive rotator cuff tears. Am J Sports Med 2010;38:619–629.

Peerbooms JC, Sluimer J, Bruijn DJ, Gosens T. Positive effect of an autologous platelet concentrate in lateral epicondylitis in a double-blind randomized controlled trial: platelet-rich plasma versus corticosteroid injection with a 1-year follow-up. Am J Sports Med 2010;38:255–262.

Randelli PS, Arrigoni P, Cabitza P, et al. Autologous platelet rich plasma for arthroscopic rotator cuff repair. A pilot study. Disabil Rehabil 2008;30:1584–1589.

Randelli P, Arrigoni P, Ragone V, Aliprandi A, Cabitla P. Platelet rich plasma in arthroscopic rotator cuff repair: a prospective randomized study. J Shoulder Elbow Surg 2011;20:518–528.

Sampson S, Gerhadt M, Mandelbaum B. Platelet rich plasma injection grafts for musculoskeletal injuries: a review. Curr Res Musculoskelet Med 2008;19:165–174.

Sánchez M, Anitua E, Azofra J, et al. Comparison of surgically repaired Achilles tendon tears using platelet-rich fibrin matrices. Am J Sports Med 2007:35:245–251.

Sánchez M, Anitua E, Orive G, Mujika I, Andia I. Platelet rich therapies in the treatment of Orthopaedic Sports Injuries. Sports Med 2009 39:345–354.

Schepull T, Kvist J, Norrman H, et al. Autologous platelets have no effect on the healing of human Achilles tendon ruptures: a randomized single blind study. Am J Sports Med 2011;39:38–47.

Spang JT, Tlscher T, Salzman GM, et al. Platelet concentration versus saline in a patellar tendon rat healing model. Knee Surg Sports Traumatol Arthroscop 2011;19:495–502.

Virchenko O, Aspenberg P. How can one platelet injection after tendon injury lead to a stronger tendon after 4 weeks? Interplay between early regeneration and mechanical stimulation. Acta Orthop 2006;77:806–812.

Visentini PJ, Khan KM, Cook JL, et al. The VISA score an index of severity of symptoms in patients with Jumpers knee (patella tendinosis). Vitorian Institute Sport Study Group. J Sci Med Sport 1998;1:22–28.

Volpi P, Marinoni L, Bait C, De Girolamo L, Schoenhuber H. Treatment of chronic patellar tendinosis with buffered platelt rich plasma: a preliminary study. Med Sport 2007;60:595–603.

Weibrich G, Hansen T, Kleis W, Buch R, Hitzler WE. The effect of platelet concentration in platelet rich plasma on peri-implant bone reintegration. Bone 2004;34:665–671.

Zhang J, Wang JH. PRP Releasate promotes differentiation of tendon stem cells into active tenocytes. Am J Sports Med 2010;38:2477–2486.

Chapter 19 Outcome measures

Umile Giuseppe Longo, Sebastiano Vasta, Nicola Maffulli, Vincenzo Denaro

KEY FEATURES

- Shoulder scores allow for the systematic evaluation of various treatment options.
- Shoulder scores are classified as generic or disease specific: the former investigate non-specific shoulder disorders that cause shoulder symptoms; the latter investigate specific conditions such as rotator cuff lesions or instability, or the outcomes of specific surgical treatments.
- Many shoulder-rating scores have not been developed following the recommended methodology.
- Cross-cultural adaptation of the various scoring systems should be validated.

INTRODUCTION

Several scoring systems have been developed to satisfy the need to assess the functional status and effectiveness of the treatment of patients with shoulder pain. These scoring systems need to be valid, reliable, and responsive, with high intraobserver agreement (Plancher et al. 2009). Different types of tools exist (many are generic and others are shoulder specific) and are available for orthopedic clinical and research practice (Longo et al. 2008a, 2010b). These tools allow for the evaluation of patients before and after a conservative or non-conservative treatment, detecting short-term or long-term clinical changes of symptoms and disabilities (Plancher et al. 2009). This chapter analyzes generic measurement tools for upper limb dysfunction and disease-specific instruments focusing on rotator cuff lesions. A description of each rating scale is reported and, when available, the psychometric evaluations are supplied.

GENERAL UPPER LIMB RATING SYSTEMS AND SHOULDER-SPECIFIC RATING SCALES

The Oxford Shoulder Score

The Oxford Shoulder Score (OSS: Dawson et al. 1996) is a patient-based questionnaire measuring shoulder pain. It is a condition-specific, self-completed questionnaire. It consists of 12 questions exploring pain (4 questions) and function (8 questions). A score ranging from 1 to 5 is attributed to each item, with a score of 12 representing minimal difficulty and a score of 5 representing severe difficulty. The scores are combined to produce a single score with a range from 12 (least difficulties) to 60 (most difficulties) (Dawson et al. 1996).

Cronbach's α was used to measure the internal consistency of this test, with 0.89 at the preoperative assessment and 0.92 at the 6-month follow-up. The coefficient of test–re-test reliability was calculated as 6.8 using the Bland and Altman method (Dawson et al. 1996).

Comparing this questionnaire with the Constant score, SF-36 (short form 36), and HAQ (Stanford Health Assessment Questionnaire), a significant correlation was found, showing good validity for this tool. The OSS is sensitive to clinical change as demonstrated by comparing scores before and 6 months after surgery. The OSS questionnaire is simple to complete, consistently reliable, and has been validated in Italian (Murena et al. 2010) and German (Huber et al. 2004).

The Shoulder Rating Questionnaire

The Shoulder Rating Questionnaire (SRQ: L'Insalata et al. 1997) consists of six domains: global assessment, pain, daily activities, recreational and athletic activities, work, and satisfaction.

The first domain (global assessment) is measured by a visual analog scale whereas the other domains are rated by a series of multiple-choice questions with five selections associated with scores from 1 (poorest) to 5 (best).

The second domain (pain) includes four questions assessing the severity of pain at rest and during activities, the frequency of pain that interferes with sleep, and the frequency of severe pain.

The third domain (daily activities), consisting of six items, includes one question that requires a general assessment of the limitation of daily activities and a series of questions that assess difficulty with typical daily activities.

The fourth domain (recreational and athletic activities) consists of three questions.

The fifth domain (work) consists of a non-rated question about the kind of work and four graded questions that assess the frequency of inability to do any work, inability to work efficiently, and the need to work a shorter day or to change the manner in which usual work is performed.

The last, non-graded, domain consists of a single question investigating the patient's grade of overall satisfaction (from poor to excellent), and finally the importance domain asks the patient to rank the two areas in which he or she most desires improvement.

The validity of the scale was assessed by comparing it with the Arthritis Impact Measurement Scales. A moderate-to-high correlation was found between the tests. A result of 0.86 was reached assessing the internal consistency using Cronbach's α. The test–re-test reliability, measured by the Spearman–Brown test–re-test analysis, showed coefficient values ranging from 0.94 (recreational and athletic activities) to 0.98 (work and overall scale). To assess responsiveness, the test showed favorable standardized response means and indices of responsiveness by comparison of the preoperative and postoperative scores.

The Flexi-level Scale of Shoulder Function

The Flexi-level Scale of Shoulder Function (FLEX-SF: Cook et al. 2003) is a shoulder-specific tool with a fixed-item index consisting of three levels of function. In this rating system, patients have to answer a single item that roughly ranks their level of function as low, medium, or high. This subsequently allows patients to answer only the items that targeted their level of function. Scores are recorded from 1 (the most limited function) to 50 (absence of limited function in the patient) (Yang et al. 2007). High test–re-test reliability (intraclass correlation coefficient [ICC] = 0.90) and validity (responsiveness index = 1.2) have been demonstrated. The internal consistency, as measured by Cronbach's α, is 0.96 for easy, 0.93 for medium difficulty, and 0.97 for hard.

Shoulder Pain and Disability Index

The Shoulder Pain and Disability Index (SPADI: Roach et al. 1991) was developed to measure pain and disability due to shoulder pathology. The SPADI is self-administered and consists of 13 items divided into two subscales: pain (5 items) and disability (8 items).

Generally, 5–10 minutes are required to complete the questionnaire. A visual analog scale (VAS) is used to rank each item and at both the extremities of each VAS there are verbal anchors, representing opposite extremes of the dimension being measured. The patient marks a line in the position corresponding to his or her pain or disability in the past week. A number ranging from 0 to 11 is attached to this segment to produce a score for each item. The subscale score is then calculated by adding the item scores for that subscale and dividing this number by the maximum score possible for the items deemed applicable by the patient. This number is then multiplied by 100. The average of scores from pain and disability subscales gives the total SPADI score.

A result of 0.9507 for the total index was reached assessing the internal consistency using Cronbach's α; in particular 0.8604 was reached for the pain scale and 0.9321 for the disability index. ICC was used to assess test–re-test reliability of the total SPADI and pain and disability subscale scores, and it showed the best result for the SPADI total score (ICC = 0.6552). Principal component factor analysis with and without varimax rotation supported the construct validity of the total SPADI and its subscales.

Shoulder range of motion (ROM) and SPADI total and subscale scores were shown to be highly negatively correlated; this confirms the criterion validity of the index. The SPADI has a high sensitivity in detecting clinical changes over short time intervals, as shown by high negative correlations among changes in SPADI scores and changes in shoulder ROM.

Disability of Arm, Shoulder, and Hand questionnaire

The Disability of Arm, Shoulder, and Hand (DASH) (Hudak et al. 1996) questionnaire was developed to assess symptoms and functional status of patients affected by different musculoskeletal pathologies of the upper limb. The questionnaire is divided into three sections: symptoms, sports and music, and work. The first one, consisting of 30 items, is about symptoms and functional status at the level of disability. The second and third are optional and contain questions about sports and music and also four about work. Each item is scored with a 5-point scale: 1 = no difficulty; 2 = mild difficulty; 3 = moderate difficulty; 4 = severe difficulty; and 5 = unable. Points reached from each module are summed, the resultant representing the total DASH score. The DASH score ranges for each section from 0 (no disability) to 100 (severe disability). Multiple tests showed high Cronbach's α (0.97) demonstrating the high internal consistency of the DASH.

QuickDASH

The QuickDASH (Beaton et al. 2005) was developed as a shorter version of the full DASH questionnaire. It consists of 11 questions that investigate symptoms and physical function in people with different upper extremity musculoskeletal disorders.

As with the full DASH, each item of the QuickDASH has five response options: 1 = no difficulty; 2 = mild difficulty; 3 = moderate difficulty; 4 = severe difficulty; and 5 = unable. The total score is reported on a 100-point scale, with 100 indicating the most disability. It is allowed to miss just one item. If two or more items are missing, the score cannot be calculated. Reliability, validity, and responsiveness of the QuickDASH are similar to the full DASH. Of note, the QuickDASH has become a popular upper extremity scoring system in North America.

Shoulder Disability Questionnaire

The objective of the Shoulder Disability Questionnaire (SDQ: van der Heijden et al. 2000) was to investigate the functional status and limitations of patients with soft-tissue shoulder disorders. It is composed of 16 items each containing 3 answer options: yes, no, and not applicable (NA); the last option has the specific meaning that the activity of the addressed item had not been performed in the previous 24 hours. The result is a percentage between 0 (no functional limitations) and 100% (affirmative answer to all applicable items), obtained by dividing the affirmative answers by the number of applicable items and then multiplying by 100. The psychometric evaluation of the SDQ showed that this rating scale has good responsiveness and is able to discriminate accurately between self-rated, clinically stable and improved patients (van der Windt et al. 1998).

Rotator Cuff Quality-of-Life measure

The Rotator Cuff Quality-of-Life measure (RC-QOL: Hollinshead et al. 2000), a disease-specific outcome rating scale, investigates patients' perceptions of the influence of the rotator cuff disorders on their quality of life. This tool consists of 34 items divided into 5 domains: symptoms and physical complaints (16 items), work-related concerns (4 items), sports and recreation (4 items), lifestyle issues (5 items), and social and emotional issues (5 items). A 100-point VAS was used to rate each item; the total score ranges from 0 (worst score) to 3400 (best score), and it has to be converted into a percentage score as suggested by the authors. The RC-QOL psychometric evaluation showed high reliability, face validity, ability to discriminate between large and massive cuff tears, and sensitivity to change (Razmjou et al. 2006).

Western Ontario Rotator Cuff Index

The Western Ontario Rotator Cuff Index (WORC: Kirkley et al. 2003) is a disease-specific quality-of-life measurement tool for patients with rotator cuff disease. The WORC has 21 items representing 5 domains: physical symptoms (6 items), sport/recreation (4 items), work function (4 items), lifestyle function (4 items), and emotional function (3 items), each with a 10-cm VAS-type response option. The total score ranges from 0 to 2100, where 0 is the best possible score, with the patient fully asymptomatic, whereas 2100 is the worst possible score, with the patient greatly symptomatic. The investigation of reliability showed an ICC of 0.96; the validity was tested by comparing WORC and 13 other tools and it showed high correlation. The sensitivity to change was tested comparing the outcomes of the WORC with five other shoulder measurement tools (including global health instruments and range of motion) at the first physical exam and 3 months later, showing that the WORC was more responsive than the others.

Constant–Murley Score

The Constant–Murley score (CMS) (Constant and Murley 1987) is one of the most often used shoulder evaluation instruments. This scoring system includes physical examination and patients' subjective judgments, allowing a functional evaluation of shoulders independently of the specific type of disturbance. The CMS is divided into four subscales: pain (15 points); activities of daily living (ADL) (20 points); range of motion (ROM) (40 points); and strength (25 points).

The pain and the ADL items are completed by patients: in the first version of the CMS, the scale of pain was marked as none (15 points), slight (10 points), moderate (5 points), and grave (0 points). In the revised 2008 version, pain is ranked by a VAS. The ADL section is separated into four elements: sleep, 2 points; work and recreational activities/sports, 4 points each; and positioning the hand in the space, 10 points. The ROM is rated as the active elevation of the arms on the sagittal and lateral planes and internal and external rotation of the shoulders, 10 points each. Finally, the force is rated as the number of pounds of pull that the patient can withstand in abduction to a maximum of 25 points. The total possible score is 100 points, pointing out an asymptomatic and healthy person, whereas the worst score is 0 points. The validity and responsiveness of CMS have been assessed in subsequent studies (Roy et al. 2009). To appraise the validity of construction, the CMS has shown a strong correlation with other scales. Evaluating reliability, ICC ranged from 0.84 to 0.87. The CMS is also responsive to noticing an improvement after intervention in a variety of shoulder disorders.

The Subjective Shoulder Rating System

The Subjective Shoulder Rating System (SSRS) (Kohn and Geyer 1997) is a clinician-independent rating system. It is founded on the subjective opinion of the patient. The questionnaire, based on CMS, is made up of five questions investigating pain, ROM, instability, activity, and work overhead. The authors emphasized the importance of pain throughout, increasing the number of points from 15 in the CMS to 35. Another difference between CMS and SSRS is that instability is not quite marked in the CMS. The items are scored as follows: pain = 35 points, ROM = 35, instability = 15, activity = 10, and work overhead = 5, so that the score ranges from 0 to 100 points, where 100 is the worst possible outcome and 0 the best. The reliability of the SSRS has been tested against the CMS and a 4-point verbal assessment scale in 200 patients. The comparison of the total points of the SSRS and the CMS using linear regression showed a highly meaningful correlation ($r = 0.83$; $p < 0.001$).

Shoulder-related Disability Questionnaire

The Shoulder-related Disability Questionnaire (van der Windt et al. 1998) has been developed "for the evaluation of the limitation in the day-to-day activities deriving from shoulder symptoms," and is self-completed by the patients themselves. The questions are based on those related to the shoulder of the Functional Limitations Profile (FLP). In addition, physiotherapists and occupational therapists have been asked to build up lists of activities that can be prevented by shoulder pain or rigidity; the questionnaire, composed of 22 items, has been constructed using these sources. The questionnaire proves to correlate with measures of clasped shoulder movement and the authors "believe that such tool has both face and content validity." It has also been validated in Turkish (Ozsahin et al. 2008).

The Simple Shoulder Test

The Simple Shoulder Test (SST) (Lippit et al. 1992) has been developed as a tool to appraise the functional limitations of the shoulder regarding the patient's ADL before or after the treatment. The SST is composed of a series of 12 "yes" or "no" questions; Kirkley et al. (2003) have published a report of shoulder result instruments suggesting that the SST is unlikely to be sensitive, even if clinically important, to the small changes in patient surgery because of the dichotomous answer options (yes or no). For the same reason, the SST will probably be unable to discriminate among patients with different degrees of the same condition. Nevertheless, a strong point for the SST is the fact that it gives a practical method for the evaluation of the after treatment outcomes. Psychometric evaluation data have been published (Godfrey et al. 2007): test-re-test reliability has an ICC >0.97; validity of construction is acceptable, and the reaction to the change is high, but there are some differences after stratification for age group and type of wound. The SST showed general acceptable psychometric performance.

The Upper Extremity Function Scale

The Upper Extremity Function Scale (UEFS) (Pransky et al. 1997) has been developed for appraising the impact of the disorders of the superior limbs on the ability to perform physical activities. The questionnaire consists of eight elements selected from an initial list of twelve that contained the common tasks involving arm or hand. So far, the eight objects are useful to investigate the common activities of daily life and they are marked by a continuous numerical scale, from the extremity of the "1 – no problem" to the other extremity "10 – great problem – can't to do it at all." The UEFS has shown excellent psychometric characteristics: internal consistency has been valued through Cronbach's α (>0.83), and the analysis of the validity has shown moderate and meaningful correlations among UEFS and other measures of self-reported pain, psychological measures, and physical examinations. Reactivity (sensibility to the changes) has been measured by the correlations among the changes in longitudinal measures of illness impact and the changes in the UEFS, showing a highly meaningful correlation.

Imatani Shoulder score (clinical evaluation system for acromioclavicular dislocation)

The Imatani Shoulder Score (Imatani et al. 1975) has been published in a 12-month follow-up study on 33 patients with an acute complete acromioclavicular dislocation, managed surgically in 11 patients and conservatively in 22. The scale has a maximum score of 100 points, 40 assigned for pain, 30 for function (covering strength), and 30 for motion. The results were classified as excellent (90–100 points), good (80–89 points), fair (70–79 points), and poor (<70 points), with satisfactory (excellent or good) and unsatisfactory (fair or poor) rating used to summarize the outcomes. Data on the development or the psychometric properties are not available.

The University of California at Los Angeles Shoulder Rating

The first edition of the University of California at Los Angeles (UCLA) Shoulder Rating (Amstutz et al. 1981) was developed to assess patients submitted to total shoulder arthroplasty for degenerative disorders of the articulations. The tool has a total score of 30 points divided into 3 sectors: the pain, function, and muscular power of movement; every sector provides a reply of 6 sentences and is marked for a maximum of 10 points. The authors consider as an excellent result if >8, as good if >6, as fair if >4, and as poor if <3.

Modified UCLA Shoulder Rating

In 1986, a more recent edition has been developed by Ellman et al. (1986) in a follow-up study of 50 patients who underwent surgical repair of a tear of the rotator cuff. The newer UCLA Shoulder Score has 5 separate sectors marked for a total of 35 points: pain (10 points), function (10 points), active forward flexion (5 points), strength (5 points), and satisfaction (5 points). The authors classify a score of 34–35 points as an excellent result, 29–33 as a good result, and <29 as poor. The following year, Ellman, in a follow-up study of the patient undergoing arthoscopic acromioplasty, adjourned the system of score so that an excellent score is 34–35 points, a good score has varied from 28 points to 33 points, a fair score is 21–27 points, and a poor score from 0 to 20 points. There are no available publications detailing the development of either versions of this tool.

The Swanson Shoulder Score System

The Swanson Shoulder Score System was developed in 1989 by Swanson et al. (Swanson et al. 1989) to appraise long-term results of a bipolar shoulder prosthesis. This scale has been used for the clinical evaluation of patients either pre- or postoperatively. It is composed of three sections, the first about pain, the second about ROM of the shoulder, and the last about the ability to develop activities of daily life. A maximum of 10 points has been assigned for every clinical category appraised, so a total score of 30 points can be reached. The results are classified as excellent (280–300 points), good (230–279), fair (180–229), and poor (<180). No data on psychometric evaluation are available.

The Wolfang criteria

The Wolfang criteria (Wolfgang 1974) were developed to postoperatively assess 65 patients' shoulders in a retrospective study. The rating system is composed of five domains. The maximum score is 17 points: pain, motion (abduction), strength, and function are scored from 0 to 4 points; the last one is satisfaction: if the patient is satisfied, a point is added to the total score. Vice versa, if the patient is unsatisfied a point is subtracted from the overall point score. The final score is ranked as excellent (14–17 points), good (11–13 points), fair (8–10 points), or poor (0–7). No data about psychometric properties are available.

The Penn Shoulder Score

The Penn Shoulder Score (Leggin et al. 2006) is a condition-specific measurement tool filled autonomously by patients. It is composed of three subscales for a total of 100 points: pain, satisfaction, and function. Pain (three items) and satisfaction (one item) are scored by a 10-point numeric rating scale. At both the extremities of the scale, verbal anchors "no pain"/"worst pain" and "not satisfied"/"very satisfied" are placed, representing opposite extremes of the dimension being measured. The function section includes 20 items, each scored using a 4-point (0–3) Likert's scale. The response options include 0 (can't do at all), 1 (much difficulty), 2 (with some difficulty), and 3 (no difficulty); a "did not do before injury" option is available for items that are not applicable. If the maximum score (100 points) is reached, the patient has high function, low pain, and high satisfaction. Data from psychometric evaluation show high reliability (ICC = 0.94), high internal consistency (Cronbach's $\alpha = 0.93$), and high validity and responsiveness.

Hospital for Special Surgery Shoulder – Rating Score Sheet

The Hospital for Special Surgery Shoulder - Rating Score Sheet (Stephens et al. 1998) was developed as a measurement tool to assess patients undergoing arthroscopic acromioplasty pre- and postoperatively. The rating system consists of 5 domains for a maximum score of 100 points: pain = 30 points; functional limitations = 28 points; tenderness = 5 points; impingement maneuvers = 32 points; range of motion = 5 points. The final score is classified as excellent (90–100 points), good (70–89 points), fair (50–69 points), or poor (<50 points). No data are available on psychometric evaluation.

Athletic Shoulder Outcome Rating Scale

The Athletic Shoulder Outcome Rating Scale (ASORS) (Tibone et al. 1992) includes subjective and objective criteria. The maximum score is 100 points: 10 points for objective testing and 90 points for the subjective section made up of pain, strength/endurance, stability, intensity, and performance. This scale is specific for athletes with shoulder disorder. No data are available on psychometric features of this instrument.

Wheelchair User's Shoulder Pain Index

The Wheelchair User's Shoulder Pain (WUSPI) Index (Curtis et al. 1995) is a condition-specific measurement tool available to evaluate and monitor because the use of wheelchairs can affect daily activities due to musculoskeletal complications of the upper limb. It is made up of a series of activities divided into four sections: transfers, focusing on patient's movements from the bed/car/tub or shower to wheelchair and vice versa, and loading wheelchair into car; wheelchair mobility, which evaluates the patient's ability to move him- or herself throughout the wheelchair; self-care, addressing the patient's ability to perform general daily activities with regard to, for example, dressing or washing, driving, work/school activities, sleeping, and household chores. Each item is scored by a 10-cm VAS anchored to "no pain" and "worst pain ever experienced."

The available data on reliability of the WUSPI show that the intraclass correlation for test–re-test reliability of the total index score is 0.99. The validity was tested comparing the results of the WUSPI administered to 64 long-term wheelchair users and the ROM measurements: the statistically significant negative correlations of total index scores to ROM of shoulder abduction, flexion, and extension shows a significant relationship of total index score to loss of ROM.

American Shoulder and Elbow Surgeons Shoulder Evaluation Form

The American Shoulder and Elbow Surgeons Shoulder Evaluation Form (ASES-S) (Richards et al. 1994) has been designed by the Research Committee of the American Shoulder and Elbow Surgeons. This measurement tool is divided into two sections: one is completed autonomously by the patient, the other by the clinician. The patient self-reported subscale is divided into three sections: pain, instability, and activities of daily living (ADL). A 10-cm VAS, ranging from 0 (no pain at all) to 10 (the worst pain possible), is used to assess pain. The second item investigates the patient's feeling of instability and a 10-cm VAS is used to measure it; the last section addressing ADL is composed of a list of 10 activities. Each item investigates an activity that is highly influenced from a pain-free range of shoulder motion, and is scored using a 4-point ordinal scale.

The clinician subscale is composed of four items addressing ROM, signs, strength, and instability. The section about ROM investigates active and passive motion in both shoulders; signs that are assessed include supraspinatus or greater tuberosity tenderness, acromioclavicular joint tenderness, and biceps tendon tenderness or biceps tendon rupture. They are graded as 0 if not present, 1 if mild, 2 if moderate, and 3 if severe. If tendon tenderness is present in other locations, the examiner is asked to note the location. Strength is measured in forward elevation, abduction, external rotation, and internal rotation, with the arm comfortably at the side. Finally instability is investigated by an ordinary 4-point scale and yes/no questions.

The shoulder score is derived by the following formula:

$$[(10 - \text{VAS pain score}) \times 5] + (5/3) \times \text{cumulative ADL score}.$$

The psychometric evaluation was performed by different authors (Kocher et al. 2005), and showed that there was acceptable test–re-test reliability for the overall ASES-S (intraclass correlation coefficient = 0.94). There was acceptable internal consistency for patients with instability (Cronbach's $\alpha = 0.61$), rotator cuff disease (0.64), and arthritis (0.62). There was good criterion validity, with significant correlations ($p < 0.05$) among the overall ASES-S and the physical functioning, role - physical, and bodily pain domains of the short form-12 scale, and non-significant correlations ($p > 0.05$) with the role - emotional, mental health, vitality, and social function domains. There were acceptable floor and ceiling effects for patients with instability (0% and 1.3%, respectively), rotator cuff disease (0% for both), and arthritis (0% for both). The ASES-S shows overall acceptable psychometric performance for outcome assessment in all subgroups. The ASES-S also has been validated in German (Goldhahn et al. 2008).

Shoulder computerized adaptive tests

A computerized adaptive test (CAT) is a method of collecting patient-reported outcomes, in which a computer algorithm tailors the selection of items administered by matching item difficulty to the patient's level of the trait being measured. A CAT administration stops when the patient's estimated trait level meets specified criteria (Hart et al. 2006). From a clinical perspective, the most important advantages of CATs are that they provide an efficient alternative to traditional paper and pencil or computer-administered tests, allow outcome data to be collected during the clinical encounter with reduced patient burden, and produce precise estimates of patient ability (Hart et al. 2006).

DISCUSSION

Outcome measures are useful to evaluate the clinical effects of surgery or improvements after non-surgical management, to compare the effectiveness of different treatment options, to easily collect data for future analysis, and to be able to follow each patient up (Williams et al. 1999; Franceschi et al. 2007a–d, 2008a–d).

Traditionally, the function of the shoulder has been assessed with objective measures such as ROM and strength. However, objective measures can be impractical in some settings. Objective measures are time-consuming, can inhibit the patient, and require the patient's presence in front of the clinician. Also, although shoulder disorders often correlate with a reduction of the ROM and muscle weakness, these measures have no direct clinical meaning to patients because they essentially expect to be free of pain and perform their daily activities unhindered.

Nowadays, the efficacy of treatment is more often evaluated using outcomes that are directly relevant to patients. The use of subjective measures assessing the ability to function in daily life ensures that the treatment and evaluations focus on the global patient functioning rather than on the disease (Longo et al. 2007, 2008b, 2009, 2010a,b).

Over time, different rating scales have been developed to assess patients with shoulder disorders, each stressing a different feature and addressing both objective and subjective criteria. Some of them are patient based (OSS), others are clinician based (CMS), and some are both clinician and patient based (ASES-S).

Usually, the shoulder measurement tools are classified as generic or disease specific; the generic ones investigate every non-specific shoulder disorders, causing symptoms and affecting patient functional status; the disease-specific tools investigate specific conditions such as rotator cuff lesions or instability, or the outcomes of specific surgical treatments.

Many shoulder rating scales lack a formal psychometric evaluation that includes assessment of validity, reliability, and responsiveness, and often the authors do not report on the process of item generation and/or reduction. There is also a great variability among the measurement tools because each of them uses specific variables or, if the same variables are evaluated, they are ranked by different weight.

The SPADI (Roach et al. 1991) is a patient-based rating scale, developed to investigate the influence of shoulder disorder focusing on pain and disability. It is composed of the pain and disability subscales; it has good internal consistency, test–re-test reliability, and criterion and construct validity. It is responsive to change over time. It has been validated in German (Angst et al. 2007) and Slovene (Jamnik and Spevak 2008).

The SRQ (L'Insalata et al. 1997) is completed by the patient and is designed to evaluate the outcome of treatment shoulder pathology. It is also available in Dutch (Vermeulen et al. 2005). Evaluation of reliability, reproducibility, and responsiveness have shown good results and the validity of the scale was demonstrated by moderate-to-high correlation of the domains and individual questions of the Shoulder Rating Questionnaire with those of the Arthritis Impact Measurement Scales 2.

The DASH (Jester et al. 2005) has been validated in several languages, whereas the evaluation of its test–re-test reliability and construct validity has been published for the original English version (Hudak et al. 1996; Davis et al. 1999; Gummesson et al. 2003), and for the Swedish (Atroshi et al. 2000), German (Offenbacher et al. 2003), Spanish (Rosales et al. 2002), Dutch (Veehof et al. 2002), Italian (Padua et al. 2003), Chinese (Lee et al. 2004), and Japanese (Imaeda et al. 2005) versions. One of the optional DASH modules, the work module, has been validated in Italian (Padua et al. 2003), Chinese (Lee et al. 2004), and Japanese (Imaeda et al. 2005).

The DASH score can be used as a rating scale for disorder of the whole upper limb, such as a shoulder, elbow, wrist, and hand (Imaeda et al. 2005). The construct validity of the DASH score has been investigated evaluating its correlation to the SF-36 (Gummesson et al. 2003); it showed good correlation to SF-36 and was demonstrated to be a valid measurement tool for patients with different disorders of the upper limbs. The DASH score was shown to be reliable for pain (Jester et al. 2005), and it is also able to detect change over time. The negative aspects of the DASH are a large number of questions and the non-organ-specific nature of the items.

The QuickDASH (Beaton et al. 2005) is a shortened version of the full DASH. Data about reliability, validity, and responsiveness showed good results when used to evaluate disorders with either a proximal or a distal upper limb. The final version of the QuickDASH contains 11 items, and is similar with regard to scores and properties to the full DASH, resulting from a "concept-retention approach." The negative aspect is that only one missing item can be tolerated, and, if two or more items are missing, the score cannot be calculated. The advantages are that, being shorter, it is easier to fill, reducing the risk of missing data.

As in the full DASH, there is an optional module (sports/performing arts and work). The QuickDASH is comparable with the full DASH (r = 0.98), and the evaluation of the construct validity and responsiveness showed that the QuickDASH scores can investigate symptoms and functional status similar to the full DASH.

The SDQ main feature is to address patient's shoulder pathologies and warn of changes in the ability to perform functional ADLs. It includes items perceived to be important by both patients and therapists, as well as questions related to psychological wellbeing, such as irritability and loss of appetite. It is simple to use in clinical practice and easy to score, taking only a short time to fill in. According to the calibrated responsiveness ratio (CRR) and the area under the receiver–operator characteristic curve (AUC), the SDQ discriminates accurately between self-rated clinically stable and improved patients (van der Heijden et al. 2000).

The CMS (Constant and Murley 1987) is one of the most used shoulder rating systems for clinicians. The CMS has both self-report and performance-based components. The developers of this tool did not publish any data about either the generating item process or responsiveness and validity, but the method for administering the rating scale is well described. In successive papers, the psychometric properties were examined. A systematic review of the psychometric properties of the CMS provides evidence to support the use of the Constant–Murley score for specific clinical and research applications, but underscores the need for greater standardization and precaution when interpreting scores. Methods to improve standardization and measurement precision are needed. Responsiveness has been shown to be excellent, but some properties still need be evaluated, particularly those related to the absolute errors of measurement and minimal clinically important difference (Roy et al. 2009).

The SSRS is based solely on the patient's own opinion, avoiding the influence (bias) that a clinician-dependent score may have. It is not time-consuming for the patient, and is suitable for evaluation of subacromial impingement, anterior instability, and frozen shoulders, and for follow-up after subacromial decompression, anterior shoulder reconstruction, and manipulation under anesthesia. The reliability of SSRS was tested against CMS, showing a high correlation (Longo et al. 2007).

The SST was developed to perceive the functional gain resulting from a specific surgical treatment of shoulder disorders but it does not address patient satisfaction. The original paper does not report on psychometric features whereas successive studies evaluated the reliability, validity, and responsiveness of the SST. The SST demonstrated overall acceptable psychometric performance; however, differences were found when data were stratified by age and injury type (Godfrey et al. 2007).

The UCLA shoulder rating scale was developed by Amstutz et al. (1981) to evaluate patients undergoing total shoulder arthroplasty pre- and postoperatively with regard to the degree of pain experienced, functional capacity of the shoulder, detailed ranges of active movement, and muscle power. A successive version, the Modified UCLA Shoulder Rating, was developed by Ellman et al. (1986) to evaluate patients before and after surgical treatment of rotator cuff lesions. There are no available papers on the development or testing of both versions of this instrument.

The ASES-S combines items of subjective evaluation with items of physical examination. The patient's subjective evaluation section contains VASs to score pain and instability, and an ADL questionnaire. This section can be filled in autonomously by patients. The section reserved for the clinician includes an area to collect demographic information and assesses ROM, specific physical signs, strength, and stability. Data from psychometric analysis are available (Kocher et al. 2005); test–re-test reliability was used to assess reliability and the results demonstrated that the score was reliable. The ASES-S also showed consistency between items (internal consistency). There were acceptable (<15%) floor and ceiling effects of the ASES-S for patients with shoulder instability, rotator cuff disease, and glenohumeral arthritis (content validity). Significant correlations were found between the ASES-S and the physical functioning, role - physical, and bodily pain domains of the SF-12 scale (criterion validity), and followed accepted hypotheses (construct validity). It can be concluded that the ASES-S demonstrated overall acceptable psychometric performance for outcome assessment in patients with shoulder instability, rotator cuff disease, and glenohumeral arthritis.

The OSS questionnaire was developed for self-completion by patients undergoing shoulder surgery other than stabilization, providing quick, practical, reliable, valid, and sensitive outcome measures and clinically important changes. The validity of the questionnaire was established by obtaining significant correlations in the expected direction with the Constant score and the relevant scales of the SF-36 and the HAQ. Sensitivity to change was assessed by analyzing the differences between the preoperative scores and those at follow-up. The main feature of the OSS is the ability to detect each improvement obtained by surgery.

The Hospital for Special Surgery's Shoulder-Rating Score Sheet (Stephens et al. 1998) was developed as an instrument to evaluate outcomes after arthroscopic acromioplasty. The preoperative results were compared with the postoperative ones with a follow-up ranging from 6 years to 10 years. It is divided into five domains (pain, functional limitation, tenderness, impingement maneuvers, and ROM); the authors did not report on the item generation process or data of psychometric evaluation, so further studies are needed to validate this questionnaire.

CONCLUSION

There are many shoulder rating scores that have not been developed following the recommended methodology. Often, such tools lack information on the item-generating process and the psychometric properties such as validity, reproducibility, responsiveness, consistency, and sensitivity to change. These properties are the most useful in a clinical setting, and need to be addressed by the authors. Otherwise, it is very difficult to compare results from different studies (Longo et al. 2012a–f).

Often, too many details are given on the content of the scales, and not enough on the psychometric properties. If the psychometric properties of the scoring systems were presented in tables detailing reliability, validity, and responsiveness, it would be easier for readers to compare the scoring systems based on these properties (Denaro et al. 2010, 2011).

Scores are not valid when used in a modified form, and the untested use of a modified scoring system should be discouraged. Also, it is necessary to formally validate cross-cultural adaptation of the various scoring systems (Longo et al. 2011a, b).

In conclusion, despite the huge availability of rating systems used to evaluate shoulder function, we are still far from a single outcome evaluation system that is reliable, valid, and sensitive to clinically relevant changes, and that takes into account both the patients' and the physicians' perspective, is short and practical to use, and allows comparison of the different management options among clinicians.

REFERENCES

Amstutz HC, Sew Hoy AL, Clarke IC. UCLA anatomic total shoulder arthroplasty. Clin Orthop Relat Res 1981;155:7–20.

Angst F, Goldhahn J, Pap G, et al. Cross-cultural adaptation, reliability and validity of the German Shoulder Pain and Disability Index (SPADI). Rheumatology (Oxford) 2007;46:87–92.

Atroshi I, Gummesson C, Andersson B, Dahlgren E, Johansson A. The disabilities of the arm, shoulder and hand (DASH) outcome questionnaire: reliability and validity of the Swedish version evaluated in 176 patients. Acta Orthop Scand 2000;71:613–618.

Beaton DE, Katz JN, Fossel AH, et al. Measuring the whole or the parts? Validity, reliability, and responsiveness of the Disabilities of the Arm, Shoulder and Hand outcome measure in different regions of the upper extremity. J Hand Ther 2001;14:128–146.

Constant CR, Murley AH. A clinical method of functional assessment of the shoulder. Clin Orthop Relat Res 1987;160–164.

Cook KF, Roddey TS, Gartsman GM, Olson SL. Development and psychometric evaluation of the Flexilevel Scale of Shoulder Function. Med Care 2003;41:823–835.

Curtis KA, Roach KE, Applegate EB, et al. Development of the Wheelchair User's Shoulder Pain Index (WUSPI). Paraplegia 1995;33:290–293.

Davis AM, Beaton DE, Hudak P, et al. Measuring disability of the upper extremity: a rationale supporting the use of a regional outcome measure. J Hand Ther 1999;12:269–274.

Dawson J, Fitzpatrick R, Carr A. Questionnaire on the perceptions of patients about shoulder surgery. J Bone Joint Surg Br 1996;78:593–600.

Denaro V, Ruzzini L, Longo UG, et al. Effect of dihydrotestosterone on cultured human tenocytes from intact supraspinatus tendon. Knee Surg Sports Traumatol Arthrosc 2010;18:971–976.

Denaro V, Ruzzini L, Barnaba SA, et al. Effect of pulsed electromagnetic fields on human tenocyte cultures from supraspinatus and quadriceps tendons. Am J Phys Med Rehabil 2011;90:119–127.

Ellman H, Hanker G, Bayer M. Repair of the rotator cuff. End-result study of factors influencing reconstruction. J Bone Joint Surg Am 1986;68:1136–1144.

Franceschi F, Longo UG, Ruzzini L, et al. To detach the long head of the biceps tendon after tenodesis or not: outcome analysis at the 4-year follow-up of two different techniques. International orthopaedics. 2007a;31:537–545.

Franceschi F, Longo UG, Ruzzini L, Rizzello G, Denaro V. Arthroscopic management of calcific tendinitis of the subscapularis tendon. Knee Surg Sports Traumatol Arthrosc 2007b;15:1482–1485.

Franceschi F, Longo UG, Ruzzini L, et al. The Roman Bridge: a "double pulley – suture bridges" technique for rotator cuff repair. BMC Musculoskelet Disord 2007c;8:123.

Franceschi F, Ruzzini L, Longo UG, et al. Equivalent clinical results of arthroscopic single-row and double-row suture anchor repair for rotator cuff tears: a randomized controlled trial. Am J Sports Med 2007d;35:1254–1260.

Franceschi F, Longo UG, Ruzzini L, et al. Circulating substance P levels and shoulder joint contracture after arthroscopic repair of the rotator cuff. Br J Sports Med 2008a;42:742–745.

Franceschi F, Longo UG, Ruzzini L, et al. Arthroscopic salvage of failed arthroscopic Bankart repair: a prospective study with a minimum follow-up of 4 years. Am J Sports Med 2008b;36:1330–1336.

Franceschi F, Longo UG, Ruzzini L, et al. No advantages in repairing a type II superior labrum anterior and posterior (SLAP) lesion when associated with rotator cuff repair in patients over age 50: a randomized controlled trial. Am J Sports Med 2008c;36:247–253.

Franceschi F, Longo UG, Ruzzini L, et al. Soft tissue tenodesis of the long head of the biceps tendon associated to the Roman Bridge repair. BMC Musculoskel Disord 2008d;9:78.

Godfrey J, Hamman R, Lowenstein S, Briggs K, Kocher M. Reliability, validity, and responsiveness of the simple shoulder test: psychometric properties by age and injury type. J Shoulder Elbow Surg 2007;16:260–267.

Goldhahn J, Angst F, Drerup S, et al. Lessons learned during the cross-cultural adaptation of the American Shoulder and Elbow Surgeons shoulder form into German. J Shoulder Elbow Surg 2008;17:248–254.

Gummesson C, Atroshi I, Ekdahl C. The disabilities of the arm, shoulder and hand (DASH) outcome questionnaire: longitudinal construct validity and measuring self-rated health change after surgery. BMC Musculoskelet Disord 2003;4:11.

Hart DL, Cook KF, Mioduski JE, Teal CR, Crane PK. Simulated computerized adaptive test for patients with shoulder impairments was efficient and produced valid measures of function. J Clin Epidemiol 2006;59:290–298.

Hollinshead RM, Mohtadi NG, Vande Guchte RA, Wadey VM. Two 6-year follow-up studies of large and massive rotator cuff tears: comparison of outcome measures. J Shoulder Elbow Surg 2000;9:373–381.

Huber W, Hofstaetter JG, Hanslik-Schnabel B, Posch M, Wurnig C. The German version of the Oxford Shoulder Score – cross-cultural adaptation and validation. Arch Orthop Trauma Surg 2004;124:531–536.

Hudak PL, Amadio PC, Bombardier C. Development of an upper extremity outcome measure: the DASH (disabilities of the arm, shoulder and hand) [corrected]. The Upper Extremity Collaborative Group (UECG). Am J Ind Med 1996;29:602–608.

Imaeda T, Toh S, Nakao Y, et al. Validation of the Japanese Society for Surgery of the Hand version of the Disability of the Arm, Shoulder, and Hand questionnaire. J Orthop Sci 2005;10:353–359.

Imatani RJ, Hanlon JJ, Cady GW. Acute, complete acromioclavicular separation. J Bone Joint Surg Am 1975;57:328–332.

Jamnik H, Spevak MK. Shoulder Pain and Disability Index: validation of Slovene version. Int J Rehabil Res 2008;31:337–341.

Jester A, Harth A, Germann G. Measuring levels of upper-extremity disability in employed adults using the DASH Questionnaire. J Hand Surg Am 2005;30:1074, e1071–1074, e1010.

Kirkley A, Alvarez C, Griffin S. The development and evaluation of a disease-specific quality-of-life questionnaire for disorders of the rotator cuff: The Western Ontario Rotator Cuff Index. Clin J Sport Med 2003;13:84–92.

Kocher MS, Horan MP, Briggs KK, et al. Reliability, validity, and responsiveness of the American Shoulder and Elbow Surgeons subjective shoulder scale in patients with shoulder instability, rotator cuff disease, and glenohumeral arthritis. J Bone Joint Surg Am 2005;87:2006–2011.

Kohn D, Geyer M. The subjective shoulder rating system. Arch Orthop Trauma Surg 1997;116:324–328.

L'Insalata JC, Warren RF, Cohen SB, Altchek DW, Peterson MG. A self-administered questionnaire for assessment of symptoms and function of the shoulder. J Bone Joint Surg Am 1997;79:738–748.

Lee EW, Lau JS, Chung MM, Li AP, Lo SK. Evaluation of the Chinese version of the Disability of the Arm, Shoulder and Hand (DASH-HKPWH): cross-cultural adaptation process, internal consistency and reliability study. J Hand Ther 2004;17:417–423.

Leggin BG, Michener LA, Shaffer MA, et al. The Penn shoulder score: reliability and validity. J Orthop Sports Phys Ther 2006;36:138–151.

Lippitt SB, Harryman DT, Matsen FA. A practical tool for evaluating function: the simple shoulder test. In: Matsen FA, Fu FH, Hawkins RJ, eds. The Shoulder: A Balance of Mobilty and Stability. Rosemont, IL: American Academy of Orthopaedic Surgeons; 1992:501–518.

Longo UG, Franceschi F, Ruzzini L, et al. Light microscopic histology of supraspinatus tendon ruptures. Knee Surg Sports Traumatol Arthrosc 2007;15:1390–1394.

Longo UG, Franceschi F, Loppini M, Maffulli N, Denaro V. Rating systems for evaluation of the elbow. Br Med Bull 2008a;87:131–161.

Longo UG, Franceschi F, Ruzzini L, et al. Histopathology of the supraspinatus tendon in rotator cuff tears. Am J Sports Med 2008b;36:533–538.

Longo UG, Franceschi F, Ruzzini L, et al. Higher fasting plasma glucose levels within the normoglycaemic range and rotator cuff tears. Br J Sports Med 2009;43:284–287.

Longo UG, Franceschi F, Spiezia F, et al. Triglycerides and total serum cholesterol in rotator cuff tears: do they matter? Br J Sports Med 2010a;44:948–951.

Longo UG, Lamberti A, Maffulli N, Denaro V. Tendon augmentation grafts: a systematic review. Br Med Bull 2010b;94:165–188.

Longo UG, Loppini M, Denaro L, Maffulli N, Denaro V. Rating scales for low back pain. Br Med Bull 2010c;94:81–144.

Longo UG, Saris D, Poolman RW, Berton A, Denaro V. Instruments to assess patients with rotator cuff pathology: a systematic review of measurement properties. Knee Surg Sports Traumatol Arthrosc 2011a Dec 20. [Epub ahead of print] PubMed PMID: 22183737.

Longo UG, Vasta S, Maffulli N, Denaro V. Scoring systems for the functional assessment of patients with rotator cuff pathology. Sports Med Arthrosc. 2011b;19:310–320.

Longo UG, Berton A, Papapietro N, Maffulli N, Denaro V. Epidemiology, genetics and biological factors of rotator cuff tears. Med Sport Sci 2012a;57:1–9. Epub 2011 Oct 4. PubMed PMID: 21986040.

Longo UG, Berton A, Papapietro N, Maffulli N, Denaro V. Biomechanics of the rotator cuff: European perspective. Med Sport Sci 2012b;57:10–7. Epub 2011 Oct 4. PubMed PMID: 21986041.

Longo UG, Franceschi F, Berton A, Maffulli N, Droena V. Conservative treatment and rotator cuff tear progression. Med Sport Sci 2012c;57:90–99. Epub 2011 Oct 4. PubMed PMID: 21986048.

Longo UG, Berton A, Marinozzi A, Maffulli N, Denaro V. Subscapularis tears.Med Sport Sci 2012d;57:114–121. Epub 2011 Oct 4. PubMed PMID: 21986050.

Longo UG, Franceschi F, Berton A, Maffulli N, Denaro V. Arthroscopic transosseous rotator cuff repair. Med Sport Sci 2012e;57:142–152. Epub 2011 Oct 4. PubMed PMID: 21986052.

Longo UG, Lamberti A, Rizzello G, Maffulli N, Denaro V. Synthetic augmentation in massive rotator cuff tears. Med Sport Sci 2012f;57:168–177. Epub 2011 Oct 4. PubMed PMID: 21986054.

Murena L, Vulcano E, D'Angelo F, Monti M, Cherubino P. Italian cross-cultural adaptation and validation of the Oxford shoulder score. J Shoulder Elbow Surg 2010;19:335–341.

Offenbacher M, Ewert T, Sangha O, Stucki G. Validation of a German version of the "Disabilities of Arm, Shoulder and Hand" questionnaire (DASH-G). Z Rheumatol 2003;62:168–177.

Ozsahin M, Akgun K, Aktas I, Kurtais Y Adaptation of the Shoulder Disability Questionnaire to the Turkish population, its reliability and validity. Int J Rehab Res 2008;31:241–245.

Padua R, Padua L, Ceccarelli E, et al. Italian version of the Disability of the Arm, Shoulder and Hand (DASH) questionnaire. Cross-cultural adaptation and validation. J Hand Surg Br 2003;28:179–186.

Plancher KD, Lipnick SL. Analysis of evidence-based medicine for shoulder instability. Arthroscopy 2009;25:897–908.

Pransky G, Feuerstein M, Himmelstein J, et al. Measuring functional outcomes in work-related upper extremity disorders. Development and validation of the Upper Extremity Function Scale. J Occup Environ Med 1997;39:1195–1202.

Razmjou H, Bean A, van Osnabrugge V, MacDermid JC, Holtby R. Cross-sectional and longitudinal construct validity of two rotator cuff disease-specific outcome measures. BMC Musculoskelet Disord 2006;7:26.

Richards RR, An K-N, Bigliani LU, et al. A standardized method for the assessment of shoulder function. J Shoulder Elbow Surg 1994;3:347–352.

Roach KE, Budiman-Mak E, Songsiridej N, Lertratanakul Y. Development of a shoulder pain and disability index. Arthr Care Res 1991;4:143–149.

Rosales RS, Delgado EB, Diez de la Lastra-Bosch I. Evaluation of the Spanish version of the DASH and carpal tunnel syndrome health-related quality-of-life instruments: cross-cultural adaptation process and reliability. J Hand Surg Am 2002;27:334–343.

Roy JS, MacDermid JC, Woodhouse LJ. A systematic review of the psychometric properties of the Constant–Murley score. J Shoulder Elbow Surg 2009;19:157–164.

Stephens SR, Warren RF, Payne LZ, Wickiewicz TL, Altchek DW. Arthroscopic acromioplasty: a 6- to 10-year follow-up. Arthroscopy 1998;14:382–388.

Swanson AB, de Groot Swanson G, Sattel AB, et al. Bipolar implant shoulder arthroplasty. Long-term results. Clin Orthop Relat Res 1989;227–247.

Tibone JE, Bradley JP. Evaluation of outcomes for athletes' shoulders. In: Matsen FA, Fu FH, Hawkins RJ (eds), The Shoulder: A balance of mobility and stability. Rosemont, IL: American Academy of Orthopaedic Surgery, 1992: 519–529.

van der Heijden GJ, Leffers P, Bouter LM. Shoulder disability questionnaire design and responsiveness of a functional status measure. J Clin Epidemiol 2000;53:29–38.

van der Windt DA, van der Heijden GJ, de Winter AF, et al. The responsiveness of the Shoulder Disability Questionnaire. Ann Rheum Dis 1998;57:82–87.

Veehof MM, Sleegers EJ, van Veldhoven NH, Schuurman AH, van Meeteren NL. Psychometric qualities of the Dutch language version of the Disabilities of the Arm, Shoulder, and Hand questionnaire (DASH-DLV). J Hand Ther 2002;15:347–354.

Vermeulen HM, Boonman DC, Schuller HM, et al. Translation, adaptation and validation of the Shoulder Rating Questi`onnaire (SRQ) into the Dutch language. Clin Rehabil 2005;19:300–311.

Williams GN, Gangel TJ, Arciero RA, Uhorchak JM, Taylor DC. Comparison of the Single Assessment Numeric Evaluation method and two shoulder rating scales. Outcomes measures after shoulder surgery. Am J Sports Med 1999;27:214–221.

Wolfgang GL. Surgical repair of tears of the rotator cuff of the shoulder. Factors influencing the result. J Bone Joint Surg Am 1974;56:14–26.

Yang JL, Chang CW, Chen SY, Wang SF, Lin JJ. Mobilization techniques in subjects with frozen shoulder syndrome: randomized multiple-treatment trial. Phys Ther 2007;87:1307–1315.

Chapter 20 Tissue engineering: the future of rotator cuff repair surgery

Scott A. Rodeo, Zakary A. Knutson

KEY FEATURES

- There are three fundamental factors in tissue engineering: cells; growth factors; and scaffolds.
- Scaffolds can be produced by either synthetic or biological materials. Each plays an important role in tissue engineering.
- The appropriate indications for PRP application are poorly defined.
- Although our understanding of tissue engineering has expanded over the last decade, many areas still need to be explored, and techniques and materials need to be improved.

INTRODUCTION

Musculoskeletal tissue engineering is rapidly expanding. Tissue engineering combines our knowledge of biology, biomechanics, and materials science to produce a biological solution to clinical problems recalcitrant to simple surgical solutions.

Repair and reconstruction of the rotator cuff is commonly performed. Recently, some have applied tissue engineering techniques in efforts to improve the results of this procedure. Although rotator cuff surgery continues to evolve and improve, we continue to see failure of the rotator cuff to heal in patients with larger tears or poor tissue quality. Scientific evidence has begun to point toward biological rather than surgical reasons for many of these failures. Rotator cuff disorders tend to be a result of degenerative tendinopathy, which is caused by attrition and inability of the tissues to heal and remodel a failed healing response. Tissue engineering seeks out a biological solution for this dilemma (Longo et al. 2010a,b).

There are three fundamental factors in tissue engineering: cells; growth factors, which provide important cellular signals; and finally scaffolds, which provide a physical substrate and function as a delivery system to support the regenerative/reparative process until incorporation can occur. A brief review of the role of each of these is outlined below.

Cells

Cell-based tissue engineering is a relatively new technique in which living tissue is used to create an environment for healing and tissue regeneration. Advances in technology have allowed scientists to produce cell-specific delivery systems. A variety of cell types can be utilized.

Mature cells can be harvested directly from unaffected areas of the body, as with autologous chondrocyte implantation. *Function-specific cells* can now be produced from stem cells or progenitor cells which, through biochemical manipulation, can become differentiated or specialized. *Autologous progenitor cells* and *stem cells* can be obtained from bone marrow, peritrabecular tissues in cancellous bone, cartilage, fat, and muscle.

Of these three cell types, stem cells have perhaps the greatest potential in tissue engineering given their capacity for self-regeneration and differentiation into specific cell types. Stem cells hold the potential, through chemical signaling and manipulation, to become specialized into cells with a specific phenotype (Muschler et al. 2004).

Chemical signals/Growth factors

Cells and tissues communicate with each other through multifunctional molecules called cytokines. The term "cytokine" includes proteins, peptides, and glycoproteins. Cytokines are produced by many different cell types, and work in concert with each other to effect cellular processes.

Cellular function is modulated by cytokines through specific cell receptors. Cytokines bind to receptors and, through a signaling cascade, stimulate either an up- or downregulation in gene expression. Enhanced cellular activity is manifested by alterations in cell proliferation, matrix synthesis, or cell differentiation.

The healing response in rotator cuff surgery is highly dependent on cytokines. At the macroscopic level, healing of a torn rotator cuff tendon involves the formation of a fibrovascular interface between the tendon and bone. Cytokine-mediated induction of cellular migration and communication enhances the formation of this fibrovascular interface and plays an important role in the healing process (Martinek et al. 2002).

Scaffolds

Scaffolds serve a variety of functions. Both cells and growth factors require a scaffold or carrier vehicle for delivery to the affected area. The scaffold material should both provide tensile strength to the repair during the healing process and serve as a physical "frame" for ingrowth of healthy tissue.

Scaffolds promote migration, attachment, proliferation, and differentiation of cells, and in turn provide a suitable environment for chemical communication between cells. Scaffolds serve as physical substrates for cell attachment. They have the ability to be incorporated and remodeled by the body into viable and functional tissue, and guide tissue regeneration (Derwin et al. 2010). Postoperative magnetic resonance imaging (MRI) and histological studies of massive rotator cuff repairs augmented with extracellular matrix (ECM) scaffolds have shown the ability of these grafts to be repopulated by living cells, and actually form a healed tendon in continuity with the humeral head (Snyder et al. 2009).

Scaffolds can be produced by either synthetic or biological materials. Each plays an important role in tissue engineering. Synthetic materials include metals (tantalum, titanium), minerals (hydroxyapatite, calcium sulfate), and polymers (polylactide, polytyrosine carbonates). Synthetics may be absorbable or non-absorbable, and are usually not remodeled into functional tissue by the body.

Biological scaffolds include bone matrix, skin (dermis), allograft tendon, submucosal tissue, polymers of collagen, hyaluronan, allograft tendon, and fibrin. When compared with synthetics, these biological tissues are more readily incorporated into the body, thereby accelerating the healing process.

Scaffold properties influence scaffold function. The architecture of the scaffold, including its porosity, pore connectivity, and infrastructure, affect the way in which the individual can revascularize and thus remodel and incorporate tissue. Scaffold designs may range from a simple geometric pattern, as seen in metals and polymers, to a complex woven sheet of collagen fibers, as seen in dermis or submucosal layers. Scaffold patterns directly affect the mechanical strength of the material. For optimal function, the scaffold pattern should be designed with the structural integrity necessary to last long enough for incorporation or healing to occur.

An ideal scaffold will gradually degrade and lose strength as it is replaced by new tissue formation. The challenge is to determine an appropriate rate of degradation to allow early protection of newly formed (and thus weaker) tissue, and then gradual stress transfer to the new tissue.

Extracellular dermal matrices have recently been used throughout the body as adjuncts or scaffolds for healing. In particular, they have been used in massive rotator cuff tears to provide a soft-tissue connection between the remaining cuff and the humeral head (Derwin et al. 2009). These tissues must withstand the complex loading environment of tensile and compressive forces present until healing can occur. Surface chemistry and the pH of the tissue affect how it interacts with its surrounding environment. Most implanted materials are rapidly covered with proteins and lipids by the body. These molecules bind preferentially to the surface based on its properties. As an example, Drobny et al. (2003) used double-quantum solid state nuclear magnetic resonance (NMR) spectroscopy to do structural studies of biomaterials. They examined salivary statherin as a mineralization protein and the way that it is incorporated into hydroxyapatite. They used this information to infer that the structure of hydroxyapatite leads to specific protein binding (statherin), and thus uses these chemical interactions to promote bone mineralization.

REVIEW OF PREVIOUS STUDIES IN TISSUE ENGINEERING

Multiple centers have investigated the aforementioned techniques as a method for improving rotator cuff repair surgery. Engineered autogenic tendons have been constructed using harvested cells from an autogenous donor site such as biceps, patellar tendon, or fascia lata. These cells are then grown in vitro for a period of time, followed by the combination of the cells with an ECM scaffold where they are cultured further to allow ingrowth on to the scaffold and production of their own ECM molecules. These engineered tendons can then be implanted into the body as a biological augmentation device.

Chen et al. (2007) tested such engineered tendons in Japanese white rabbits. Tenocytes from the patellar tendons of these animals were harvested and then implanted onto xenogenic and synthetic extracellular matrices. The combination was cultured for 5 days to allow time for cellular matrix production and incorporation. Defects were created in the rabbit infraspinatus tendon, and were subsequently repaired with the engineered tendon, ECM alone, or autogenous tendon. The engineered tendon was superior to the ECM alone with better incorporation into the host tendon, as well as increased production of collagen types I and III. The engineered graft was comparable to the autogenous grafts.

Other options besides autogenous tissue harvest have been explored as well. Dines et al. (2007) used gene therapy to transduce tenocytes harvested from Sprague–Dawley rats. The gene for either platelet-derived growth factor β (PDGF-β) or insulin-like growth factor 1 (IGF-1) were transduced into these cells using retroviral plasmid vectors. PDGF-β mediates many processes responsible for chemotaxis, proliferation of fibroblasts, ECM production, and vascularization. IGF-1 promotes healing by increasing the production of collagen and glycosaminoglycan, and decreasing inflammation. The genetically altered cells were then isolated and placed on to synthetic scaffolds made of polyglycolic acid (PGA). The engineered grafts were implanted into rotator cuff repairs, compared with a control group with no augmentation, and a repair augmented with PGA scaffold alone. At 6 weeks, the grafts were harvested and tested. Histologically, the engineered grafts showed more cellularity at the healing sites. Mechanical testing showed improved toughness and mechanical load to failure in the IGF-1 group when compared with the controls.

An argument could be made that augmentation with a scaffold that adds mechanical strength to a rotator cuff repair is unnecessary, or at least of minor importance if the correct mixture of cells and signaling/growth factors is present. Some studies have investigated the addition of growth factors alone, as the only augmentation to large rotator cuff defects. Rodeo et al. (2007) produced infraspinatus lesions in 72 adult sheep which immediately received one of three repairs: augmentation of the repair with a collagen sponge impregnated with an osteoinductive bone protein extract, augmentation with the collagen sponge alone, and no augmentation. The collagen sponge provided no mechanical strength to the repair, but included the following growth factors: bone morphogenetic proteins (BMPs) BMP-2–BMP-7, TGF-β1 to TGF-β3, and fibroblast growth factor (FGF). The animals were then euthanized at either 6 or 12 weeks, and the rotator cuffs were evaluated histologically and mechanically. All specimens showed a gap filled with scar tissue between the rotator cuff tendon and the bone. The growth factor-treated animals showed more scar tissue, fibrocartilage, and new bone formation compared with control animals. The repairs treated with growth factors also showed significantly greater failure loads at both 6 and 12 weeks. However, when the data were normalized by tissue volume, the differences were not significant.

The authors concluded that the augmentation with growth factor led to increased strength and stiffness of the construct (structural properties), but perhaps not a better quality of tissue (material properties). This study examined several growth factors working together (Rodeo et al. 2007). Future research will focus on isolation of these growth factors and the timing of their application to healing tissues.

CURRENTLY AVAILABLE PRODUCTS FOR USE IN ROTATOR CUFF HEALING

Scaffolds

Scaffolds comprise the largest and oldest group of products available for surgical use. They consist of devices primarily used as structural support for the tendon or to augment poor quality/attenuated tissue. As described above, these devices can be either synthetic or biological. There are many different products available, all with differences in tissue source, tissue processing, sterilization, packaging, and storage. Fundamental aspects of tissue processing and sterilization have important effects on the products' structural and chemical properties. These different processing methods have led to some significant alterations in the biomechanical properties of the various products (Valentin et al. 2006). A list of some of the commercially available scaffold products and their characteristics are included in **Table 20.1**.

One of the primary differences between the products is the tissue source. Many of the scaffolds are based primarily on collagen, which can be obtained from multiple different species of animal and different organs. Some of the first biological scaffolds were produced from porcine small intestinal submucosa (SIS). The Restore Orthobiologic Implant (Depuy) was among the first to be studied in humans. In 2006, Iannotti et al. performed a randomized clinical study examining rotator cuff repairs augmented with SIS xenograft patch. MRI results showed healing in only 4 of 15 shoulders in the augmentation group, compared with 9 of 15 in the control group. The functional outcome scores were on average lower in the SIS group as well. Although these results were not statistically significant, they were concerning enough for the authors to recommend against the use of porcine SIS grafts for rotator cuff augmentation (Iannotti et al. 2006). Since that time, further analysis of these implants has pointed toward residual cellular material containing porcine DNA that remained after processing as an immunological stimulus and an important reason for failure. The genetic material remaining from the porcine DNA led to a significant inflammatory reaction in humans and subsequent failure of the grafts (Zheng et al. 2005).

After the failure of the Restore SIS patch, focus shifted from the type of materials harvested to their post-harvest processing. The Permacol or Zimmer Collagen Repair device (Zimmer) is also a xenograft, but is made from porcine dermis rather than SIS. Processing techniques include removal of the cellular material from the implant, reducing the risk of immune response, as well as chemically cross-linking the collagen fibers. This results in a slower degradation in humans and perhaps a decrease in the amount of tensile strength loss that occurs in more rapidly absorbed products. The collagen cross-linking results in very slow graft incorporation and a foreign body response: the graft is encapsulated and effectively "walled off" by the host. Literature on the clinical implantation of this device remains mixed. Badhe et al. (2008) used the Zimmer Collagen Repair device to augment cuff repairs in 10 patients. At MRI or ultrasound follow-up, 8 of 10 grafts were intact, and clinical outcome measures were improved. They also reported no episodes of inflammation or immune response as seen in other xenograft products. A later study by Soler et al. (2007), however, found 100% graft failure rate between 3 and 6 months in a study involving four patients. Other xenografts, including the CuffPatch (Arthrotek), TissueMend (Stryker), OrthADAPT (Pegasus), and Matristem (ACell) are available for commercial use. There is essentially no clinical data available on these implants.

Human skin or dermis scaffolds have been popularized as allografts that avoid some of the immunogenic concerns of xenografts. The GraftJacket (Wright Medical) is a single layer of acellular human dermis that has been evaluated in several clinical trials for augmentation of rotator cuff repair. Bond et al. (2008) used an all-arthroscopic implantation technique to augment massive rotator cuff tears in 16 patients in whom they were unable to bring the native cuff tendon back to the humeral footprint. After 1–2 years of follow-up, the patients had improvements in the mean UCLA and Constant scores, pain, strength, and range of motion. Patients did not experience any inflammatory reactions, and 13 patients showed full incorporation of the graft.

Synthetic grafts are also commercially available. Sportmesh (Biomet, Warsaw, IN) is a degradable poly(urethane urea) implant designed as a load-sharing device with the repaired cuff. A porous surface allows vascular and soft-tissue ingrowth into the mesh. The tensile strength of this device is reported to be 50% intact at 4 years by the company. The major advantage of a synthetic graft is that there is no risk of immunological reaction or rejection and no risk of disease transmission, as there is in xenografts and allografts. However, the clinical data on these grafts are limited.

Platelet-rich plasma

Platelet-rich plasma (PRP) has been popularized as a method of delivery of multiple different types of growth factors to healing tissues. The platelets themselves bring multiple types of cytokines, proteins, and bioactive factors to the affected area in a more efficient manner and potentially in higher amounts than would be possible through natural healing. Cytokines are contained within the α granules of the platelets and are released when the platelets are activated. These factors include TGF-β, PDGF, IGF-1, FGF, vascular endothelial growth factor (VEGF), epidermal growth factor (EGF), and epithelial cell growth factor (ECGF) (Foster et al. 2009). These cytokines play a role in chemotaxis, cell proliferation, cell differentiation, and angiogenesis. De Mos et al. (2008), showed that PRP positively affects gene expres-

Table 20.1 Commercially available extracellular matrix patches and their characteristics

Product	Species/Tissue of origin	Device composition	Processing methods	Sterilization method
GraftJacket	Human Dermis	Single Layer	Cryogenic, proprietary	None (regulated as tissue transplant)
Restore (Depuy)	Porcine small intestinal submucosa (SIS)	10 layers (dehydrated)	Peracetic acid, vacuum dried	Electron-beam radiation
CuffPatch (Biomet Sports Medicine)	Porcine SIS	8 layers (hydrated)	Vacuum-dried, chemically cross-linked carbodiimide	25 kGy gamma irradiation
TissueMend (Stryker)	Fetal bovine skin	Single layer	Proprietary	Ethylene oxide
Zimmer Patch (Permacol)	Porcine dermis	Single layer (hydrated)	Chemically cross-linked: isocyanate	Gamma irradiation
Sportmesh (Biomet Sports Medicine)	Synthetic	Poly(urethane urea)	Proprietary	Proprietary
Allopatch HD (MTF)	Human skin	Single layer	Epidermal layer and cells removed	None (regulated as transplant)
Orthadapt (Pegasus)	Horse pericardium	Single layer	Decellularized, cross-linked	Liquid chemicals
Matristem (ACell)	Porcine urinary bladder	Single layer with basement membrane	Decellularized, non-cross-linked	Electron-beam irradiated

sion and matrix synthesis in tendon cells. The potential negative side of PRP is that the multiple chemotactic factors may have differing effects based on the location and timing of their delivery. There is tremendous variability in the use of PRP based on different commercial PRP products, with differences in platelet recovery, white blood cell inclusion, platelet activation, and kinetics of cytokine release. New advances in technology have allowed scientists to isolate individual growth factors known to be beneficial.

Various commercial systems are available to make PRP. Blood is usually harvested from the patient at the time of the procedure. Single-use blood collection systems and desktop centrifuges are now marketed by several different companies and can be used within the operating room during the procedure. Preparation of the PRP involves centrifugation first to remove the red and white blood cells, and second to concentrate the platelets to two to eight times the physiological levels. Further manipulation of the plasma results in either a fibrin matrix containing platelets, or a liquid form that is then applied directly to the repair as an adjunct for healing (**Fig. 20.1**) (Gamradt et al. 2007). The augmentation does not require any alteration in the normal rehabilitation process, but does not in itself provide structural integrity to the repair.

Studies reporting the efficacy of PRP continue to emerge. At this point there is very little evidence to support its use in rotator cuff surgery. More information is needed to evaluate the appropriate use of PRP because many questions remain concerning the timing, processing, and patient selection for this product.

FUTURE OPTIONS/AREAS OF FURTHER RESEARCH

Although there have been significant gains in the body of knowledge concerning tissue engineering over the last decade, there are still many areas that need further exploration, techniques that need improvement, and materials that can be made more effective.

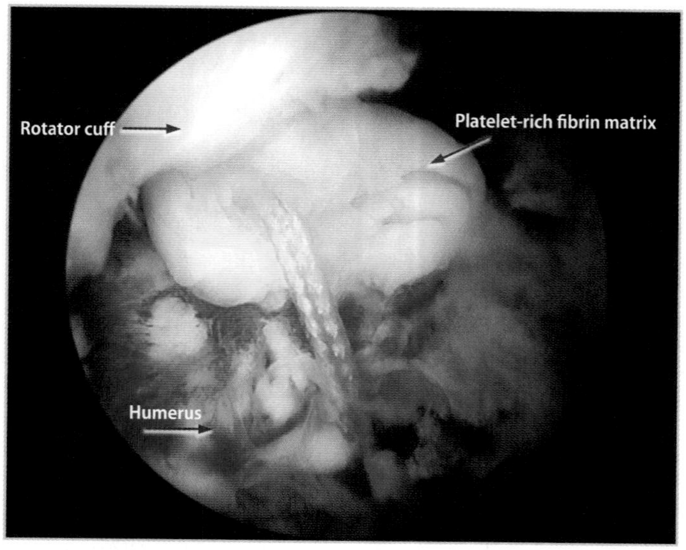

Figure 20.1 Platelet-rich plasma surgical application. The platelet-rich fibrin matrix, once formed into a solid clot, is passed into the subacromial space using a suture from a suture anchor. This is accomplished through a cannula with the diaphragm removed. The implant is incorporated into the repair with the rotator cuff tied down superiorly, securing the PRP implant against the tendon–bone interface.

Cellular engineering

Scientists have grown cells from human tissue for some time now. However, the discovery of stem cells and their possible role in tissue regeneration has led to attempts to differentiate these cells into a tendon phenotype. This can be performed through chemical means such as growth factors, or through mechanical stimulation. Transduction of the cells can be performed using gene therapy approaches. This approach introduces active genes into the cell to induce appropriate differentiation. Certain cell lineages can be induced by mechanical stimulation, which simulates the in vivo stress that occurs biologically in humans. Kupesick et al. (2010) recently attempted to induce chondrocyte differentiation in stem cells through the use of mechanical stimulation. They used mesenchymal stem cells that had been transduced with the *SOX9* gene, and found an increased production of sulfated glycosaminoglycans (GAGs) as well as type X collagen and lubricin. As we understand more about cellular and molecular signals that govern tenocyte development and function, our ability to direct the growth and structure of the resulting tissues will increase: for example, scleraxis is a transcription factor that has an important role in tendon development during embryogenesis, and is thus a promising factor for further study.

Growth factors/Cellular signaling

The normal bone–tendon interface is complex, made up primarily of type I collagen fibers arranged in an organized pattern of four specific zones. There is a longitudinal organization of these four zones of tissue: tendon, non-mineralized fibrocartilage, mineralized fibrocartilage, and bone. The structure and composition of this complex organ function to transfer stress from hard to soft tissue. After rotator cuff repair, in normal tendon-to-bone healing, the zone of insertion involves a fibrovascular scar made up primarily of type I and III collagen. Current research is focused on improving the quality of this healing interface to help decrease the failure rates and perhaps shorten healing times in rotator cuff repair.

Bone-derived growth factors known as BMPs have been extensively studied in recent years since the discovery of their beneficial role in bone growth and fracture healing. Many types of BMPs have been discovered, as scientists continue to explore the functions of each on bone, and even the potential effects on tendon and soft tissue healing. Seeherman et al. (2008) used a sheep model to show that collagen carriers treated with recombinant human BMP-12 (rhBMP-12) accelerated and strengthened healing of full-thickness rotator cuff tears as measured by mechanical testing, histological evaluation, and imaging. BMPs play a role in chemotaxis to promote the migration of healing progenitor cells to the injured area. They aid in the proliferation of these progenitor or stem cells to increase the number of cells in the area that could affect growth of new tissue. BMPs then promote differentiation of these cells into the appropriate mature cell line. BMP-12 induces the production of tendon and fibrocartilage which may aid tendon-to-bone healing, whereas BMP-2 induces new bone formation.

Neurochemicals have emerged as a new area of focus in the recent literature as their role in the pathobiology of bone, ligament, and even cartilage has been elucidated. Serotonin, oxytocin, and glutamate are among the neurochemicals being evaluated, in particular because of the discovery that their effects are direct, occurring through the activation of receptors and/or the excretion of the neurochemicals by osteoblasts, osteoclasts, chondrocytes, and tenocytes. These pathways can occur independently of direct peripheral or central nervous system influence. With regard to their potential role in rotator cuff healing, Mammoto et al. (2008) reported on the neurotropin nerve growth factor (NGF) and its role in rat medial collateral ligament healing. The chemical, when implanted exogenously, resulted in an increase in nerve density and a decreased amount of the angiogenesis inhibitor thrombospondin-2. The ultimate result was increased tissue vascularity, which was thought to be the reason for the observed increase in tensile strength and stiffness of the healing ligament.

Nanofiber materials

Nanofibers, or fibers measuring <1000 nm, are now being produced using organic polymer materials, and hold tremendous promise as scaffolds for tissue engineering. As nanofibers partly mimic the ultrastructure of the native extracellular matrix, cell function may be optimized on these materials (Mendes et al. 2010). Living progenitor cells can be added to the nanofiber scaffolds, which closely mimic the normal extracellular matrices and allow their proliferation in an in vitro environment. These cultured cells can then be implanted with the scaffold to the desired area for healing in a human. Lu and co-authors (2009, 2010) have been very active in pioneering these compounds and examining their capabilities as tissue scaffolds to aid in tissue regeneration and healing. Recently, they reported a method of endothelial cell outgrowth on a scaffold made of poly-L-lactic acid nanofibers.

Hydrogels represent another class of materials used to guide cell and tissue ingrowth, with a potential use for human implantation. These scaffolds are highly hydrophilic, a property that can be used to create a three-dimensional lattice to allow multidirectional ingrowth and organization of desired cells. Suri and Schmidt (2010) have recently described a hydrogel composed of collagen, hyaluronic acid, and laminin which has allowed them to culture and observe the growth of Schwann cells in multiple planes. So-called neural tissue engineering could play an important role in the re-innervation of damaged and denervated tissue in the future. Manipulation of the composition of multiple types of scaffold could lead to the development of methods to grow and implant other types of cells, including chondrocytes and tenocytes, in the future.

CLINICAL ASPECTS/CONCLUSION

Although many clinical applications resulting from tissue engineering investigations are already in regular use today, scientists will continue to discover new techniques in tissue engineering to optimize the use of cells, cytokines, and scaffolds to ultimately reduce failures and improve patient outcomes in rotator cuff surgery. Great strides have been made in the discovery and isolation of the cytokines involved in soft-tissue and tendon healing. Although still in its infancy, use of tissue grown in vitro will continue to be explored with the goal of producing safe, effective, and affordable engineered tissues for human patients. Human dermal matrices have been popularized for augmentation of rotator cuff repairs when surgeons feel that the tissue is weakened to the point of a high likelihood of failure, or the rotator cuff is unable to be reapproximated to its native footprint. Surgeons are using combinations of cellular products, growth factors, and ECM scaffolds to help improve the quality of their rotator cuff repairs. When used together, these three aspects of tissue engineering may lead to increased tendon healing after repair, with improved clinical outcomes.

REFERENCES

Badhe SP, Lawrence TM, Smith FD, Lunn PG. An assessment of porcine dermal xenograft as an augmentation graft in the treatment of extensive rotator cuff tears. J Shoulder Elbow Surg 2008;17:35S–39S.

Bond JL, Dopirak RM, Higgins, J, Burns, J, Snyder SJ. Arthroscopic replacement of massive, irreparable rotator cuff tears using a GraftJacket allograft: technique and preliminary results. Arthroscopy 2008;24:403–409.e1.

Chen JM. Autologous tenocyte therapy using porcine-derived bioscaffolds for massive rotator cuff defects in rabbits. Tissue Engin 2007;13:1479–1491.

de Mos M, van der Windt AE, Jahr H, et al. Can platelet-rich plasma enhance tendon repair? A cell culture study. Am J Sports Med 2008;36:1171–1178.

Derwin KA, Codsi MJ, Milks RA, et al. Rotator cuff repair augmentation in a canine model with use of a woven poly-L-lactide device. J Bone Joint Surg Am 2009;91:1159–1171.

Derwin KA, Badylak SF, Steinmann SP, Iannotti JP. Extracellular matrix scaffold devices for rotator cuff repair. J Shoulder Elbow Surg 2010;19:467–476.

Dines JS, Grande DA, Dines DM. Tissue engineering and rotator cuff tendon healing. J Shoulder Elbow Surg 2007;16(suppl):S204–S207.

Drobny GP, Long JR, Karlsson, T, et al. Structural studies of biomaterials using double-quantum solid-state NMR spectroscopy. Annu Rev Phys Chem 2003;54:531–571.

Foster TE, Puskas BL, Mandelbaum BR, Gerhardt MB, Rodeo SA. Platelet-rich plasma: from basic science to clinical applications. Am J Sports Med 2009;371:2259–2272.

Gamradt SC, Rodeo SA, Warren RF. Platelet rich plasma in rotator cuff repair, techniques in orthopaedics. Biologics Shoulder Surg 2007;22:26–33.

Iannotti JP, Codsi MJ, Kwon YW, et al. Porcine small intestine submucosa augmentation of surgical repair of chronic two-tendon rotator cuff tears. A randomized, controlled trial. J Bone Joint Surg Am 2006;88:1238–1244.

Kupcsik, L, Stoddart MJ, Li, Z, Benneker LM, Alini, M. Improving chondrogenesis: potential and limitations of SOX9 gene transfer and mechanical stimulation for cartilage tissue engineering, Tissue Engin Part A 2010;16:1845–1855.

Longo U, Lamberti A, Maffulli N, Denaro V. Tendon augmentation grafts: a systematic review. Br Med Bull 2010a;94:165–188.

Longo U, Lamberti A, Maffulli N, Denaro V. Tissue engineered biological augmentation for tendon healing: a systematic review. Br Med Bull Adv Access 2010b;94:1–29.

Lu H, Feng Z, Gu Z, Liu C. Growth of outgrowth endothelial cells on aligned PLLA nanofibrous scaffolds. J Mater Sci: Mater Med 2009;20:1937–1944.

Lu H, Ko YG, Kawazoe N, Chen G. Cartilage tissue engineering using funnel-like collagen sponges prepared with embossing ice particulate templates. Biomaterials 2010;312:5825–5835.

Mammoto, T, Seerattan RA, Paulson KD, et al. Nerve growth factor improves ligament healing. J Orthop Res 2008;26:957–964.

Martinek, V, Latterman, C, Usas, A, et al. Enhancement of tendon-bone integration of anterior cruciate ligament grafts with bone morphogenetic protein-2 gene transfer: a histological and biomechanical study. J Bone Joint Surg Am 2002;84:1123–1131.

Mendes RM, Silva GA, Caliari MV, et al. Effects of single wall carbon nanotubes and its functionalization with sodium hyaluronate on bone repair. Life Sci 2010;87:215–222.

Muschler GF, Nakamoto, C, Griffith LG. Engineering principles of clinical cell-based tissue engineering. J Bone Joint Surg Am 2004;86:1541–1558.

Rodeo SA, Potter HG, Kawamura, S, et al. Biologic augmentation of rotator cuff tendon-healing with use of a mixture of osteoinductive growth factors. J Bone Joint Surg Am 2007;89:2485–2497.

Seeherman HJ, Archambault JM, Rodeo SA, et al. rhBMP-12 accelerates healing of rotator cuff repairs in a sheep model. J Bone Joint Surg Am 2008;90:2206–2219.

Snyder SJ, Arnoczky SP, Bond JL, Dopirak, R. Histologic evaluation of a biopsy specimen obtained 3 months after rotator cuff augmentation with GraftJacket Matrix. Arthroscopy 2009;25:329–333.

Soler JA, Gidwani, S, Curtis MJ. Early complications from the use of porcine dermal collagen implants (Permacol) as bridging constructs in the repair of massive rotator cuff tears. A report of 4 cases. Acta Orthop Belg 2007;73:432–436.

Suri, S, Schmidt CE. Cell-laden hydrogel constructs of hyaluronic acid, collagen, and laminin for neural tissue engineering. Tissue Engin Part A 2010;16:1703–1716.

Valentin JE, Badylak JS, McCabe GP, Badylak SF. Extracellular matrix bioscaffolds for orthopedic applications. A comparative histologic study. J Bone Joint Surg Am 2006;88:2673–2686.

Zheng MH, Chen, J, Kirilak, Y, et al. Porcine small intestine submucosa (SIS) is not an acellular collagenous matrix and contains porcine DNA: possible implications in human implantation. J Biomed Mater Res B Appl Biomater 2005;73:61–67.

Index

Note: Page numbers with suffix *f* and *t* refer to figures and tables respectively.

92-kDa gelatinase, 119

Abduction torque, 29, 31, 33, 34
"Acetabularization," 117, 124*t*
Achilles tendon ruptures
  and ABO blood groups, 26
Acromial keel spurs, 6
Acromial spur, 7, 21, 38, 41
  classification, 6
Acromioclavicular (AC) joint, 4, 6, 10, 22, 39, 41, 57
  degenerative changes of, 59
  dislocation
  in Imatani Shoulder Score, 169
  pathology of, 42*f*
  pseudoganglion of, 123
Acromioclavicular joint tests, 52
Acromion, 10, 16
  abnormalities, 21
  classification of, 20
  impingement syndrome, 64
  morphology types, 6, 59, 64
  in rotator cuff tears, 20
Acromioplasty, 20, 35, 36, 69, 70
Activities of daily living (ADL), 15, 163
  in American Shoulder and Elbow Surgeons Shoulder Evaluation Form, 171
  in Constant–Murley score (CMS), 169
  and rotator cuff lesions, 25
  in symptomatic glenohumeral arthritis, 121
Acute tendon injuries, PRP usage of, 159–160
Aging
  and degeneration, 15*t*, 20, 91
  and rotator cuff lesions, 25, 26
  and rotator cuff overload, 83
Allografts
  acellular non-cross-linked human dermal matrix, 146–147
  of human skin, 177
  for rotator cuff repair, 152
  scaffold augmentation, 151
Allopatch, 152, 177*t*
American Shoulder and Elbow Surgeons Shoulder Evaluation (ASES-S) Form, 170–171, 172
Anterior L tears, 12
Anteroinferior shoulder dislocation, 22*f*
Arthrodesis, 125
Arthrography, 65–66
Arthroscopic and surgical evaluation
  subscapularis tears, diagnosis of, 110–111
Arthroscopic debridement
  for elderly, 125
  pain relief, 152
  with or without subacromial decompression, 68*t*, 69, 72
Arthroscopic joint debridement, 117
Arthroscopic repair, 99
  of partial-thickness tears, 70
  conversion to full-thickness tears, 68*t*, 70, 71
  intratendinous repair, 68*t*, 71, 72
  mini-open technique, 69*t*, 72
  transtendon repair, 68*t*, 70–71, 71–72
Arthroscopic rotator cuff repair, 99
Arthroscopy, 65*t*, 110–111, 125, 161
  benefits of, 89
  See also Diagnostic arthroscopy
Articular surfaces, 76
  biceps tendon, 78
  capsuloligamentous complex, 76
  inferior glenohumeral ligament complex, 77
  labrum, 76
  middle glenohumeral ligament, 77
  rotator cuff, 77–78
  rotator cuff interval, 76–77
Articular-sided rotator cuff tears, 75
  partial-thickness rotator cuff tears, 18
Asymptomatic tears, 25, 99
Athletic Shoulder Outcome Rating Scale (ASORS), 170
Autologous progenitor cells, 175
Avascularity, 15*t*, 19

Basic fibroblastic growth factor (basic FGF)
  in tendon healing, 139
Bear hug test, 109, 111, 112*t*
Belly press sign, 48
Belly press test, 109, 110*f*
Belly-off test, 109, 112*t*
Bennett's lesions, 39*f*, 75, 84
  See also Posterior glenoid exostosis
Biceps tendinopathy, surgical management of, 93–94
Biceps tendon, 78, 84
  examination, 51
  Speed's test, 51–52
  pathology of, 75
Biceps tenodesis, 87, 93
  versus tenotomy, 95, 113
  and transfer, 95–96
Bigliani classification, 35*f*
  acromion morphology, 6, 10, 65
Biological scaffolds, 145, 176
  features of, 149*t*
  from porcine small intestinal submucosa, 177
Body mass index
  and rotator cuff lesions, 26
Bone morphogenetic proteins (BMPs), 137, 176
  in tendon healing, 139
Bovine dermis, 148
Buford complex, 88, 91
Bursae, 7, 36–37
Bursal-sided rotator cuff tears, 18
Bursitis, of rotator cuff, 75
Bursography, 65–66

Calcium phosphate crystal, 118
Capsular laxity, 75, 84, 91, 117
Capsuloligamentous complex, 76, 77
Cellular engineering, 178
Cellular hyperplasia, 119
Cellular mitogenesis, 137
Chemotaxis, 137, 176, 177, 178
Cholesterol, 15*t*, 20
Chronicity, and tears, 12
Collagen Repair patch, 148, 151–152, 177
Collagen, 37–38, 119, 138, 147, 176, 179
Collagenase, 119
Collagen–glycosaminoglycan analog, 38
Combined subscapularis tears, prevalence of, 108*t*
Complex tears, 12–13
  extent of, 13*f*
Computed tomography (CT) arthrography, 20, 55, 60, 110, 114, 134
"Concavity–compression" mechanism, 77
Constant–Murley score (CMS), 169, 172
Contrast MR arthrography, 66
Conversion to full-thickness tears, 68*t*, 70
Coracoacromial arch, 6, 35
  anatomy of, 10
  cadaveric dissection of, 16*f*
Coracoacromial ligament, 10, 35–36
Coracohumeral ligament (CHL), 77
  with rotator cuff and scapula glenoid, 3*f*
  with superior glenohumeral ligament and long biceps tendon, 4*f*
Coracoid impingement, 6, 15*t*, 21, 36, 113*t*
Coracoid process, 6, 21, 35, 36, 108, 119, 122
Cortisone injections, 124
Crepitation, 122
Crescent-shaped tears, 11*f*, 12, 100
Critical zone, 3, 19, 38, 56, 64, 66
  See also Hypovascular zone
Crystal-mediated theory, 118–119
Cuff interval, 57
  and shoulder girdle anatomy, 26*f*
  See also Rotator interval; Rotator cuff interval
Cuff tears, etiology
  extrinsic, 38
  intrinsic, 39
Cuff ultrastructure, 37
CuffPatch (Arthrotek), 152, 177

Debridement
  See Arthroscopic debridement; Subacromial decompression
Delta III prosthesis, 128
Deltoid muscle, 3, 5, 7, 16, 34
Deltoid rehabilitation program, 125
Dermal matrix, 145, 149
  acellular, non-cross-linked, 146–147
Diabetes mellitus, 25
  and rotator cuff lesions, 25, 26
  and traumatic type II SLAP tear, 95

Diagnostic arthroscopy, 66
Differentiation, in embryology, 7
Disability of Arm, Shoulder, and Hand (DASH) questionnaire, 168, 171
Double-row, suture anchor, 133*t*, 135*t*
Drop-arm sign, 44, 47, 49, 65
Dropping lag sign, 49
Dynamic restraints, 34, 76, 78
"Dysfunctional symptomatic" rotator cuff tear, 32

Eccentric glenospheres, 127, 128*f*
Ecchymosis, 51, 122
Elevation, 43–44
 drop-arm sign, 44
 painful arc, 44
 shrug sign, 44–45
"Empty can" exercise, 30, 31*f*, 32*f*, 33, 34, 48*f*
Endogenous tissue inhibitors of MMPs (TIMPS), 145
Epidermal growth factor (EGF), 137, 138*f*, 177
Equine pericardium, 146, 148, 149*t*
 See also OrthADAPT bioimplant
External rotation (ER), 16, 29, 31, 33, 34, 78, 79
 in Constant–Murley score, 169
 and strength testing, 47–48, 100
 weakness in, 52
 See also "Full can" exercise
External rotation lag sign (ERLS), 31, 49
Extracellular dermal matrices, 176
Extracellular matrix (ECM) patches, 145
 commercially available, 177*t*
 considerations, 146–147
 contraindications, 148–149
Extracellular matrix (ECM) scaffold
 for autogenic cells, 153
 rotator cuff repair, FDA approved, 151*t*
Extrinsic impingement, 29, 38

Family history, and rotator cuff lesions, 26
Fatty infiltration, 64
 Goutallier grade, 113*t*
 and muscle atrophy, 112
 of muscle belly, 110, 111
 of muscles, 56, 100, 110, 133, 145
Favard classification, 122
"Femoralization," 117, 124*t*
Fibroblast growth factor (FGF), 138*f*, 152, 176
Flexi-level Scale of Shoulder Function (FLEX-SF), 167–168
Flexion exercises, 164*t*
Footprint contact pressure, 133
Footprint restoration, 131–132
Force couple theory, 120–121
"Full can" exercise, 30, 31*f*, 32*f*, 33, 34, 48*f*
Full DASH questionnaire, 172
Full-thickness rotator cuff tears, 17*f*
 classification, 12*t*, 100
 clinical presentation, 100
 diagnosis, 99–100
 epidemiology, 99
 etiology, 99
 and healing, 99
 treatment
 conservative, 100
 surgical, 100–101
Functional tears, 32
Function-specific cells, 175

Germ layers, 7
Geyser sign, 123
Glenohumeral abduction, 29, 78
Glenohumeral biomechanical stability, 75–76
Glenohumeral internal rotation deficit (GIRD), 46, 78, 80, 81, 82, 84
Glenohumeral joint, 5–6
 subacromial or suprahumeral space, 6
Glenohumeral ligaments (GHLs), 6, 76, 77*f*, 91, 100
Glenohumeral synovium, 7
 See also Bursae
Glenoid labrum, 76*f*
 See also Labrum
Global resistance exercises, 164*t*
Goutallier fatty infiltration classification, 112*t*
GraftJacket, 146–147, 151*t*, 152, 177*t*
Grammont's device, 126
Growth factors, and tendon healing, 137–138
 basic fibroblastic growth factor, 139
 bone morphogenetic proteins, 139
 healing phases, 138*f*
 insulin-like growth factor, 139
 platelet-derived growth factor, 139–140
 and rotator cuff, 141–142
 transforming growth factor, 138, 140–141
 vascular endothelial growth factors, 141

Hamada classification system, 122
Hemiarthroplasty, 125–126
Hepatocyte growth factor (HGF), 137, 138*f*, 157
Hospital for Special Surgery Shoulder – Rating Score Sheet, 170
Humeral head, superior subluxation of, 30, 49
Humeroscapular motion interface, smoothness, 118
Humerus, 5, 11*f*, 15, 16*f*, 141
 "femoralization," 117
 and rotator cuff overuse, 21
 shoulder bone, 4
 subscapularis, 1–2
Hyaluronic acid, 179
Hydrogels, 179
Hygroma, 117, 122
Hypercholesterolemia, 20, 22
Hypovascular zone, 3, 19, 64
 See also Critical zone

Imatani Shoulder Score, for acromioclavicular dislocation, 169
Inferior glenohumeral ligament complex, 77
Inflammatory biceps pathology, 88–89
Infraspinatus, 3, 9, 15, 16, 33
 function of, 16
 and teres minor, 33
Infraspinatus atrophy, 43*f*
Instability-related biceps pathology, 89
Insulin, 137
Insulin-like grow factor (IGF), 101, 139, 153, 157, 176
 in tendon healing, 139
Internal impingement, 18, 38, 39, 79, 81
Internal rotation (IR), 16, 29, 32*f*, 33, 34, 69
 in athletes, 75
 in range of motion, 79
 in strength measurement, 171
 weakness of, 48, 107, 109
 See also "Empty can" exercise
"Internal rotation lag" variation, 109
Intra-articular injections, 124
 for pain control, 69
Intraoperative tensioning, 103*f*
Intratendinous partial-thickness rotator cuff tears, 18–19
Intratendinous repair, 68*t*, 71, 72
Intrinsic degeneration, 29, 39
Isolated subscapularis tears, prevalence of, 108*t*

Jobe's strength testing, 43*t*, 47, 52, 65

Kennedy–Hawkins sign, 50–51
"Kissing" lesion, of rotator cuff, 18

"L'arthropathie destructrice rapide de l'epaule," 117
"L'epaule senile hemorragique," 117
Labrum, 76, 84
Lafosse classification scheme, 112*t*
Lag signs
 dropping lag sign, 49
 external rotation lag sign, 49
 lift-off lag sign, 49
Laminin, 179
Lift-off lag sign, 49
Lift-off test, 48, 109, 112*t*
Ligamentum semicircular humeri, on intact rotator cuff, 1
Long head of biceps tendon (LHBT), 10, 37, 41
 anatomy of, 88
 clinical presentation, 90
 conservative management, 91
 diagnosis, 90–91
 pathology, 88
 biceps instability, 89
 of inflammatory biceps, 88–89
 traumatic biceps, 89
 postoperative management, 94
Lubricin, 178

Magnetic resonance imaging (MRI), 66
 of shoulder, 56
 contraindications of, 56–57
 fundamentals of, 56
 sequences of, 56
Mason–Allen rotator cuff repairs, 132, 134
Massive rotator cuff tears, 58–59, 60*f*, 117
 augmentation of, 151
 allografts, 152
 ECM scaffold for autogenic cells, 153
 postoperative management, 154
 synthetic ECM grafts, 152–153
 xenografts, 151–152
Matristem (Acell), 177
Matrix metalloproteases (MMPs), 138*f*, 145
Mature cells, 175
Microinstability
 anterior laxity, 81–82
 and over-rotation, 82
Microtrauma
 and aging, 20
 in athletes, 75, 158
 degenerative changes in, 64, 157
 rotator cuff overload, 83
 tendon injuries, 137
Middle glenohumeral ligaments, 77
"Milwaukee shoulder," 117, 118, 125
Mini-open technique, 69*t*
 partial-thickness rotator cuff tears, 72
 for tendon-to-bone repair, 100
Modified UCLA Shoulder Score, 170
MR arthrography, 56, 58–59, 60, 90, 100, 110
Muscle atrophy, 56, 59, 60, 65, 112, 149, 153
Muscle strength and balance
 rotator cuff, 81
 scapular, 81

Muscles
 See Rotator cuff muscles
Musculoskeletal disorders, 25, 26
 See also Shoulder diseases
Musculoskeletal tissue engineering, 175
 See also Tissue engineering

Nanofibers, 179
Napoleon's sign, 109, 112t
 See also Belly press test
Neer's sign, 49–50
Neurotropin nerve growth factor (NGF), in rat medial collateral ligament healing, 178
Nocturnal pain, 65
Non-steroidal anti-inflammatory drugs (NSAIDs)
 healing rate, effect on, 99, 163, 164
 for pain control, 69, 124
 type II SLAP tear, 91

OrthADAPT (Pegasus), 177
OrthADAPT bioimplant, 148, 149t, 151t
 See also Equine pericardium
Orthobiologics, 145
Os acromiale, 7, 15t, 21, 22f
 composition of, 16
Osseous adaptations, 80
Overhead athlete, 75
 articular surfaces, 76
 biceps tendon, 78
 capsuloligamentous complex, 76
 inferior glenohumeral ligament complex, 77
 labrum, 76
 middle glenohumeral ligament, 77
 rotator cuff, 77–78
 rotator cuff interval, 76–77
 biomechanics, 75
 glenohumeral stability, 75–76
 injuries in, 83–85
 muscle strength and balance
 rotator cuff, 81
 scapular, 81
 osseous adaptations, 80
 pathological processes, internal impingement, 81
 pathomechanics, 81–83
 pitching motion, 78–79
 phases of, 79f
 posterior capsular tightness, 80–81
 range of motion, 79–80
 sports, 75
Overhead athletes, pathomechanics
 anterior capsular laxity, 81–82
 microinstability and/or over-rotation, 82
 posterior capsular contracture, 82
 rotator cuff overload/tensile failure, 83
Overhead athletes, injuries in, 83
 biceps tendon, 84
 full thickness rotator cuff, 83–84
 labrum, 84
 partial-thickness rotator cuff, 83
 posterior glenoid exostosis, 84–85
 scapular dyskinesia, 85
 subcoracoid impingement, 85
Oxford Shoulder Score, 167

Painful arc, 43, 44
Paralabral ganglion cysts, 89
Partial tears, pathophysiology of, 17
Partial-thickness rotator cuff tears (PTRCTs), 17f
 articular sided, 18
 classification of, 10t, 63t
 clinical presentation, 65
 definition of, 63
 diagnosis, 65–66
 extrinsic factors, 64
 versus full-thickness tears, 25
 incidence and prevalence, 63–64
 intratendinous, 18–19
 pathogenesis, 64
 physical examination, 65
 risk factors of, 64t
 traumatic factors, 64–65
Passive range of motion exercises, 154, 164t
"Peel-back mechanism", 84, 90, 91, 92
Penn Shoulder Score, 170
Permacol, 148, 149t, 151, 152, 177
Pfirrmann classification scheme, 113t
Physical therapy
 for adhesive capsulitis, 102
 for muscle strength, 69, 100
 for postoperative pain, 60, 114
 for rotator cuff tear, 66, 83, 99
 for shoulder pain, 55, 124
 for SLAP tears, 91
 for subscapularis tears, 112
Pitching motion, 78–79
 phases of, 79f
Placenta growth factor (PIGF){AQ: Should this read PlGF? Please check}
 in tendon healing, 138f, 141
Plain film radiography, 55
Platelet-derived growth factor (PDGF), 101, 137, 157
 in tendon healing, 138f, 139–140
Platelet-derived growth factor β (PDGF-β), 176
Platelet-rich plasma (PRP), 177–178
 benefits of, 158
 in postoperative management, 163
 preparation process
 injection technique, 161–162
 methods of, 159–160
 post-injection treatment, 162–163
 after repairing injured tendon, 159
 during surgery, 163
 in tendon healing, 157
 indications for, 159
Platelets, in tendon healing, 101
Pluripotency, 7
Polyglycolic acid (PGA), 152, 176
"Popeye" deformity
 biceps tendon rupture, 51, 93
 tenodesis, 95
Porcine dermal collagen, 148
Porcine small intestinal submucosa (porcine SIS), 177
Posterior capsular tightness, 80–81
Posterior cuff
 See Infraspinatus; Teres minor
Posterior glenoid exostosis, 84
 See also Bennett's lesions
Posterior glenoid lesions, 75, 84–85
Posterior L tears, 12
Preparation rich in growth factors (PRGF), 157, 161f, 162f
Primary bicipital tenosynovitis, 88
Pseudolaxity, 82
Pyrophosphate metabolism, 119

QuickDASH questionnaire, 168, 172

Range of motion (ROM), 79–80
Recurrent blood-tinged effusions, 122
"Reflection pulley," 108
Reinforcement patches, 145
Relocation, for subscapularis tears, 113
Repetitive microtrauma, 64
 capsular laxity, 84
Restore Orthobiologic Implant (Depuy), 177
Retracted tears, 10, 12, 100
Reverse total shoulder prosthesis, 126–128
 biomechanical advantages, 126–127
"Rocking horse" phenomenon, 125
Rotation test, 45–46
Rotator cable, on intact rotator cuff, 1
Rotator cuff anatomy, 15–17
 bones and subacromal space, 4
 humerus, 5
 scapula, 4–5
 embryology, 7
 joints
 glenohumeral joint, 5–6
 coracoacromial arch, 6
 subacromial or suprahumeral space, 6
 acromion, 6
 coracoid process, 6
 os acromiale, 7
 bursae, 7
 muscles, 1
 subscapularis, 1–2, 9
 supraspinatus, 2–3, 10
 infraspinatus, 3, 9
 teres minor, 3, 9–10
 and tendon-to-bone healing, 131
 vessels, 3–4
Rotator cuff and related structure, pathology
 infraspinatus, 58
 long head of biceps tendon, 58
 massive rotator cuff tears, 58–59
 subscapularis, 58
 supraspinatus, 57–58
Rotator cuff arthropathy, 117
Rotator cuff arthropathy theory, 119–120
Rotator cuff biomechanics
 bursae, 36–37
 coracoacromial arch, 35
 coracoacromial ligament, 35–36
 coracoid process, 36
 cuff muscles, 30–34
 deltoid muscle, 34
 functions of, 16
 long head of biceps, 37
 rotator interval, 37
 of tear development, 38f
Rotator cuff complex
 bony and soft tissue anatomy of, 16f
Rotator cuff disease
 AC joint pain, 42f
 biceps tendon examination, 51
 acromioclavicular joint tests, 52
 Speed's test, 51–52
 combined tests, 51
 etiology of, 15t, 25
 epidemiology of, 25–26
 genetics of, 26–27
 lag signs, 49
 dropping lag sign, 49
 external rotation lag sign, 49
 lift-off lag sign, 49
 provocative maneuvers
 Kennedy–Hawkins sign, 50–51
 Neer's sign, 49–50
 shoulder examination, 41–43

basic muscle testing, 43*t*
basic nerve testing, 43*t*
elevation, 43–45
rotation, 45–46
strength testing, 46
in abduction, 46–47
in external rotation, 47–49
visceral pain, 42*f*
Rotator cuff failure, extrinsic causes, 19
coracoid impingement, 21
os acromiale, 21, 22*f*
overuse, 21
subacromial impingement, 20–21
trauma, 21–22
Rotator cuff failure, intrinsic causes, 19
aging and degeneration, 20
avascularity, 19
cholesterol, 20
smoking, 19
Rotator cuff healing, scaffolds, 176–177
Rotator cuff interval, 76–77
Rotator cuff muscles, 29–30
functions of, 1
infraspinatus, 33
subscapularis, 33–34
supraspinatus, 30–33
teres minor, 33
Rotator cuff overuse, 15*t*, 21
Rotator cuff orthobiologics
See Orthobiologics
Rotator Cuff Quality-of-Life (RC-QOL) measure, 168
Rotator cuff, 77–78
force-tension relationship, 17
in glenohumeral stability, 81
and growth factors, 141–142
images, 57
normal anatomy, 57–58
imaging of
CT arthrography, 55
magnetic resonance imaging, 55–56–57
plain film radiography, 55
related structure pathology, 58
ultrasonography, 55
pathoanatomy
collagen, 37–38
cuff ultrastructure, 37
secondary impingement, 78*f*
Rotator cuff repair
biological augmentation of, 145–146
FDA approved
extracellular matrix scaffold, 151*t*
synthetic scaffold, 152*t*
single-row versus double-row, 131
biomechanics of, 131–133
clinical outcomes of, 134
structural integrity, 134
Rotator cuff repair failures
and complications, 102
Rotator cuff repair surgery
tissue engineering, 175
Rotator cuff scaffolds
features of, 146
Rotator cuff tear arthropathy, 117, 118
clinical manifestation, 121
mechanical factors, 118
reverse total shoulder prosthesis, 126–128
shoulder arthroplasty
hemiarthroplasty, 125–126
surgical treatment, 124
arthrodesis, 125
arthroscopy, 125
Rotator cuff tears, 10–11, 39*f*
articular-sided, 18
bursal sided, 18
classification of, 10
diagnostic tools, features of, 65*t*
intratendinous, 18–19
risk factors associated with, 19*t*
Rotator cuff tears, management of, 66
non-surgical management, 69, 71
surgical management, 69
arthroscopic debridement, 69, 71
arthroscopic repair, 70
Rotator cuff tendons, 2*f*
Rotator interval, 37, 76–77
See also Cuff interval
Ruptured Achilles tendons, PRP injections, 158

Scaffolds, 145, 175–176
See also Rotator cuff scaffold; Biological scaffold
Scapula, 4–5
Scapular dyskinesia, 44, 75, 81, 85
Scapular winging, 42, 43*f*
Seebauer classification system, 122, 124*t*
Semi-constrained reverse ball-and-socket design, 126
See also Reverse total shoulder prosthesis
Short-tailed interference knotted (STIK) sutures, 154
Shoulder arthropathy, 117
Shoulder arthroplasty, 151
Shoulder bones, 4
humerus, 5
scapula, 4–5
Shoulder comparison, with arthritis, 123
Shoulder computerized adaptive tests, 171
Shoulder Disability Questionnaire (SDQ), 168, 172
Shoulder diseases, 25–26
Shoulder joint replacement, 117
Shoulder joint resurfacing, 117
Shoulder muscles, physiology of, 9*t*
Shoulder Pain and Disability Index (SPADI), 168, 171
Shoulder pain, and tear, 15
Shoulder physiology
articular cartilage integrity, 118
motion, 117
stability, 117–118
strength, 118
Shoulder radiographs, 65–66
Shoulder Rating Questionnaire (SRQ), 167, 171
Shoulder score, formula, 171
Shoulder severity index (SSI), 134
Shoulder-related Disability Questionnaire, 169
Shrug sign, 44–45
Simple Shoulder Test (SST), 169, 172
Single- versus double-row repairs, biomechanics
footprint contact pressure, 133
footprint restoration, 131–132
mechanical strength, 132–133
Single-row, suture anchor, 133*t*, 135*t*
Sling immobilization, 102
Small intestine submucosa, 147–148
Smoking
in rotator cuff tears, 15*t*, 19, 26, 38
and tendon healing, 99, 102
Smooth joint surfaces, for shoulder function, 118
Smooth muscle actin (SMA), 37–38
Speed's test, 51–52
Spinoglenoid notch cysts (SGNCs), 89
Sports, overhead motion, 75
biomechanics, 75
Spurs, types of, 5*f*
Static restraints, 5, 34, 75–76
Stem cells, 175
Steroid injections
in damaging tissues, 158
in tendon healing, 99
Strength testing, 46
Strengthening exercises, 164*t*
Stromelysin mRNA, 119
Subacromial bursa, 10, 36
Subacromial decompression
with or without arthroscopic debridement, 69
Subacromial extrinsic impingement, 39
Subacromial impingement, 15*t*, 20–21
Subacromial region, structures in, 10
Subacromial space, 6
Subacromial space hygroma, 117
Subcoracoid bursae, 36
Subcoracoid impingement, 85, 108
Subdeltoid bursae, 36
Subjective Shoulder Rating System (SSRS), 169, 172
Subscapsularis tears, 107
etiology and mechanism, 108
Goutallier fatty infiltration classification, 112*t*
Lafosse classification scheme, 112*t*
Pfirrmann classification scheme, 112*t*
surgical management
arthroscopic technique, 114
open surgical technique, 113–114
postoperative care, 114
Subscapularis, 1–2, 9, 33–34
fibers, 2*f*
into humerus, 15
muscles, 16
muscular anatomy of, 107*f*
tendon, tests of, 48
belly press sign, 48
lift-off test, 48
tendons of, 2*f*
Sulfated glycosaminoglycans (GAGs), 178
Superior deltoid-splitting approach, 113
Superior glenohumeral ligament (SGHL), 77
Superior labral anteroposterior (SLAP) lesions, 39*f*, 75
See also Superior labrum anterior and posterior (SLAP) lesions
Superior labral lesions, 87
Superior labrum anterior and posterior (SLAP) lesions, 87, 95
clinical presentation, 90
conservative management, 91
diagnosis, 90–91
pathogenesis of, 88
postoperative management, 94
surgical management of, 91–93
Suprahumeral space
See Subacromial space
Supraspinatus tendon
full-thickness tendon, MR image, 56*f*, 57*f*
mechanical properties of, 38
partial-thickness tendon, 57*f*
Supraspinatus testing, 47–48
Supraspinatus wasting, 43*f*
Supraspinatus, 2–3, 10, 16–17, 30–33
tendons of, 2*f*
Suture bridge, 133, 135*t*
Suture-holding properties, 12
Swanson Shoulder Score System, 170
Symptomatic glenohumeral arthritis, 121
Synthetic ECM grafts, 152–153
Synthetic extracellular matrices, scaffold augmentation, 151

Tear pattern, morphological classification, 12–13
Tears
chronicity, 12
extent of, 12
of complex tears, 13*f*
mobility of, 11–12
shapes of, 11
size of, 11
tissue quality, 12
"Tendinitis," 137
"Tendinopathy," 137
"Tendinosis," 137
Tendon healing, 101
Tendon injuries, 137
healing, growth factors in, 138
basic fibroblastic growth factor, 139
bone morphogenetic proteins, 139
insulin-like growth factor, 139
platelet-derived growth factor, 139–140
transforming growth factor, 138, 140–141
vascular endothelial growth factors, 141
healing phases, 138*f*
tendon repair, 137–138
Tendon thickness, 12
Tendon transfers, 151
"Tendonitis," 137
of rotator cuff, 75
Tenocyte apoptosis, 145
Tenodesis for subscapsularis tears, 113
Tenotomy
for subscapsularis tears, 113
versus tenodesis, 94
Teres minor, 3, 9–10, 16
fibers from, 2*f*
and infraspinatus, 33
Tissue engineering
previous studies in, 176
Tissue quality, and tears, 12
TissueMend (Stryker), 148, 149*t*, 151*t*, 152, 177
Tobacco smoking, 25
and rotator cuff lesions, 25, 26
Tongue-shaped tears, 12
Transforming growth factor β (TGF-β)
in BMPs, 139
in collagen, 158, 176
and GraftJacket, 147
and platelets, 101
in PRP concentrate, 157
in tendon healing, 138*f*, 140–141
Translation control, of humeral head, 29
"Transosseous equivalent" repairs, 133
Transosseous repair, 133, 135*t*
Transtendon repair, 68*t*, 70–71
Transverse band, on intact rotator cuff, 1
Transverse ruptures, 10, 100
Transverse tear, 12
Transverse-plane force couple, 120
Trauma, 15*t*, 21–22
in athletes, 83
in biceps tendon rupture, 59, 89
infraspinatus tendon tears, 59
subscapular tendon tears, 59
Traumatic factors, 64–65
Traumatic biceps pathology, 89
Triangular space, 2
Type I acromion, 6, 16, 59, 65
Type II acromion, 10, 16, 65
Type III acromion, 6, 10, 16*f*, 20, 35, 65
Type X collagen, 178
Tyrosine kinase receptors, 141

Ultrasonography
for arm elevation evaluation, 52
for dislocated biceps tendon, 110
for full cuff tears, 100
for partial cuff tears, 66, 100
for rotator cuff tars, 25, 55, 65*t*
in rehabilitation program, 164
University of California at Los Angeles (UCLA)
Shoulder Rating, 169–170, 172
Upper Extremity Function Scale (UEFS), 169
Upper limb rating systems
shoulder computerized adaptive tests, 172
shoulder-specific rating scales
American Shoulder and Elbow Surgeons
Shoulder Evaluation Form, 170–171, 172
Athletic Shoulder Outcome Rating Scale, 170
Constant–Murley score, 169, 172
Disability of Arm, Shoulder, and Hand
questionnaire, 168, 171
Flexi-level Scale of Shoulder Function, 167–168
Hospital for Special Surgery Shoulder – Rating
Score Sheet, 170
Imatani Shoulder Score, 169
Modified UCLA Shoulder Score, 170
Oxford Shoulder Score, 167
Penn Shoulder Score, 170
QuickDASH questionnaire, 168, 172
Rotator Cuff Quality-of-Life measure, 168
Shoulder Disability Questionnaire, 168, 172
Shoulder Pain and Disability Index, 168, 171
Shoulder Rating Questionnaire, 168, 171
Shoulder-related Disability Questionnaire, 169
Simple Shoulder Test, 169, 172
Subjective Shoulder Rating System, 169, 172
Swanson Shoulder Score System, 170
UCLA Shoulder Rating, 169–170, 172
US Food and Drug Administration (FDA)
Western Ontario Rotator Cuff Index, 168
Wheelchair User's Shoulder Pain Index, 170
Wolfang criteria, 170
approved scaffolds, for rotator cuff repair, 151
U-shaped tear, 11*f*, 12

Vascular endothelial growth factor (VEGF), 137
in endothelial cell proliferation, 158
in PRP concentrate, 157, 177
in tendon healing, 138*f*, 141
Vascularity, 38
VEGF receptors (VEGFRs), 141
in tendon healing, 141
See also Tyrosine kinase receptors
Vertical splits, 10, 100
Vessels, of rotator cuff, 3–4
Visual analog scale (VAS), 125, 134, 167, 168
Vitorian method, 157
V-shaped tears, 12

Western Ontario Rotator Cuff Index (WORC), 168
Wheelchair User's Shoulder Pain (WUSPI) Index, 170
Wolfang criteria, 170

Xenograft
bovine dermis, 148
porcine dermal collagen, 148
for rotator cuff repair, 151–152
scaffold augmentation, 151
small intestine submucosa, 147–148

Zimmer Collagen Repair patch, 148, 149*t*, 151, 177
See also Collagen Repair patch; Permacol
Zone of anastomoses, 4
See also Critical zone